HEALTH AND HU...

INTERNATIONAL ASPECTS OF CHILD ABUSE AND NEGLECT

HEALTH AND HUMAN DEVELOPMENT

JOAV MERRICK - SERIES EDITOR –

NATIONAL INSTITUTE OF CHILD HEALTH
AND HUMAN DEVELOPMENT,
MINISTRY OF SOCIAL AFFAIRS, JERUSALEM

Living on the Edge: The Mythical, Spiritual, and Philosophical Roots of Social Marginality
Joseph Goodbread
2009. ISBN: 978-1-60741-162-8

Alcohol-Related Cognitive Disorders: Research and Clinical Perspectives
Leo Sher, Isack Kandel and Joav Merrick (Editors)
2009. ISBN: 978-1-60741-730-9 (Hardcover)
2009. ISBN: 978-1-60876-623-9 (E-book)

Child Rural Health: International Aspects
Erica Bell and Joav Merrick (Editors)
2010. ISBN: 978-1-60876-357-3

Advances in Environmental Health Effects of Toxigenic Mold and Mycotoxins- Volume 1
Ebere Cyril Anyanwu
2010. ISBN: 978-1-60741-953-2

Children and Pain
Patricia Schofield and Joav Merrick (Editors)
2009. ISBN: 978-1-60876-020-6 (Hardcover)
2009. ISBN: 978-1-61728-183-9 (E-book)

Conceptualizing Behavior in Health and Social Research: A Practical Guide to Data Analysis
Said Shahtahmasebi and Damon Berridge
2010. ISBN: 978-1-60876-383-2

Chance Action and Therapy. The Playful Way of Changing
Uri Wernik
2010. ISBN: 978-1-60876-393-1

Adolescence and Chronic Illness. A Public Health Concern
Hatim Omar, Donald E. Greydanus, Dilip R. Patel and Joav Merrick (Editors)
2010. ISBN: 978-1-60876-628-4 (Hardcover)
2010. ISBN: 978-1-61761-482-8 (E-book)

Adolescence and Sports
Dilip R. Patel, Donald E. Greydanus, Hatim Omar and Joav Merrick (Editors)
2010. ISBN: 978-1-60876-702-1 (Hardcover)
2010. ISBN: 978-1-61761-483-5 (E-book)

International Aspects of Child Abuse and Neglect
Howard Dubowitz and Joav Merrick (Editors)
2010. ISBN: 978-1-60876-703-8

**Positive Youth Development: Evaluation and Future
Directions in a Chinese Context**
Daniel T.L. Shek, Hing Keung Ma and Joav Merrick (Editors)
2010. ISBN: 978-1-60876-830-1 (Hardcover)
2010. ISBN: 978-1-61668-376-4 (E-book)

**Positive Youth Development: Implementation of a Youth Program
in a Chinese Context**
Daniel T.L Shek, Hing Keung Ma and Joav Merrick (Editors)
2010. ISBN: 978-1-61668-230-9

**Pediatric and Adolescent Sexuality and Gynecology:
Principles for the Primary Care Clinician**
*Hatim A. Omar, Donald E. Greydanus, Artemis K. Tsitsika, Dilip R. Patel
and Joav Merrick (Editors)*
2010. ISBN: 978-1-60876-735-9

**Understanding Eating Disorders: Integrating Culture,
Psychology and Biology**
Yael Latzer, Joav Merrick and Daniel Stein (Editors)
2010. ISBN: 978-1-61728-298-0

Advanced Cancer Pain and Quality of Life
Edward Chow and Joav Merrick (Editors)
2010. ISBN: 978-1-61668-207-1

Bone and Brain Metastases: Advances in Research and Treatment
Arjun Sahgal, Edward Chow and Joav Merrick (Editors)
2010. ISBN: 978-1-61668-365-8 (Hardcover)
2010. ISBN: 978-1-61728-085-6 (E-book)

Environment, Mood Disorders and Suicide
Teodor T. Postolache and Joav Merrick (Editors)
2010. ISBN: 978-1-61668-505-8

Social and Cultural Psychiatry Experience from the Caribbean Region
Hari D. Maharajh and Joav Merrick (Editors)
2010. ISBN: 978-1-61668-506-5 (Hardcover)
2010. ISBN: 978-1-61728-088-7 (E-book)

Narratives and Meanings of Migration
Julia Mirsky
2010. ISBN: 978-1-61761-103-2 (Hardcover)
2010. ISBN: 978-1-61761-519-1 (E-book)

Self-Management and the Health Care Consumer
Peter William Harvey
2011. ISBN: 978-1-61761-796-6

Sexology from a Holistic Point of View
Soren Ventegodt and Joav Merrick
2011. ISBN: 978-1-61761-859-8

**Principles of Holistic Psychiatry: A Textbook on
Holistic Medicine for Mental Disorders**
Soren Ventegodt and Joav Merrick
2011. ISBN: 978-1-61761-940-3

HEALTH AND HUMAN DEVELOPMENT

INTERNATIONAL ASPECTS OF CHILD ABUSE AND NEGLECT

HOWARD DUBOWITZ
AND
JOAV MERRICK
EDITORS

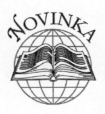

Nova Science Publishers, Inc.
New York

For permission to use material from this book please contact us:
Telephone 631-231-7269; Fax 631-231-8175
Web Site: http://www.novapublishers.com

NOTICE TO THE READER

The Publisher has taken reasonable care in the preparation of this book, but makes no expressed or implied warranty of any kind and assumes no responsibility for any errors or omissions. No liability is assumed for incidental or consequential damages in connection with or arising out of information contained in this book. The Publisher shall not be liable for any special, consequential, or exemplary damages resulting, in whole or in part, from the readers' use of, or reliance upon, this material. Any parts of this book based on government reports are so indicated and copyright is claimed for those parts to the extent applicable to compilations of such works.

Independent verification should be sought for any data, advice or recommendations contained in this book. In addition, no responsibility is assumed by the publisher for any injury and/or damage to persons or property arising from any methods, products, instructions, ideas or otherwise contained in this publication.

This publication is designed to provide accurate and authoritative information with regard to the subject matter covered herein. It is sold with the clear understanding that the Publisher is not engaged in rendering legal or any other professional services. If legal or any other expert assistance is required, the services of a competent person should be sought. FROM A DECLARATION OF PARTICIPANTS JOINTLY ADOPTED BY A COMMITTEE OF THE AMERICAN BAR ASSOCIATION AND A COMMITTEE OF PUBLISHERS.

LIBRARY OF CONGRESS CATALOGING-IN-PUBLICATION DATA

International aspects of child abuse and neglect / [edited by] Howard Dubowitz, Joav Merrick.
  p. cm.
  Includes index.
  ISBN 978-1-61122-049-0
  1. Child abuse. 2. Child welfare. 3. Abused children--Services for. 4. Social work with children. I. Dubowitz, Howard. II. Merrick, Joav, 1950-
  HV6626.5.I58 2009
  362.76--dc22
  2009051309

Published by Nova Science Publishers, Inc. ✦ *New York*

CONTENTS

FOREWORD

Although child abuse and neglect (physical abuse, emotional or psychological abuse, neglect and sexual abuse) have attracted attention over the past thirty years, violence towards infants and children has unfortunately always been part of our history (1-8). In international medical literature, intentional injuries to a child was mentioned in the year 900 by a Persian physician working in the harems of Baghdad (2). Greek physicians in the early second century also seemed aware of newborn babies at high risk for later abuse and neglect, and even advocated infanticide in some circumstances (2).

Throughout the 16th, 17th and 18th centuries, children were raised under the rule of the "Schwarze Paedagogik" (8), with parents as the supreme masters of their children. Parents made all decisions, had complete power and ruled with a firm hand. Tradition and child rearing instructions cautioned parents to begin ""breaking in " their children at a very early stage in order to gain complete control over them. This tradition has unfortunately continued to this very day.

During the 18th century, poverty, violence and alcohol abuse were part of daily life in London and indeed in all of Europe. The English artist William Hogarth (1) made the well-known engraving "Gin Lane" in 1751, showing the total disintegration of society, children with the characteristics of fetal alcohol syndrome, neglect and even fatal child abuse.

The 19th century brought more understanding for children's rights, as well as the acknowledgement of child maltreatment. In Paris, Ambrois Tardieu (2,3,5,6), professor of forensic medicine, reported on 32 cases of child abuse in 1860: nine cases of brutality and ill-treatment, five cases of severe injuries and torture and 18 cases of fatal child abuse. In New York in 1871, a church worker discovered that 8 year old Mary-Ellen was beaten and starved by her foster family. Appeals to the police and department of charity were unsuccessful (3,6). However contact with the American Society for Prevention of Cruelty to Animals brought the matter before the Court on the grounds that Mary-Ellen was a member of the animal kingdom and she was subsequently removed and replaced in an orphanage.

The American Society for Prevention of Cruelty to Children was founded in 1875. The first English Society was founded in Liverpool in 1883 and the London chapter the following year. During the first three years, the London Society dealt with 762 cases of assault, starvation, dangerous neglect, desertion, cruel exposure to excite sympathy, other wrongs and 25 deaths (2). In Israel the Association for Child Protection (ELI) was established in 1979.

In the first half of the 20th century, sometimes called "the century of the child", there were several papers published on subdural hematoma in infants (2), but it was first in 1946 that John Caffey (9), from Babies and Children's Hospital of New York, associated subdural hematoma with multiple fractures. He described six infants born between 1925 and 1942, who had chronic subdural hematoma with 23 fractures and four contusions of the long bones.

After publication of that article, several papers on subdural hematoma associated with fractures and bruises were written in both the United States (10) and France (2). In each case no etiological explanation was offered, because the parents denied trauma.

In 1953, Frederic Silverman from the Children's Hospital in Cincinnati was the first to state that caretakers of children "may permit trauma and be unaware of it, may recognize trauma, but forget or be reluctant to admit it, or may deliberately injure the child and deny it" (11).

In 1955, Woolley and Evans (12) from Detroit reviewed cases from 1946-54 at the Children's Hospital and found that "the general environmental factors surrounding infants who suffer osseous discontinuity range from "unavoidable" episodes in stable households through what we have termed an unprotective environment, to a surprisingly large segment characterized by the presence of aggressive, immature or emotionally ill adults".

Subsequently, articles and books on maltreatment appeared by pediatricians, radiologists, orthopedic surgeons, medical examiners and social workers around the world, but the response of the medical world and the media was rather reserved at first.

Charles Henry Kempe (1922-84) became chairman of the Department of Pediatrics at the University of Colorado Medical School in Denver in 1956. In 1959, Kempe, together with a medical student, William Droegemueller, tried to determine the extent of the phenomenon of inflicted injuries in childhood in the United States. They surveyed 71 hospitals and 77 district attorneys across the country and found 749 cases of maltreated children; 78 had died and 114 suffered permanent brain damage. When Droegemueller graduated in 1960, he left the data in two shoeboxes for Kempe to retrieve and collate. Together with the pediatric radiologist Frederic Silverman, the psychiatrist Brandt Steele and the pediatrician Henry Silver, they published the landmark article "The battered –child syndrome" in 1962 (13). Soon popular press, radio and television presented case-histories and scientific papers appeared from all over the world. From 1965, the Cumulated Index Medicus featured a heading on child abuse and today several hundred articles are published each year.

The National Center for the Prevention and Treatment of Child Abuse and Neglect (today the Kempe Center) in Denver was established in 1972, the International Society for the Prevention of Child Abuse and Neglect in 1976 and the International Journal "Child Abuse and Neglect" published its first issue in 1977.

Helen Keye (1849-1926), a Swedish author and educator devoted to the welfare of children, wrote a book in 1900 entitled "The Century of the Child" claiming that in the twentieth century the nations of the world would finally begin to understand that the life of a nation, indeed the life of the world, depends upon the breath of children. We believe that the 20th century discovered family violence, child abuse and neglect. Let us make sure that the next century will really be "the century of the child".

Child abuse and neglect must be seen as a major public health problem, but it seems that the lay and professional community have not been able to view this problem with the same seriousness as cancer, heart disease and AIDS.

A coordinated effort must be sought world wide to increase the level of funding for prevention, treatment, education and research in this important field of child health and development. We hope this book will give a small window of what is happening around the world and the issues that each country struggles with. Somehow it is not so different from country to country as one might think.

Joav Merrick, MD, MMedSci, DMSc
National Institute of Child Health and Human Development, Office of the Medical Director, Health Services, Division for Mental Retardation, Ministry of Social Affairs, Jerusalem and Kentucky Children's Hospital, Department of Pediatrics, University of Kentucky College of Medicine, Lexington, United States.
E-Mail: jmerrick@zahav.net.il
Website: http://jmerrick50.googlepages.com/home

REFERENCES

[1]   Rodin AE. Infants and gin mania in 18th-century London. JAMA 1981;245:1237-9.
[2]   Lynch MA. Child abuse before Kempe: An historical literature review. Child Abuse Negl 1985;9:7-15.
[3]   Heins M. The battered child revisited. JAMA 1984;251:3295-3300.
[4]   Kroll J, Bachrach B. Child care and child abuse in early medieval Europe. J Am Acad Child Psychiatr 1986;25:562-8.
[5]   Knight B. The history of child abuse. Forensic Sci Int 1986;30:135-41.
[6]   Radbill SX. Children in a world of violence: A history of child abuse. In Helfer RE, Kempe RS, eds. The battered child. Chicago: Univ Press, 1987:3-22.
[7]   Aries P. L`enfant et la vie familiale sous l`Ancien Regime. Paris: Editions du Seuil, 1973.
[8]   Miller A. For your own good. Hidden cruelty in child rearing and the roots of violence. New York: Farrar Straus Giroux, 1985.
[9]   Caffey J. Multiple fractures in the long bones of infants suffering from chronic subdural hematomas. AJR 1946;56:163-73.
[10]   Lis EF, Frauenberger GS. Multiple fractures associated with subdural hematoma in infancy. Pediatrics 1950;6:890-2.
[11]   Silverman FN. The roentgen manifestations of unrecognized skeletal trauma in infants. AJR 1953;69:413-27.
[12]   Woolley PV, Evans WA. Significance of skeletal lesions in infants resembling those of traumatic origin. JAMA 1955;158;539-43.
[13]   Kempe CH, Silverman FN, Steele BF, Droegemueller W, Silver HK. The battered-child syndrome. JAMA 1962;181:17-24.

INTRODUCTION

CHILD PROTECTION AROUND THE WORLD. SIMILARITIES AND DIFFERENCES, ADVANCES AND CHALLENGES

Howard Dubowitz

Department of Pediatrics, University of Maryland School of Medicine,
Baltimore, Maryland, United States of America

INTRODUCTION

It is very clear that children in every country experience abuse and neglect (1,2). The descriptions of the child welfare systems in different countries in this book illustrate several common themes: the lack of clear definitions, ambiguous policies, laws not being implemented, limited data on the extent and nature of the problem, and inadequate resources for addressing child maltreatment. Challenges facing Argentina are remarkably familiar to someone in the United States. At the same time, there are also striking differences in approaches and resources. The field of child protection is relatively young; in many areas optimal policies and practice remain uncertain. A goal of this book is to promote dialogue across borders to learn from each other and advance this multifaceted field, and to better serve children and families. This commentary highlights some of the main themes evident in the descriptions of the different child welfare systems.

NEED FOR SPECIFIC LAWS RELATED TO CHILD MALTREATMENT

A legal framework is critical for guiding policies and practice concerning child maltreatment. It is possible that laws indirectly related to children's welfare may also help protect them. However, it appears important to have laws that specifically address child maltreatment and the many related issues. Such laws allow for a focus and clarity this problem requires, that may otherwise be missing. Specific laws also play an important role in establishing what a society deems unacceptable, and thereby constitutes a valuable means for public education.

For example, in the USA, an increasing number of states now hold parents responsible, when a young child accesses a gun and a tragedy ensues. The legal system can play a vital role in protecting children; advocacy is needed to develop and refine this role - via sound law.

There have been striking advances in the legal arena in several countries. It is encouraging to learn, for example, of the many laws concerning child protection passed in Russia since the 1990s. The vital role that civil society can and should play in formulating such laws is a promising development. Yet, the experience in South Africa, despite all the enthusiasm of forging a new society, illustrates how difficult this can be (3). It is also noteworthy how the United Nations Convention on the Rights of the Child (CRC) has provided the impetus for reformulating laws affecting children in several countries (4). It serves as a valuable blueprint for what is needed to ensure children's health, development and safety.

THE CHASM BETWEEN LAWS ON PAPER AND REALITY ON THE GROUND

Even when there are good laws "on the books," there are often huge barriers to implementing them. For example, reporting child abuse is mandatory in the Phillipines, but there are no consequences for professionals failing to so. This likely contributes to few physicians carrying out this duty (5). The gap between the promising language in the CRC and the pitiful predicament of so many children in so many countries also illustrates the gap between countries' legal obligations and prevailing conditions. There is a clear challenge in translating such "aspirational" laws or policies into reality.

Another issue is that laws are often necessarily broad; it is impossible, for example, for legal definitions to precisely cover all possible manifestations of abuse and neglect. Thus, it falls on the responsible agencies to operationalize laws with specific policies and procedures that provide clear guidance to professionals and the public. This remains a serious weakness in countries where the public agencies are poorly developed or non-existent.

THE NEED FOR DATA ON CHILD ABUSE AND NEGLECT

Laws, policies and programs pertaining to child protection require political and public support and funding. There are often powerful political and personal interests for denying the problem of child maltreatment. The media can play a valuable role bringing stories of abused and neglected children to public attention. However, many countries still need basic epidemiological research to demonstrate the extent and nature of maltreatment. Such data is crucial for drawing attention to the problem, for developing suitable approaches and interventions, and for monitoring progress. Some countries gather information on reported cases – always the tip of the iceberg. Community or population-based surveys are another useful approach, with some advantages over "official" reports.

Measurement begins with defining that which one aims to measure. Thus, the field needs clear definitions regarding the problems of interest. Definitions provided by the World Health Organization, for example, offer useful guidance (6), but these will likely be modified to fit with local culture and circumstances. Regarding definitions of sexual abuse, there is much in common across countries. It is interesting, in contrast, to note the definition of psychological maltreatment in Brazil (7), far broader than in most other countries, and a problem seldom addressed by the child welfare system in the USA (8). Clearly, differences in definitions, laws, policies and practice preclude simple comparisons across countries. Even within the USA, there are enough differences among states making comparisons quite difficult (8). Only in the realm of research are common definitions across countries realistic (9). In sum, there are a variety of approaches for probing the extent and nature of child maltreatment in a country and across borders.

THE NEED FOR A CHILD WELFARE SYSTEM(S)

Most industrialized countries have developed child welfare systems for addressing child maltreatment. There remains, however, considerable variability in how these are designed and function. In England, the national government has established the processes, roles and responsibilities for all professionals and agencies when there are concerns about possible child abuse or neglect (10). In the United States, there are extensively developed but decentralized systems; different counties within a state often have considerable autonomy. Despite all the advances in such countries, there has been considerable criticism by advocates aiming to improve these systems (11).

Yet countries without any system face enormous challenges in responding to abused and neglected children. A patchwork of local efforts and non-governmental programs may help, but typically fall terribly short of being adequate solutions. While systems inevitably vary, useful principles such as having a lead agency coordinate the response have been identified. In Pakistan and the Philippines, hospitals play the key role, with special units for addressing child abuse (5,12). In the former, however, the focus is on the medical care, with little available in terms of social and mental heath resources. Advocacy to develop and improve child welfare systems is much needed – everywhere. An international endeavor to establish optimal core principles, policies and practice could be fruitful, while recognizing that these would surely need to be adapted to fit local circumstances.

WHAT PRINCIPLES SHOULD GUIDE THE DEVELOPMENT OF CHILD WELFARE SYSTEMS?

It is beyond the scope of this Commentary to detail such principles, but the different approaches described in the special issue do illustrate some fundamental philosophical differences in the field of child protection. For example, the Belgian approach focuses on working with families engaged in incest, attempting to avoid involvement in the judicial system (13). Other countries are very concerned with the punishment of perpetrators. What approach best protects a child remains unclear. The adversarial approach inherent in many child welfare systems may limit their ability to engage and help families. This can be an immense challenge; the alternatives to enabling families to better protect their children are often limited. A promising development in the USA are the Alternative Response Systems offering a more collaborative approach, working with families – in cases involving neglect and less serious physical abuse (8). The Israeli approach appears similar; addressing families' needs is the priority (14). Interestingly, Argentina prioritizes removing offenders rather than child victims of sexual abuse (15). These are all inherently complex issues; much remains to be learned regarding best practices.

The nature and scope of child welfare practice clearly varies greatly. In most countries, there appears to be a relatively narrow focus on protection or ensuring safety. In contrast, other countries such as England accept a broader role including for example a developmental assessment of children (10). It appears to be a good goal to embrace a broader concern for children's development, health and safety, issues that are naturally intertwined. As a practical matter, public agencies are often overwhelmed and under resourced. Adding to their mission requires adding to their resources, or, good collaboration with other systems and agencies (eg, healthcare).

The field of child protection demands good collaboration; it is a necessity, not simply a nice idea. Bureaucratic barriers, however, loom large everywhere. In the USA the importance of collaboration across agencies is too often still a "buzz word," difficult to achieve. Even within the same agency, communication, coordination and collaboration are often inadequate - compromising the care children and families receive. Such dysfunction within and among agencies may mirror or exacerbate the dysfunction of families they are serving. There appear to be advantages having policymaking being highly centralized as in France, although that may not be possible politically in some countries. There are no quick fixes to this endemic challenge, but the need for good collaboration and communication among all involved in child protection is critical to effectively helping children and families.

MANDATORY REPORTING – FOR OR AGAINST?

Mandatory reporting of suspected abuse and neglect to a public agency remains a hotly debated issue (16-18). One view holds that mandatory reporting is necessary to ensure that appropriate steps are taken to protect as many children as possible who are in danger. Mandating reporting also conveys the seriousness with which the state considers maltreatment. Others argue that reporting should be voluntary and that mandating it imposes an undue and rigid burden on professionals (and sometimes citizens) who may have better ways to approach the problem. It does seem important that mandated reporters be immune from liability, if a report is made in good faith.

Even within countries that have mandatory reporting, there is considerable variability as to who needs to report (eg, professionals only, all citizens). The Belgian model, without mandatory reporting (unless the child cannot be protected), offers an interesting model for engaging families in cases of incest, attempting to minimize the stigma and adversarial context often associated with child protective services (13). Once again, it is difficult to know what approach is optimal. It is clear, however, that mandatory reporting places an ethical and legal obligation upon the state to help ensure a child's protection.

THE NEED TO ENHANCE PROFESSIONAL CAPABILITIES

A good child welfare system requires having well-trained and skilled staff to perform this difficult work. This is a major challenge for most countries. The inherent complexity of the work and its often lowly status do not help attract professionals. There is also a broader need to develop the capabilities of all professionals who have contact with children, especially those engaged in health care, child care and education, law enforcement and the judicial system. For example, considerable efforts have been made in the USA to ensure that physicians are educated to diagnose and report suspected maltreatment. Some states require training in child maltreatment as a prerequisite for medical licensure. Here too, however, there is much room for improvement - across all disciplines. This issue of enhancing professionals' capabilities is central to the mission of the International Society for the Prevention of Child Abuse and Neglect (ISPCAN) (19).

THE NEED FOR GREATER RESOURCES

In addition to bolstering the capabilities of professionals, an array of services are needed to address the problems underpinning child maltreatment. Funding for child protection and related services is typically woefully inadequate. Available resources seldom come close to matching the needs of children and families. Even in the USA, for example, there is a terrible dearth of mental health resources for children, and the unmet needs are great (20). Clearly, a far greater financial commitment is needed to better address child maltreatment and its associated problems.

A related problem concerns the burdens of poverty and the harm resulting to children. For example, 22% of families in the Philippines reported regularly experiencing "moderate to severe hunger" (5). Inequality in income distribution is a major problem in Brazil (7). In addition to the direct impact on children, there is little mystery how such conditions can impede the ability of families and parents to care for their children. In some countries, such as South Africa, poverty is further compounded by the HIV/AIDS epidemic (3). It seems clear that it not enough to narrowly focus our efforts on parenting problems without helping address the underlying systemic problems that contribute to child maltreatment. The social safety net in relatively affluent Belgium offers an enviable model for what can be in place to ensure decent conditions for children and families (13).

CULTURAL ISSUES

Aside from economic factors, cultural and historical issues may hinder, or help, optimal approaches to child protection. It goes without saying that cultural issues are not easy to change. Cultural issues emerge through each of the papers. One common theme is the importance attached to the family unit, with a high threshold for removing children. This should translate to extensive efforts to support the family to better protect a child. In the USA, the trend has been to prioritize placement with relatives (ie, kinship care) when a child is in danger of imminent harm (8). Even when children are placed in regular foster care, the initial goal is to reunite them with their families. It is curious that in Russia parental rights are more often terminated than restricted (21). And in Lebanon, many maltreated children are placed in institutions, rather than with family members (ie, kinship care) or in foster care (22). These differences may reflect varying resources rather than philosophical preferences.

There is also striking variation in the recognition of a child's identity and rights. This is strong in some countries, such as France (23). Yet a child's unexplained death in other countries is not clear cause for investigation. No doubt there may be deeply rooted cultural factors at play. Parental rights, long prioritized over those of children, may be predominant. A related issue concerns the direct involvement of children and youth in helping develop policies and programs concerning their own welfare. Lebanon is an example of where this does occur; the extent to which children are directly involved in most countries is unclear (22). Probing, understanding and addressing cultural attitudes and practices should be integral to advancing this field and the wellbeing of children.

Addressing underlying cultural issues is a daunting challenge, but the advances made in many countries provide encouraging evidence of what is possible. The recent surge in public awareness in Israel concerning the rights of children is a good example (14). In a world with increasing mobility, the need for child welfare professionals to be competent working with families from different cultures has become important (23). This is also true for working with different cultural groups that have long lived in a country – Australia being a prime example (25).

PREVENTION

Preventing child maltreatment may appear to be a luxury when resources for responding to child maltreatment are so limited in many countries. But the human and economic costs of maltreatment provide a compelling case for preventive efforts (26). The moral issue of respecting children's rights and the legal implications of signing the CRC are an added impetus for preventing child maltreatment and promoting their health, development and safety. Russia provides a useful example of having a tradition of providing a "safety net' ensuring children's basic needs are met (21). As mentioned earlier, Belgium offers an impressive model (13), and England's "Staying Safe" program offers a comprehensive set of actions for ensuring children's safety (10).

There is a need for creatively filling inevitable gaps in governmental programs. All countries have excellent examples of private and non-governmental agencies providing much needed services. As laudable and necessary as this is, it is doubtful that they can realistically address the broader systemic issues such as poverty that contribute to child maltreatment. Much remains to be learned and to be done in the realm of prevention – the need for feisty advocacy is clear.

NEED FOR RESEARCH

The authors in this Special Issue were not asked to provide the evidence base for child welfare policies and practice in their countries. Nevertheless, the variations in child protection systems raise an important question. What evidence is there to help guide our field? In general, limited research and evidence hinder child welfare policies and practice - in all countries. Instead, we have to rely on philosophical preferences and practice experience.

There are many examples where research and program evaluations can play a critical difference. In the USA, evaluations of home visiting programs led to the development of many such preventive programs (27). Evaluation of children removed from their parents and placed in kinship care drew attention to the need to better support these families (28). England offers a useful example where monitoring and evaluation of agencies and services are built into the system (10). Public inquiries have helped develop specific recommendations for improvements as well as galvanizing public attention to the problem. Understandably, the limited resources available for desperately needed services make research and evaluation appear to be another luxury. But, without investing in this area, it remains very difficult to know what works, and what does not.

COMMON CHALLENGES

There are many challenges that likely apply in all countries. Roylance in his paper on Australia articulated these well (25). They include: finding the appropriate balance between respecting family autonomy and state intervention to protect a child, finding an optimal means of oversight for child welfare without being unduly burdensome, seeking optimal interventions to prevent and address child maltreatment, developing sound alternatives for children who need to be placed away from their home, and balancing the possibly conflicting goals of strengthening a family with holding offenders accountable. Other countries face more basic challenges, developing a legal framework and child welfare infrastructure for protecting children. Each of these is a complex issue with profound ramifications for children and families. A sustained commitment by dedicated professionals is needed to help address these and other important challenges.

REFERENCES

[1]   ISPCAN World Perspectives on Child Abuse, 6th and 7th ed, www.ISPCSAN.org
[2]   Pinheiro SP. World report on violence against children. Secretary General's study on violence against children. Geneva: United Nations, 2006.
[3]   van Niekerk J. Child protection in South Africa. Int J Child Health Hum Dev 2009;2(3):239-247.
[4]   United Nations. Convention on the rights of the child. Geneva: United Nations, 1990.
[5]   Madrid BJ. Child protection and the Philippines. Int J Child Health Hum Dev 2009;2(3):47-53.
[6]   World Health Organization. World report on violence and health. Geneva: WHO, 2002.
[7]   Lidchi VD, Eisenstein E. Child protection in Brazil: Challenges and opportunities. Int J Child Health Hum Dev 2009;2:217-229.
[8]   Dubowitz H, DePanfilis D. Child welfare in the USA: In theory and practice. Int J Child Health Hum Dev 2009;2(3):179-187.
[9]   Straus MA, Savage SA. Neglectful behavior by parents in the life history of university students in 17 countries and its relation to violence against dating partners. Child Maltreat 2005;10:124-35.
[10]   Gray J. Protecting children form abuse and neglect in England. Int J Child Health Hum Dev 2009;2(3):129-139.

[11]   US Advisory Board on Child Abuse and Neglect, 1993 US Advisory Board on Child Abuse and Neglect, Neighbors helping neighbors: A new national strategy for the protection of children. Washington, DC: US Gov Printing Office, 1993.

[12]   Muhammad T. Child protection in Pakistan. Int J Child Health Hum Dev 2009;2(3):42-46.

[13]   Adriaenssens P. From protected object to lawful subject. Practical applications of the Belgian model of child protection. Int J Child Health Hum Dev 2009;2(3):115-128.

[14]   Szabo-Lael R, Zemach-Marom, T. Child protection in Israel. Int J Child Health Hum Dev 2009;2(3):65-73.

[15]   Intebi I. Child maltreatment in Argentina. Int J Child Health Hum Dev   2009;2(3):208-216.

[16]   Melton GB. Mandated reporting: a policy without reason. Child Abuse Neglect 2005;1:9-18

[17]   Brett D, Johnson-Reid M. A response to Melton based on the best available data. Child Abuse Neglect 2007;31:343-360.

[18]   Ben M, Bross DC. Commentary: Mandated reporting is still a policy with reason: Empirical evidence and philosophical grounds. Child Abuse Neglect 2008;32:511-516.

[19]   International Society for the Prevention of Child Abuse and Neglect (ISPCAN). www.ISPCSAN.org

[20]   US Department of Health and Human Services. Mental health: a report of the surgeon general-executive summary. Rockville, MD: US Dept Health Hum Serv, Subst Abuse Ment Health Serv Adm, Center Ment Health Serv, Natl Inst Health, Natl Inst Ment Health, 1999.

[21]   Balachova TN, Bonner BL, Alexeeva IA Child maltreatment in Russia. Int J Child Health Hum Dev 2009;2(3):167-178.

[22]   Gerbaka B. Child protection in Lebanon. Society and strategy: More than one? Int J Child Health Hum Dev 2009;2(3):74-81.

[23]   Taub G. Child protection in France. Int J Child Health Hum Dev 2009;2(3):140-148.

[24]   Korbin J, Spilsbury J. Cultural competence and child neglect. In: Dubowitz H, ed. Neglected children: Research, practice and policy. Thousand Oaks, CA: Sage, 1999:69-88.

[25]   Roylance R. A snap-shot of child protection systems in Australia. Int J Child Health Hum Dev 2009;2(3):259-273.

[26]   World Health Organization. Preventing child maltreatment: a guide to taking action and generating evidence. Geneva: WHO, 2006.

[27]   Olds DL, Kitzman H, Hanks C, Cole R, Anson E, et al. Effects of nurse home visiting on maternal and child functioning: Age-9 follow-up of a randomized trial. Pediatrics 2009;120:832-45.

[28]   Dubowitz H, Feigelman S, Harrington D, Starr R, Zuravin S, Sawyer R. Children in kinship care: How do they fare? Children Youth Serv Rev 1994;16:85-106.

In: International Aspects of Child Abuse and Neglect   ISBN: 978-1-60876-703-8
Editors: H. Dubowitz, J. Merrick pp. 1-10   © 2010 Nova Science Publishers, Inc.

Chapter 1

CHILD PROTECTION SYSTEM IN HONG KONG

Patricia LS Ip

United Christian Hospital, Hong Kong, China

Hong Kong has developed a multidisciplinary response to child abuse and neglect over the last three decades involving mainly the social, medical and allied health, education and law enforcement sectors. Management is based on the Procedural Guide for Handling Child Abuse Cases which delineates the roles of various disciplines. It covers reports and referrals, investigations, case conferences and follow-up action. There is a Child Protection Registry that records names of abused children and those at high risk of abuse as concluded in case conferences. Establishment of specialized units within the different disciplines has improved service provision but the system is plagued with work overload and staff turnovers. Many issues are still under discussion such as mandatory reporting and treatment, sex offender register, and the prohibition of corporal punishment and the leaving of young children unattended by law. Remedial services always seem to demand urgent attention but primary and secondary prevention need higher priority if eventually it is hoped the demand could be reduced.

INTRODUCTION

Although Kempe drew widespread attention from professionals towards the abuse of children through his historic paper in 1962 (1), it took Hong Kong nearly another twenty years to start looking into child abuse and neglect (CAN) seriously. The response had been incident driven followed by service development and legislative support.

In 1978, a 10-year old emaciated girl with multiple injuries walked into a police station in Hong Kong to seek help. The media publicity brought a group of professionals together to form a non-government organization (NGO), Against Child Abuse, in 1979. In 1983, a corresponding specialized service in the government Social Welfare Department (SWD) was set up. A multidisciplinary child protection system developed progressively modeled on that of western countries, especially the United Kingdom. Hong Kong was a British colony till the handover to Chinese rule in 1997 under one country, two systems. The legal system in Hong Kong continues to be based on the common law system.

DEFINITION OF THE DIFFERENT FORMS OF CAN

According to SWD's Procedural Guide for Handling Child Abuse Cases (2), child abuse is defined as any act of commission or omission that endangers or impairs the physical / psychological health and development of an individual under the age of 18. Four types of abuse are generally recognized. The following are their working definitions.

Physical abuse is a physical injury or physical suffering to a child where there is a definite knowledge, or a reasonable suspicion that the injury has been inflicted non-accidentally.

Sexual abuse is the involvement of a child in sexual activity which is unlawful or to which a child is unable to give informed consent.

Neglect is severe or a repeated pattern of lacking of attention to a child's basic needs that endangers or impairs the child's health or development.

Psychological abuse is the repeated pattern of behavior and attitude towards a child or extreme incident that endangers or impairs the child's emotion or intellectual development.

EXTENT OF THE PROBLEM

A Child Protection Registry was set up in Hong Kong in 1986. For each child suspected to have been abused, a multidisciplinary case conference is held to decide whether abuse is established. The names of abused children or those at high risk of abuse are recorded in the Registry. There were 944 new cases of CAN registered in 2007 (3). As 1.12 million of the 6.7 million population in Hong Kong in 2007 were children, 0.8 /1,000 children were on the Registry. Statistics of newly registered cases over the previous four years summarized in Table 1 demonstrates a rising trend in total numbers and that for neglect (4).

Table 1. Types of cases registered in Child Protection Registry 2004 – 2007 (5)

	2004		2005		2006		2007	
	No.	%	No.	%	No.	%	No.	%
Physical	345	55.5	413	54.1	438	54.3	499	52.9
Sexual	189	30.2	234	30.7	233	28.9	270	28.6
Neglect	40	6.4	41	5.4	77	9.6	114	12.1
Psychological	9	1.5	23	3.0	12	1.5	20	2.1
Multiple	39	6.3	52	6.8	46	5.7	41	4.3
Total	622	100	763	100	806	100	944	100

These were children brought to the notice of professionals. Chan's territory-wide survey gave prevalence rates of various forms of child abuse as reported by children aged 12 to 17 years (5). Fourteen percent and 4% of the children reported severe and very severe physical assault respectively by one or both parents in the 12 months prior to enumeration. The figure for psychological aggression was 58% and that for neglect was 27%. For child sexual abuse, Tang reported an overall prevalence rate of 6% among college students under 17 years of age (6).

SYSTEM THAT ADDRESSES CAN

The Child Protection System in Hong Kong adopted a multidisciplinary approach with the involvement of the social, medical and allied health, education and law enforcement sectors.

Integrated Family Service Centers are managed by SWD or NGOs on a regional basis (7). These centers attend to all levels of prevention of social problems of clients of all ages. Children with severe CAN or those requiring statutory protection are referred to SWD's specialized Family and Child Protective Services Units (FCPSUs). Against Child Abuse is the NGO that provides remedial services and prevention programs for all forms of CAN but statutory cases are referred to FCPSUs. Medical social workers are stationed in public hospitals and school social workers in primary and secondary schools.

CAN are generally referred to and managed in the medical sector by pediatric units of public hospitals all having Medical Coordinators on Child Abuse. They may be consulted by other professionals on CAN and can arrange direct admissions for children suspected of abuse without having to go through Accident and Emergency Departments. Clinical psychological service is provided through the public hospitals or through SWD.

In the police force, there are regional Child Abuse Investigation Units responsible for investigating child sexual abuse when the perpetrator is known to the child, severe physical abuse and organized child abuse (e.g., pedophilia). Other cases are investigated by the local criminal investigation departments.

There is no child abuse law, but a number of ordinances can be used to protect children. Offences Against the Person Ordinance is used in wilful assault, ill treatment, neglect, and exposure to unnecessary suffering and injury to a child's health including mental health. The Crimes Ordinance covers various forms of sexual abuse. A Care or Protection Order can be applied if necessary so that social workers can have access to supervise the care of a child or commit a child to an alternate placement. An assessment order can also be made without first having to remove a child from home. The same Ordinance can be used to detain a child who requires medical attention in hospital.

In the mid 1990's specifically for child sexual abuse and severe cases of physical abuse, legislations were amended to allow children up to 14 years old to give unsworn evidence in court. Corroboration of a young child's unsworn evidence is not required. The video record of a forensic interview can be used as evidence in court. The child can also testify via a television link. A witness support program was started to assist children who have to testify in court. In 2003, the Prevention of Child Pornography Ordinance was passed to make the production, possession and publication of child pornography whether photographs or computer generated a crime, as is participation in sex tourism.

REPORTING OF SUSPECTED CAN AND RESPONSE

CAN may be reported to any welfare agency, clinic/hospital, school or the police directly or through hotlines of the SWD and the police which are generic or that of Against Child Abuse which is specific for CAN. Professionals will assess the risk and decide on the urgency for investigation and action required.

Children requiring medical assessment are referred to Medical Coordinators on Child Abuse. Pediatricians and medical social workers work jointly with social workers of other agencies, if they have been involved with the child previously or with FCPSU if it is a new case. Whether a report is made to the police depends on the nature/severity of the CAN, any past record and the attitude of the suspected perpetrator. A forensic interview will be arranged by the police for a child with suspected sexual abuse or severe physical abuse if his/her physical and mental status is suitable for such an interview. The forensic examination for sexual abuse can be done by a forensic pathologist at the request of the police or, especially for pre-pubertal children with non-acute abuse, done by trained pediatricians. Other medical specialties are involved as necessary.

A multidisciplinary case conference of involved professionals who have significant information about the child and the family whether inside or outside the hospital e.g. school teachers, is held within 10 working days of hospital admission. The parents and/or the child as appropriate are invited to participate unless there are specific contraindications. A decision is made as to whether child abuse is established, the need to enter the child's name into the Child Protection Registry, nature of the abuse, services required for the child and other family members, division of labor in the follow-up and whether a subsequent review report or meeting is required. Whether legal action is warranted is decided by the police after consulting the Department of Justice.

STRENGTHS OF THE SYSTEM

When child protection work took off in Hong Kong some 30 years ago, it was rapidly recognized that professionals could not work in isolation. Communication and co-operation are important elements to avoid children in need slipping through the net. The Procedural Guide has been helpful in role delineation and is a good reference for professionals new to the field. Joint training of different disciplines was carried out especially in the early days and update briefings are conducted whenever the procedures were revised. With professionals within the social, medical and law enforcement sectors designated to manage CAN, expertise has built up. Regular regional meetings are held by these professionals to iron out operational concerns while individual disciplines like the Medical Co-ordinators on Child Abuse have group meetings to share experiences and provide mutual support (8).

Having a NGO, Against Child Abuse, which accepts reports and referrals on CAN provides the community with a choice of government or non-government service which some people feel less threatening. Although the NGO has no statutory power of access or supervision, a working relationship with government units has built up so that referrals or transfers are made at the appropriate time.

The Child Protection Registry, which allows registered professionals to check if a child is known to social service agencies, speeds up the initial investigation. The agency who entered a child's name can take the name off the Registry after two years if there is no further concern.

On the medical side, the electronic patient record system of public hospitals facilitates doctors who want to find out if a child has attended other public hospitals for whatever reason even if the history is not offered by the parents. Further enquiries directed at the previous healthcare team can be made easily. Hong Kong government works on the principle that no citizen is denied medical treatment because of lack of means. Public hospital fees currently at US$13 a day is inclusive of consultation fees, medication, investigations, and surgery required. Fees are waived for needy families. This gives medical staff a free hand to provide care considered best for the child whether the parents who are the majority of perpetrators, are able or willing to cover the medical expenses. Social work services or therapy by clinical psychologists of the SWD is free.

CHALLENGES TO THE SYSTEM

Definition of child abuse

A procedural guide is a guide. Its value depends on the people who carry out the procedures. Definitions of child abuse are broad and open to interpretation. As Hong Kong does not clearly prohibit corporal punishment at home, the line between excessive discipline and abuse can be difficult to draw. Even professionals have a variable tolerance of physical punishment of children. There is also no law to define at what age or circumstances a child left unattended constitutes neglect. Children continue to be at risk till they are physically harmed, such as falling off high-rise buildings, a common form of housing in Hong Kong. Awareness of psychological abuse is low as is psychological neglect like that suffered by children left alone for prolonged periods or being looked after by other slightly older siblings. Thus there is variable sensitivity amongst professionals from the recognition of CAN to what action is to be taken. Ip outlined the factors that influence decision making by different disciplines all using the same guideline in Hong Kong (9).

Recruitment and retention of workers

CAN work is labor intensive and stressful especially when risk assessments go astray. Recruitment and retention of professionals for child protection work is not easy. Apart from staff resignations, the practice of a number of service units of rotating workers through different areas of work every few years for staff development disrupts continuity of care for children and families. How to balance the enhancement of workers' future promotional prospect with the need of service users is a challenge. Children appear to be particularly at risk during "handover periods" of their regular attending worker.

Workload

Although social and medical services to children and families with CAN are free or low-cost, workload of all professionals is a concern. The one-stop-service of Integrated Family Service Centers, a restructuring adopted territory-wide in 2002, is ideal in theory with each centre being responsible for the population of its jurisdiction. Unfortunately with rising caseloads not matched by corresponding increase in resources, manpower is channeled towards remedial work at the expense of primary or even secondary prevention. Social workers in these centers are managing on average 50 cases at any one time going up to 70 in busy districts. Although counseling and therapy are available, the waiting time and the limited intensity of services are concerns.

Availability of alternate placements

A pediatric ward is a relatively safe place for children with suspected CAN requiring physical assessment and treatment while the social investigation is being carried out. Unfortunately, due to the lack of alternate emergency placement, many who do not need in-hospital treatment remain unnecessary long in hospital pending the case conference being held. The children end up having febrile illnesses before the end of their stay. Similarly when the decision is that return to the child's home is not feasible, there is a lack of suitable placements. While a home environment is desirable, there are only 960 foster care places (emergency or long-term) for the over one million childhood population in Hong Kong, the children requiring the service for different reasons of which CAN is only one. Many, especially older children, or those with behavior problems, end up in larger institutions.

Timely investigations

There is a tendency for the police to arrange video recorded interviews for not only child sexual abuse when the system started but increasingly for physical abuse as well. Trained SWD social workers and clinical psychologists and the police are authorized to do the interviews. Social workers are not keen to be interviewers when there is a high chance of prosecution. Interviewing children at different stages of development also requires much skill. The recent practice is to designate SWD clinical psychologists as the interviewer of children with developmental problems as well as children less than 7 years old. Because clinical psychologists also do assessment and treatment, the forensic interviews are not necessarily timely, by which time the child may have been influenced by family members to recant. A non-informative interview affects the subsequent action that can be taken to protect the child.

Cross-border families

With the handover of the sovereignty of Hong Kong to China, there are more cross border population movements with currently 40 percent of marriages of Hong Kong residents being cross border marriages. Although children born to these couples have Hong Kong residential status, the mainland spouse, often the mother, who wishes to reside permanently in Hong Kong takes years of application before approval is granted. There may be prolonged periods of separation of parents creating marital and adjustment problems. The children may be living in the mainland or Hong Kong at different times. With the "one country, two system" principle, investigation of CAN that is reported in Hong Kong but occurred in the mainland is near impossible. Should parents decide to take their child who has been abused to live in the mainland, there could be neither supervision nor provision of treatment for the child and other family members while they are in the mainland.

MAJOR CONTROVERSIES IN THE SYSTEM

Mandatory reporting

Reporting of CAN is not mandatory. There are incidents where employers such as school boards dismiss employees suspected of child abuse without reporting to the responsible authority, and the employees move to other employment with access to children. The government argues against mandatory reporting because of the concern that valuable resources may be used for the investigation of unsubstantiated reports. For professionals, this is to some extent addressed by individual professional codes of conduct but failure to report is often only apparent when re-abuse is brought to light.

Mandatory treatment

Currently a Care or Protection Order can be applied for a child, but there is no provision that the perpetrator has to receive counseling or treatment. A debate is ongoing as to whether non-voluntary treatment is effective although an amendment of the Domestic Violence Ordinance is considering mandating treatment of abusers who are under an injunction order for threatening behavior towards their spouse and children.

Sex offender register

Reports of pedophiles repeating their offence after release from prison terms prompted a public consultation exercise on the setting up of a sex offender register. The proposed mechanism is a voluntary checking by employers with the consent of potential employees in work situations involving children and mentally incapacitated persons. The community responses are still being analysed.

Zero tolerance of violence

Zero tolerance of violence is what the society claims, but there are diversified opinions as to how to achieve this: by more education or by clearly stating in law that violence anywhere, including the home in the form of corporal punishment, is unacceptable so that children do not model this behavior for conflict resolution.

Specific or broad legislations

For children left unattended, the government argues that there is already legislation against neglect. A specific law against young children being left unattended is unnecessary. The law as it is gives more flexibility in interpretation. The community is concerned that parents who leave their children unattended going to work to make ends meet will be criminalized. Advocates for a clear cut law stresses the educational value of legislation giving a clear message to the community what parental behavior is not tolerated. The penalty need not involve imprisonment in the first instance. It is difficult to prove "willful" neglect as stated in the current legislation.

Prevention of CAN

Tertiary preventive efforts have already been discussed. A two-year Child Fatality Review pilot project was launched early 2008. Whether lessons can be learnt waits to be seen as there is the review panel is not a statutory body. Submission of information by agencies that has been involved is on a voluntary basis. For non-fatal but serious child abuse cases, the review is mainly intra-agency.

Secondary prevention directed towards at risk families is undertaken through various programs one of which introduced by the government in 2005 is the Comprehensive Child Development Service being piloted in a few districts in Hong Kong. The program targets at risk pregnant women who are teenagers or have substance abuse or mental illness, families with psychosocial needs, mothers with postpartum depression and pre-school children with developmental problems. Its first evaluation report showed promising results so that the program will be extended to the entire territory in time (10).

NGOs like Against Child Abuse also runs programs like Healthy Start targeting first time mothers and Good Parenting Project for new parents whose fathers are Hong Kong residents but the mothers are mainland Chinese residents (11).

The government Department of Health has an Integrated Child Health and Development Program for 0 to 5 year olds that includes a parenting program started in 2002 with two components – universal parenting program for all expectant parents or child carers of pre-school children and the Positive Parenting Program (Triple P) for parents having difficulties in parenting (12).

Family Life Education also as primary prevention is the responsibility of Integrated Family Service Centers. As explained above, there is high competition for resources in the same centres to address remedial services.

LOOKING FORWARD

Although tertiary prevention always seems more urgent, when hardly one percent of children who suffer severe physical abuse in the community are reported, there will never be enough resources to manage all the potential cases. Resources have to be devoted to primary and secondary prevention despite results needing a longer period of time to achieve. As Hong Kong is facing constant changes with the closer ties with mainland China, prevention has to address changing needs of families and reach the population most at risk. There is awareness that any new program should incorporate evaluative research so that scarce resources can be directed towards programs of proven value. It is hoped that funding bodies will cover not only the service, but also the research element to help ensure that evidence-based services are being provided. Apart from individual programs, Hong Kong needs a child policy and a child commission which can put into practice the principle stated in the Convention on the Rights of the Child which has been extended to Hong Kong since 1994 - "the best interests of the child shall be a primary consideration". For children to be protected, a system is only part of the jigsaw puzzle.

REFERENCES

[1]   Kempe CH, Silverman FN, Steele BF, Droegemueller W, Silver HK. The battered-child syndrome. JAMA 1962;181:17-24.

[2]   Social Welfare Department, Hong Kong Special Administrative Region. Procedural guide for handling of child abuse cases (Revised 2007). [cited 2009 Mar 10] . Available from: http://www.swd.gov.hk/en/index/site_pubsvc/page_family/sub_fcwprocedure/id_childabuse1998/

[3]   Social Welfare Department, Hong Kong Special Administrative Region. Child Protection Registry Statistical Report 2007. Hong Kong: Social Welfare Department.

[4]   Social Welfare Department, Hong Kong Special Administrative Region. Statistics on child abuse, battered spouse and sexual violence cases. [cited 2009 Mar 10]. Available from: http://www.swd.gov.hk/vs/english/stat.html

[5]   Chan KL. Study on child abuse and spouse battering: report on findings of household survey. 2005. Hong Kong: Department of Social Work and Social Administration, the University of Hong Kong. [cited 2009 Mar 10]. Available from: http://www.swd.gov.hk/vs/doc/Report on Findings of Household Survey.pdf

[6]   Tang CS. Childhood experience of sexual abuse among Hong Kong Chinese college students. Child Abuse Negl 2002;26:23-37.

[7]   Social Welfare Department (2005). Integrated Family Service [homepage on the Internet]. C2005[updated 2009 Feb 18:cited 2009 Mar 10]. Available from http://www.swd.gov.hk/en/index/site_pubsvc/page_family/sub_listofserv/id_228/

[8]   Hong Kong Medical Co-ordinators on Child Abuse. Medical management of child abuse in Hong Kong: results of a territory-wide inter-hospital prospective surveillance study. Hong Kong Med J 2003;9:6-9.

[9]   Ip P. Multi-disciplinary decision-making. In: O'Brian C, Cheng CYL, Rhind N, editors. Responding to child abuse: procedures and practice for child protection in Hong Kong. Hong Kong: Hong Kong Univ Press, 1997.

[10]   Family Health Service, Department of Health, Hong Kong. Evaluation Report of the Comprehensive Child Development Service (CCDS). 2007. Available from http://www.fhs.gov.hk/english/reports/files/ccds_full.pdf

[11]   Against Child Abuse. [homepage on the Internet]. [cited 2009 Mar 10]. Available from http://www.aca.org.hk/menu/ef_menu.html?2

[12]   Leung SSL. Child health service in Hong Kong: the child health programme for Hong Kong. HK J Paediatr (new series) 2008;13:275-8.

In: International Aspects of Child Abuse and Neglect   ISBN: 978-1-60876-703-8
Editors: H. Dubowitz, J. Merrick pp. 11-23   © 2010 Nova Science Publishers, Inc.

Chapter 2

CHILD PROTECTION: SCENARIO IN INDIA

Sibnath Deb

Department of Applied Psychology, Calcutta University, India

The broad objective of this chapter is to outline the current scenario related to child protection in India. The chapter clearly highlights the definition of child abuse and neglect (CAN) used in different legal measures in India and describes the strategies and approaches for combating the problem and their advantages and disadvantages. The Government of India has created a new ministry called The Ministry of Women and Child Development for ushering and implementing a prevention and intervention program for protection of child rights. Further impetus to CAN has come from the National Commission for Protection of Child Rights Act 2005 and formation of the National Commission for Protection of the Child Rights in subsequent years; all the States and Union Territories in India are in the process of setting up of State Commissions for Protection of Child Rights. Regarding reporting and redressal of CAN issues, laws like Juvenile Justice (Care and Protection) Act 2000 (amended in 2006) are implemented across the country along with a number of social measures. In general, over population resulting in poor service delivery, poverty, illiteracy, abandonment of children, poor reporting, cultural beliefs and practices pertaining to parenting style and child development are the biggest challenges in addressing the issue of child abuse and neglect in India. Although the main problem lies with the implementation of the laws in reality, in the truest sense, it is expected that close monitoring of the programs will change the situation over time.

INTRODUCTION

India, one of the largest democracies in the world, ranks second in terms of population (about 1.2 billion) in the world, surpassed only by China (1). The peculiarity of India lies in its cultural diversity. Geographically, India is an amalgam of 28 States and seven Union Territories, each with its own set of cultural beliefs and practices with regard to child rearing, social and linguistic identity. Statistically speaking, the children form about 44.4% of the total population (1), but yet form a minority in terms of legal protection, governmental policy and benefits as a citizen. They are almost always at the mercy of their immediate caregivers.

However, ongoing works of academicians, social activists and community-based organizations are helping to mobilize the popular concern for these sections of the society in forming legislative protection. One out of every two children in India are deprived of the opportunity of basic primary education although the Government of India has come out with a National Policy on Education (1986, modified in 1992).

In the ensuing introduction certain facets of child abuse prevalent in different sections of Indian society are discussed along with core issues. Violence against children in Indian society is linked to socio-economic and demographic variables operating at each stratum of the society. The Indian society can be divided into three broad groups in terms of income viz., low, middle and high-income groups. Each group has its unique beliefs, regarding child rearing and parenting practices - converging on certain issues but divergent in others.

Dimensions of child abuse in low socio-economic sections of the society are different from the other two income groups. Most pressing issues in the low-income group are related to literacy and economic factors. The highest rates of school dropout, petty crimes, juvenile delinquency (2), and child mortality and morbidity are found among the children. A peculiar feature of the people of the low income group is related to the size of the family which is seen to be influenced by the belief system that the larger the family, the greater would be its chances of survival in the society. The parents use the children for economic support, and have a high preference for the male child. The discrimination in terms of gender is caused by multiple social and cultural factors. The girl child is considered an expense and liability to the family and is discriminated against in terms of nutrition, education, and medical care. Issues of child marriage among girls and adolescent pregnancy are avid in this section of the society, endangering not only the mother but also the child in the process. Premarital pregnancy is also on the rise, leading to child abandonment and infanticide. Lack of family supervision and disturbed family environment leads to high number of school dropouts, lowering the literacy rate and increasing the crime rate. Another fallout of this issue is the increase in the number of street children and their exploitation as domestic and commercial help.

Trafficking of children and commercial exploitation are issues that are overlooked in spite of border security and patrol. Parents sell off their children for meager sums of money - mostly daughters - who are then trafficked to cities or across the border as labours, domestic help, or for other commercial purposes (3). Lack of available modes of entertainment in the lower income groups, especially in the rural areas, increase the dependence of young males on pornography, the brunt of which is bore by young females who are taken advantage of. A prevalent belief among the men in the rural areas is that one may cure oneself of sexually transmitted diseases through intercourse with a minor. Disciplinary procedures in the rural areas are mostly through corporal punishment - girls are more likely to be verbally and psychologically abused than boys.

In this discussion, the people of the upper and middle-income group are grouped since they have some similarities. Issues of abuse relate mostly to the parenting styles and unrealistic expectations of the parents regarding the child's education and career (4). Parents psychologically pressurize the children and also apply corporal punishment for better academic performance, which leads to high rates of depression and anxiety among the youth (5). The fear of examination, and specific phobias associated with the same, mark the lackluster life of the youths of this section of the society. Often suicide is the only option they see available to them. Lack of role models and identity crises are some of the pressing issues that children have to combat with.

THE DEFINITION OF CHILD ABUSE AND NEGLECT (CAN)

There are a number of laws pertaining to prevention of exploitation of children in India that provide definitions of child abuse and neglect. Child abuse and neglect have various dimensions and rights of the children have been violated in different forms. Therefore, situation-specific definitions have been used in different legislations. For example, Articles 23 and 39 of the Constitution of India guarantee the Right to Freedom from all forms of Exploitation. Article 23 of the Constitution of India particularly prohibits trafficking in human beings and forced labour. The Constitution of India also directs all the States to provide free and compulsory education to all children of the age of six to fourteen years (Article 21A). Through the National Policy for Children, 1974, the Government of India is committed to provide adequate services to children, both before and after birth, and throughout the period of growth, to ensure their full physical, mental and social development.

The Indian Penal Code (IPC), 1860, is meant for the victims of various kinds of crimes, including crimes committed in the course of trafficking a child. It provides for criminal liability and prosecution of offenders for simple and grievous hurt (sections 319 to 329); wrongful restraint and wrongful confinement (sections 339, 340-346); criminal force and criminal assault (sections 350 and 351); import/export/removal/buying, selling/disposing/ accepting/receiving/detaining of any person as a slave (section 370). Section 372 and 373 of the IPC set punishment for selling and buying of minors for purposes of prostitution while section 376-2C spells out the punishment for rape.

The Juvenile Justice (Care and Protection of Children) Act, 2000 (amended in 2006) helps ensure care and protection for trafficked children and their reintegration with their families and the community. The law also recognizes certain offences against children as special offences and provides for punishment. These include cruelty against a juvenile (section 23), using a child for begging (section 24), giving liquor or drugs to a child (section 25), and procuring a child for employment (section 26).

The Immoral Traffic (Prevention) Act, 1956, has been passed by the Indian Parliament, for addressing the immoral trafficking of women and children. Section 6 of the Immoral Traffic (Prevention) Act, 1956, sets punishment for detaining a person (woman or girl) in premises where prostitution is carried on. The Child Marriage Restraint Act, 1929, prohibits marriage of a male child below twenty-one years of age, and that of a female child who is yet to reach eighteen years of age. The Child Labour (Prohibition and Regulation) Act, 1986, defines the child as a person who has not completed his fourteenth year of age. This Act prohibits employment of children in certain occupations and processes.

The National Charter for Children (2003) states (article 9) that all children have a right to be protected against neglect, maltreatment, injury, trafficking, sexual and physical abuse of all kinds, corporal punishment, torture, violence and degrading treatment. The National Institute for Public Cooperation and Child Development (NIPCCD) (1988) has come out with a definition. According to NIPCCD, child abuse and neglect is the intentional and non-accidental injury or maltreatment of children by parents/caretakers, employers or others, including those individuals representing Government/NGO bodies, which may lead to temporary or permanent impairment of their physical, mental, psycho-social development, disability or death (6).

Apart from these, different definitions related to the issue are used by different researchers. The WHO definition of child abuse is one commonly cited. For example, child abuse and maltreatment constitutes all forms of physical and/or emotional ill-treatment, sexual abuse, neglect or negligent treatment or commercial or other exploitation, resulting in actual or potential harm to the child's health, survival, development or dignity - in the context of a relationship of responsibility, trust or power (7).

THE EXTENT OF CHILD ABUSE AND NEGLECT IN INDIA

In India, child maltreatment is a little recognized phenomenon. In addition to the horrors of feticide, many children are subjected to violence, discrimination and abuse and neglect, which affect their physical and mental development. There is no accurate estimation of the extent of these problems in India (8).

Some of the latest study findings carried out in India have been reviewed and presented in this section. The worst form of violence against children in India is the killing of a child guided by religious and cultural beliefs (8).

A national level study on child abuse carried out by the Prayas Institute of Juvenile Justice during 2006 and 2007, in collaboration with the Ministry of Women and Child Development, Government of India, revealed widespread abuse of girls and boys in India. Both boys and girls are equally at risk of abuse. The persons in trust and authority are major abusers. Five to twelve year old children are in the high-risk category. About one-third (70%) of the children have not reported the abuse to anyone. Two out of every three children have been physically abused. Two out of every three school-going children are victims of corporal punishment; half of these incidents occur in government-run schools. More than half of the child respondents reported facing one or more forms of sexual abuse. Half the children reported facing emotional abuse, and in more than 80% this was by their parents (9).

In another article on ethics in research on child abuse, the authors reviewed the national level study on child abuse carried out by Prayas Institute of Juvenile Justice and recognized the need for ethical inquiry in this area. Certain concerns about the conduct of the study were raised. Core ethical issues pertaining to consent and refusal, risk and benefit, effects of the study process on the researcher and the researched and the reporting of adverse events were discussed. The ethical implications of the study and ethical responsibilities of the researcher were emphasized (10).

In a study in an observation home in Delhi covering 189 boys, the author found that only 38.1% of the sexual abuse cases were reported (11). Further, on clinical examination, among the sexually abused children (n=72) physical signs were seen in 23.8% and behavioural signs were seen in 16.3%. Sexual abuse was found to be significantly associated with domestic violence (p=0.016), solvent/ inhalant use (p=0.0002) and working status (p=0.017).

In a Kolkata-based study, Deb (12) found that 30.0% of the male and 16.7% of the female teachers still believe in applying physical punishment to discipline the students in school. On the contrary, when it comes to practice, 33.3% of male and 40.0% of female teachers reportedly confessed that they punished students physically, although a good number of them did condemn this practice. Findings also revealed that 60.0% of the male teachers and 53.4% of the female teachers had been physically punished during their childhood. In another study, Deb (4) revealed that 4.55% of the mothers openly stated that it is necessary to use physical punishment to discipline children or to make them obedient.

A study covering a group of 120 migrant child laborers working in households, tea stalls, garages and shops in South Kolkata revealed that an overwhelming number of the children were abused (13). A study of 35 trafficked children and young women found that trafficking is usually conducted through offers of false marriages and jobs, or through outright abduction and sale (3). In another study, the authors (14) found that six out of 41 trafficked children were affected by HIV/AIDS.

In the recent past, the media has reported a number of cases related to violence against children. The latest incidence in the village of Nithari, Noida, UP, revealed a horrifying picture of death of many children after they have been sexually abused. Perhaps the media coverage brought such practices to the attention of the public and that might have made them alert to the possibility of such horrible crime taking place in their backyard. The Judge of a special court of Criminal Bureau of Investigation (CBI) has given death sentence to the two perpetrators, one-aged 55 years and the other 38, for rape and murder of a 14-year-old girl - one of 19 victims in the sensational Nithari serial killings (15).

Laws banning child marriages were introduced in India as early as 1929. But 80 years down the line, this gravest of all social ills continues to thrive. Nearly half of (45.0%) the women in India are married off before they reach the age of 18, a joint Indo-American study reported the same in the Lancet. The report further states that more than 40.0% of the world's child marriages take place in India (16).

Malnutrition is another important issue, which affect a large number of children in India. According to the National Family Health Survey-3 (2006), more than 56.0% of the teenaged girls in India are anaemic with a haemoglobin count of less than 12g/deciliter, the world standard. But what is worrying is the increasing incidence of iron-deficiency among the city-bred teens (17).

THE SYSTEMS AND INFRASTRUCTURE TO ADDRESS CAN IN INDIA

The Government of India (GOI) acceded to the UN Convention on the Rights of the Child on December 11, 1992, which reflects the seriousness of the government in addressing the CAN within the broad framework. The Ministry of Women and Child Development and the Ministry of Social Justice and Empowerment, GOI, are mainly responsible for ushering and implementation of the prevention and intervention program for protection of child rights.

The Child Protection Programs of the two aforesaid Ministries focus on the group namely, children in crisis situation such as street children, children who have been abused, abandoned children, orphaned children, children in conflict with the law, and children affected by conflict or disasters, etc. Some of the programs of the government include An Integrated Program for Street Children, Chidline Services, Government of India – UNICEF Work Plan on Child Protection, Central Adoption Resource Agency, The National Institute of Public Cooperation and Child Development and so on.

The National Charter for Children (2003) states: The State shall take legal action against those committing such violations against children even if they be legal guardians of such children; (c) The State shall, in partnership with the community, set up mechanisms for identification, reporting, referral, investigation and follow-up of such acts, while respecting the dignity and privacy of the child; (d) The State shall, in partnership with the community, take up steps to draw up plans for the identification, care, protection, counselling and rehabilitation of child victims and ensure that they are able to recover, physically, socially and psychologically, and re-integrate into society.

One of the latest initiatives of the Government of India for ensuring child rights is bringing new legislation i.e., the Commissions for Protection of the Child Rights Act, 2005. Therefore, the National Commission for Protection of Child Rights has been established in 2006 and all the States and the Union Territories are in the process of setting up State Commissions for Protection of Child Rights. The objective of these National and State Commissions is to ensure proper enforcement of children's rights and effective implementation of laws and programs relating to children. The Commission has a Chairperson and six other members, including two women members, a Member Secretary and other supporting staff. The functions of the commission:

- Examine and review the safeguards provided by Constitution or any law for the protection of child rights and recommend measures for their effective implementation
- Present to the Central Government, annually, reports upon the working of those safeguards.
- Examine all factors that inhibit the enjoyment of rights of most vulnerable children and children in need of special care and protection
- Study treaties and other international instruments and undertake periodical review of existing policies, programs and other activities on child rights and make recommendation for their effective implementation in the best interest of children.
- Undertake and promote research in the field of child rights
- Spread child rights literacy among various sections of the society and promote awareness
- Inspect any juvenile custodial home, or any other place of residence or institution meant for children for the purpose of treatment, reformation or protection and take up with these authorities for remedial action
- Inquire into complaints and take suo motu notice of matters relating to deprivation of child's rights, non-implementation of laws for protection and development of children, non-compliance of policy decisions, take up the issues arising out of such matters with appropriate authorities and such other functions as may be considered necessary for the promotion of child rights

The powers of the commission include:

- Summoning and enforcing the attendance of any person and examining him on oath;
- Requiring the discovery and production of any document;
- Receiving evidence on affidavits;
- Requisitioning any public record or copy thereof from any court or office; and
- Issuing commissions for the examination of witnesses and documents;

- Forwarding any case to a magistrate having jurisdiction to try the same and the magistrate to whom any such case is forwarded shall proceed to hear the complaint against the accused;
- Recommending to the concerned government or authority the initiation of proceedings for prosecution or such other action as deem fit against the concerned person/s;
- Approaching the supreme court or the high court concerned for such directions, orders or writs as that court may deem necessary;
- Recommending to the concerned government or authority for the grant of such interim relief to the victim or the members of his family, as the commission consider necessary.

The Bill also provides that State Governments may constitute State Commissions for Protection of Child Rights in their State and designate a State level and other district level children's Court in their respective State.The Bill has similar provisions for State Commissions with respect to their constitution, report functions and powers.

With the alleviation of the status of Department of Women and Child Development to an independent Ministry headed by the Minister of State having independent charge, it was necessary to change the above provision to make the Minister in charge of the Ministry of Women and Child Development as the Chairperson of the Selection Committee for the selection of the Chairperson of the National Commission for Protection of Child Rights. The Commissions for Protection of Child Rights (Amendment) Bill 2006 have been passed by both the Houses of Parliament for the same.

The Juvenile Justice (Care and Protection of Children) Act, 2000 (amended in 2006) is an Act to consolidate and amend the law relating to juveniles in conflict with law and children in need of care and protection, by providing for proper care, protection and treatment by catering to their development needs, and by adopting a child-friendly approach in the adjudication and disposition of matters in the best interest of children and for their ultimate rehabilitation through various institutions established under the enactment. Under this Act, two committees are supposed to be established, the Juvenile Justice Board and Child Welfare Committee in each district or for a group of districts for dealing with juvenile cases in conflict with the law.

The Juvenile Justice Board shall consist of a Metropolitan Magistrate or a Judicial Magistrate of the first class and two social workers of which at least one shall be a woman. The Magistrate should have clear knowledge or training in child psychology or child welfare while social workers should al least seven years working experience in the field of health, education and/or child welfare activities. This board is empowered to deal exclusively with all proceedings under this Act relating to juvenile in conflict with law.

The Child Welfare Committee under the Juvenile Justice (Care and Protection) Act 2006 is empowered to ensure care and protection to children in need. The Committee shall consist of a Chairperson and four other members. At least, one of the members of the committee shall be a women and an expert on matters concerning children. A non-judicial person can become a Chairperson of the Child Welfare Committee. A child in need of care and protection may be produced before an individual member for being placed in safe custody or otherwise when the Committee is not in session. The Committee shall have the final authority to dispose of cases for the care, protection, treatment, development and rehabilitation of the children as well as to provide for their basic needs and protection of human rights. The Committee has the power to deal exclusively with all proceedings under this Act relating to children in need of care and protection.

REPORTING OF POSSIBLE CAN

Although reporting is mandatory (sections 176, 177, 197 and 201 of IPC, 1860), in general, reporting of CAN cases in Indian society is very low owing to a number of factors like social stigma, perceived harassment, unwillingness of parents, disbelief of parents and threat by perpetrators. For example, in a recent study in Kolkata, India only 1.7% of sexually abused cases were reported to the police (18) while in case of another study carried out in Agartala, Tripura (India), 15.5% of the sexually abused cases were reported to the police (19). The causes behind non-reporting are similar as stated above. Reporting of cases of sexual abuse is always very low across the geographical boundaries because of a number of factors (20).

As per Juvenile Justice (Care and Protection) Act 2000 (amended in 2006), any child in need of care and protection may be produced before the Child Welfare Committee by any of the persons like any police officer or special juvenile police unit or a designated police officer; any public servant; childline, a registered voluntary organization or by such other voluntary organizations or an agency as may be recognized by the State Government; any social worker or a public spirited citizen authorized by the State Government; or by the child himself. On receipt of a report under section 32 of JJ Act 2000, the committee or any police officer or special juvenile police unit or the designated police officer shall hold an inquiry in the prescribed manner and the Committee, on its own or on the report from any person or agency as mentioned in sub-section (1) of section 32, may pass in order to send the child to the children's home for speedy inquiry by a social worker or child welfare officer.

When professionals such as doctors, social workers and teachers identify a suspected case of family violence against children, they may be required by law to report their suspicions to the responsible authorities, or are expected to do so, irrespective of legal obligation. To be effective, reporting structures must always be matched with equally well-developed structures for protection, support and treatment for the children and their families. Countries with mandatory reporting laws, including India, should consider systems reforms that allow the children and their families' access to confidential services where they can receive support on a voluntary basis.

In India, in general, most of the police stations do not have a confidential space to conduct interviews with the child, and the lack of female police officials is a huge impediment in investigating and recording of the incident. Sometimes, the children are coerced to describe in-detail the traumatic incident over and over again, with no guarantee of confidentiality of the information they render. This subsequently may make them more vulnerable to the perpetrators who had abused them in the first place. Most importantly, the greatest hindrance to the female child's disclosure comes from her immediate family. Sexual abuse being perceived, as it is in India, family members often find it difficult to acknowledge the incident, accept the child and extend unconditional affection and co-operation. In the Indian society, the female, however young and helpless, is tarnished for life by this experience and is socially despised as if guilty of a crime. This has enormous importance, especially when it comes to arranging the girl's marriage.

STRENGTHS IN THE APPROACH/SYSTEM

Recently, the Government of India realized the extent of the problem of child abuse and neglect in India, and created a separate ministry called the Ministry of Women and Child Development (2005) to look into child protection issue more seriously. Thereafter, the Commission for Protection for Child Rights Act 1995 has been passed by the parliament and also established the National Commission for Protection of Child Rights in 1997. As per the Commission for Protection of Child Rights Act, 1995 every state should constitute Commission for Protection of Child Rights. The beauty of this Act is its wide coverage of issues relating to Child Protection i.e., every district should appoint a child protection officer to closely monitor and work with the grass-root level organizations. Further, looking into the various dimensions of child abuse in India, such as, sexual exploitation, economic exploitation, domestic violence, trafficking for prostitution, corporal punishment and so on, the Ministry of Women and Child Development prepared a draft called Offenses against Children (Prevention) Bill and circulated among experts at various levels for comments and suggestions. In this proposed Bill the corporal punishment has been banned. The Bill is still under discussion and awaiting approval by the Cabinet.

Presently, there is no law for prevention of corporal punishment in schools. However, the government has issued instructions to States to stop its use in schools and the National Policy on Education (1986, modified in 1992) states in section 5.6 that "corporal punishment will be firmly excluded from the educational systems".

Increasing collaboration between government and non-government organizations in some of the States in India is another positive aspect for implementation of the Child Protection Policy of the Government at the district level. A good number of districts have already appointed Child Protection Officer and they are working closely with the grass-root organizations for child protection.

Some of the professional agencies are trying to bring together certain educational institutions for forming Child Protection Team comprising of teacher, guardians, psychologists and students. At the same time, some NGO's have adapted Child Protection Policy for rendering effective services to the children.

It is relevant to mention here the positive gesture of senior Police Officials as well as authorities of different Medical Colleges and Hospitals for organizing multidisciplinary training programmes on Child Protection funded by OAK foundation and ISPCAN implemented during 2003 to 2007, which sensitized professionals, developed and fine tuned their skills in identification, diagnosis and treatment of abused children in addition to developing strong network among the professionals.

THE WEAKNESSES AND CHALLENGES OF THE SYSTEM

Although there are a number of laws for protecting children's rights in India, the main problem lies with its implementation across the country. For example, section 63 of the Juvenile Justice (Care and Protection) Act 2000 clearly states that every police station should have at least one 'juvenile or the child welfare officer' for handling juvenile cases, and they should be properly trained. However, in reality the said provision in law could not been implemented across the country. Secondly, lack of allocation of fund for adequate services and lack of trained professional manpower for dealing with abused and maltreated children, lack of coordination among the NGOs and between government and NGOs especially in the rural areas are some of the major weaknesses of the system in addition to lack of government accommodation facilities for safe custody of the rescued children from the red light areas and for the children in need of care especially orphan and destitute children. Since there is no provision for systematic documentation of reported cases of abuse in the police stations and in the hospitals, organisations find it difficulty to develop evidence-based comprehensive intervention programme for child protection. On the other hand, there are no family-based services to identify the high-risk families for prevention of child abuse and neglect. Most of the educational institutions especially the primary schools do not have child protection policy. As compared to need, very few workshops, orientation and/or sensitization programmes have been undertaken in the community for creating awareness among the parents on the issue.

Overpopulation resulting in poor service delivery, poverty, illiteracy, abandonment of children, cultural beliefs, poor reporting and practices pertaining to parenting style and child development are some of the biggest challenges in addressing the child abuse and neglect issue in India. For example, corporal punishment, early girl child marriage, gender discrimination, not giving colostrums to a new-born out of a feeling that it might upset the stomach of the infant are some of the common cultural beliefs and practices prevalent in some communities in India. Child trafficking is another problem increasing alarmingly, since India shares its boarder with Bangladesh, Pakistan, Nepal, Mayanmar and Bhutan. A good number of children from the said countries cross the boarder and finally land up in commercial sex trade. Even, within the country, a good number of girl children from poor families are becoming the victim of child trafficking. In general, Indians do not consider children as an individual who should have freedom of expression of views and opinions. Therefore, changing the mindset of Indian population towards the children is essential for creating child friendly environment across the society.

MAJOR CONTROVERSIES IN THE APPROACH/SYSTEM

A number of issues sometime create problems in implementing the laws. For example, when a question of rescue of newborn abandoned child comes, there is always a controversy about the jurisdiction between two police stations. As a result, in most of the cases the newborn abandoned child dies. Few month back a newborn abandoned child was laying on the bank of Ganga. After noticing the child few people informed the local police station and were informed that the area concerned does not fall under their jurisdiction so they cant take any action. Then the same group of people informed another police station as suggested by former police station and the same explanation was issued. Finally, after settling the issue when police from one of the stations came, the child had already died. This is not an isolated incidence. There are so many such incidences that have happed in the past.

The dilemmas related to acceptance of rescued child from the red light areas by the family members create a major problem for the mental health of the child. Red light areas are those areas from where commercial sex workers operate their business. On the other hand, a good number of family members do not come forward to receive their missing child when they come to know that the child has been rescued from the red light areas because of social stigma. There is a fear that if the family members have received the child, it could affect the social relation of another girl child of the same family.

In the Juvenile Justice (Care and Protection) Act 2000, a person up to 18 years of age is considered as a juvenile while in case of The Child Labour (Prohibition and Regulation) Act, 1986 a person up to 14 years of age is considered as child.

Another important issue which often bothers researchers, child rights activists and policy makers is how to prevent marriage of people suffering from major mental health problems of varying degrees. Child abuse and neglect has a direct relation with the mental health problems of the parents. The children coming from disturbed family or broken families have to bear the brunt of the family violence. At the same time, as per the Human Rights Law every individual has a right to marry, that cannot be prevented. Since there is a stigma attached to being diagnosed with mental health problems in the developing countries like India, instead of seeking professional help from the psychologists and/or psychiatrists, parents arrange marriage of their children secretly with an expectation that after marriage the mental health problems of their chidren will be solved automatically - which is absolutely a mistaken notion. Marriage does not solve the problem, rather it creates a major life-long problem for the spouse and other family members.

There should be a stringent law in any society to penalise the guardians who arrange marriage of their children with mental health problems and/or with other serious problems like alcoholism/addiction without informing the spouse clearly about the same. The progenies coming from such union are invariably born with mental health problems and the disturbed family environment cultivates delinquency, neglect, maltreatment and other social adjustement problems in the children.

PREVENTION EFFORTS

After adoption of the Commission for Protection for Child Rights Act 1995, local governments and some NGOs are working together, especially in the urban and semi-urban areas, along with international NGO's such as UNICEF, DFID, Save the Children, CARE and Goal (Ireland) on primary prevention education campaign on issues such as gender discrimination, violence against children, primary health care and education, child trafficking and labour. Local/State Governments identified a number of NGOs as safe custody for destitute, orphan and trafficked children. Some of those NGOs have arrangements for vocational training programs for the children along with individual and group counseling for the traumatic children. A good number of children get the opportunity to become self-sufficient and start living independently. Some of the NGOs also try to establish contact with the family members and ask them for visiting the child periodically so that child feels better. Children are also encouraged to go back to their own family to avoid re-victimization. However, the efforts, which have been made for prevention of child abuse and neglect by different agencies, are not adequate as compared to the need. More preventive efforts should be made in the interior rural belts.

CONCLUSIONS

The Government of India recognizes the seriousness of child abuse and neglect in India. To combat the same, a new ministry with independent charge has been created and the government has come out with a number of new legislations for protection of child rights followed by formation of the National Commission. All the States and the Union Territories are in the process of setting up of State Commissions for Protection of Child Rights. There is a serious need to look into some of the core issues like population control, poverty, illiteracy, unemployment and primary health issues at the national program of the Government of India, which are directly linked with child abuse and neglect. Otherwise, whatever efforts are being made, they may not have expected results.

REFERENCES

[1]   Census of India. Office of the Registrar General, India, Ministry of Home Affairs, Government of India, New Delhi, 2001.
[2]   Sibnath D, Kathakali M. Deviance among disadvantaged children in kolkata and reasons thereof. Indian J Criminol Criminalistics 2001; 22(1):41-53.
[3]   Sibnath D, Srivastava N, Chatterjee P, Chakraborty T. Processes of child trafficking in West Bengal: A qualitative study. Social Change 2005;35(2):112-23.
[4]   Sibnath D, Pooja C. Styles of parenting adolescents: The Indian scenario. New Delhi: Akansha Publ House, 2008.
[5]   Sibnath D. Corporal punishment of children at home and in the school: A comparative study of attitude, perception and practice of parents and teachers. Paper presented in the 15th International Congress on Child Abuse and Neglect, held during Sept. 19-22, 2004 in Brisbane, Australia.
[6]   National Institute of Public Cooperation and Child Development (NIPCCD) workshop report on child abuse and neglect, 1988.
[7]   World Health Organisation Report, 1999.
[8]   Sibnath D. Chidlren in agony. New Delhi: Concept Publ, 2006.
[9]   Report on Child Abuse and Neglect. New Delhi: Min Women Child Dev, 2007.
[10]   Veena AS, Chandra Prabha S. A review of the ethics in research on child abuse. Indian J Med Ethics 2007;3:25-34.
[11]   Deepti P. A study of physical and sexual abuse and behavioural problems amongst boys from an observation home in Delhi. Dissertation. New Delhi: Univ Delhi, 2003.
[12]   Sibnath D. Defining child maltreatment in India. World perspectives on child abuse, 6th ed. Chicago: ISPCAN, 2004:63-7.
[13]   Sibnath D. Child abuse and neglect in a metropolitan city: A qualitative study of migrant child labour in South Kolkata. Social Change 2005;35(3): 56-67.
[14]   Pooja C, Tanusree C, Neerajakshi S, Sibnath D. Short and tong-term problems faced by the trafficked children: A qualitative study. Soc Sci Int 2006;22(1):167-82.
[15]   Death sentence for Pandher and Koli. Assam Tribune 2008 Feb 14:71 (43):1.

[16] Eighty years after it has been banned, 45% of the girls are still married off before 18. Times of India 2009 Mar 13:11.

[17] Girls, interrupted: Anaemia hits cities. Times of India 2009 March 13:11.

[18] Sibnath D, Aparna M. Impact of sexual abuse on mental health of children. New Delhi: Concept Publ, 2009.

[19] Subhasis M. Violence against children in Tripura and its impact. Dissertation. Calcutta: Calcutta Univ, 2009.

[20] Csorba R, Lampe L, Borsos A, Balla L, Poka R, Olah E. Female child sexual abuse within the family in a Hungarian county. Gynecol Obstet Invest 2006;61(4):188-193.

In: International Aspects of Child Abuse and Neglect   ISBN: 978-1-60876-703-8
Editors: H. Dubowitz, J. Merrick pp. 25-29   © 2010 Nova Science Publishers, Inc.

Chapter 3

CHILD PROTECTION IN PAKISTAN

Tufail Muhammad

Child Rights and Abuse Committee, Pakistan Pediatric Association,
Hyatabd, Peshawar, Pakistan

Pakistan does not have a legal definition of child abuse and neglect (CAN) and professionals usually follow the definition put forward by the World Health organization. Mandatory reporting does not exist and there is very little data on the prevalence of child abuse. The government has approved a "National Plan of Action for Children" and a draft "Child Protection Bill" await parliamentary action. The Plan of Action calls for the prevention of CAN at all levels, protection of children from all forms of abuse and exploitation, and the recovery and rehabilitation of victims. Although some steps have been taken in that direction, the implementation of the plan is rather weak. The Child Protection Bill calls for the establishment of child protection bureaus, a child protection fund for legal and social support and the appointment of child protection officers at the community level.

INTRODUCTION

There are no legal definitions of the forms of child abuse and neglect (CAN) in Pakistan. Professionals usually follow the WHO (World Health Organization) definitions of physical, emotional and sexual abuse (1). There is still ambiguity and poor understanding regarding the non-contact forms of sexual abuse, such as exposure to pornography. There are no agreed upon definitions of neglect.

WHAT IS KNOWN ABOUT THE EXTENT OF THE PROBLEM?

In Pakistan, there is no system of mandated reporting of child abuse and neglect. Although CAN exists in several overt and covert ways, there is a paucity of reliable statistics and published data on its prevalence in Pakistan. Like other major public health and social problems, it is not easy to document the actual incidence or prevalence of child abuse. It is always difficult to obtain information on sensitive and highly stigmatized issues, and even more difficult when the victims are children, who often cannot or do not disclose their experiences. In such a socio-cultural setting, most cases of child abuse remain hidden and unreported.

Professionals working in the field of CAN have tried to construct a picture of CAN in Pakistan, based on small studies, situational analyses, clinical experience, limited medico-legal records and newspaper reports. The overall picture that emerges shows that most of the reported cases are for sexual abuse and exploitation. A study conducted by the Child Rights and Abuse Committee, Pakistan Pediatric Association (CRAC-PPA) and NGOs Coalition on Child Rights in the North West Frontier Province (NWFP) showed that physical abuse was the most common form of CAN in the province (2). Crimes such as murder, severe beatings, kidnapping, trafficking, rape, sodomy, gang rape, severe neglect, emotional abuse and other forms of violations of children are being frequently reported. Similar information subsequently was found another UNICEF sponsored study conducted by CRAC-PPA (2).

A recent study by CRAC-PPA (3) showed that newspapers alone reported 2,447 cases of violent forms of child sexual abuse. There were an alarming number of cases (10 %) of CSA, who had been killed during or soon after the assault by the perpetrators. A community-based study in NWFP showed that almost all children are subjected to some form of physical abuse at home (4). Slapping on the face or back, hitting with a stick, kicking, and pulling hair are the most common forms of abuse - in that order. The most common reasons for corporal punishment at home, as stated by parents, are "naughty" behavior, disobedience to elders and poor school performance. Most of these behaviors are not seen as abusive by parents and society at large.

WHAT SYSTEM(S) OR INFRASTRUCTURE EXISTS TO ADDRESS CAN?

Pakistan does not have a structured child protection system. Some major hospitals in the country have hospital Child Protection Committees (HCPC). The aim of a HCPC is to promote the health and wellbeing of children in distress through the optimal management of abused children by using a multidisciplinary approach at healthcare centers. All hospitals at district and sub-district levels have emergency and medico-legal sections to mange cases of child abuse, if reported for abuse or identified during regular health care. Some NGOs in the major cities have established psychosocial rehabilitation services for victims of sexual abuse and trafficking. Others have established shelters, drop in centers and help lines. By and large, there are no services in the rural areas and even in urban areas, the access to quality services is extremely limited.

How Does the System Work Regarding Reporting of Possible CAN? Laws?

As stated, the reporting of CAN is not mandatory in Pakistan (5). Most of the reported cases fall under the category of child sexual abuse or other violent crimes (e.g., severe physical injuries, kidnapping, etc.) against children. A case of CAN may be reported directly to the nearest police station or to the emergency room of a hospital, where parents or other caregivers have taken the victim for medical help. A child may also report him/herself, even in the absence of a legal guardian, depending on the circumstances. Similarly, the hospitals may also report abuse, suspected or diagnosed.

Describe the Nature of the "Typical" Response by the Responsible Agency(ies).

A typical response after the registration of a CAN case is that the victim is examined by a doctor, trained in medico-legal examination, and provided immediate medical services. The nature of harm is recorded after a complete medical examination. Forensic tests are also performed when needed. The police officers investigate the case, and may arrest the perpetrator under the relevant laws. In some cases, the victim is also provided psychological counseling and free legal aid. There is no system for follow-up and preventing the recurrence of abuse. The only intervention on the part of the hospital is to counsel the care providers to protect the child from further harm.

What Are the Strengths in Your Approach/System?

The only strength is that victims, in most cases, are provided free medical services. There are few provisions for social and legal support by the state. The existing institutes of joint and extended family systems provide most of the emotional and social support to the victims. This may partly compensate for the highly inadequate social support services by the state agencies.

What Are Weaknesses/Challenges in Your Approach/System?

The system is inconsistent, unstructured and the workforce has limited capacity. Different professionals follow different approaches, based on the availability of resources and their own likes and dislikes. Most of them would limit themselves only to medical services and refer the victim to NGOs for further help. The legal and social components of the response are extremely weak. The police and court system is not very sensitive to the needs of children and the victims are always in danger of further victimization. Lack of strategic planning and leadership is another major challenge facing the system.

WHAT ARE THE MAJOR CONTROVERSIES IN YOUR APPROACH/SYSTEM?

There is still a lack of consensus on what constitutes child abuse and neglect, not only among professionals, but also among the general public. Children are perceived as the property of their parents and families and the state and society should not question what they do to their children. The family unit is considered a strictly private domain and no one from outside should ever interfere in its affairs. With a few exceptions, most professionals lack expertise to properly manage the victims of CAN.

WHAT PREVENTION EFFORTS (PRIMARY, SECONDARY, TERTIARY) ARE IN PLACE AND TO WHAT EXTENT?

The government has approved a "National Plan of Action for Children" and a draft "Child Protection Bill" awaiting parliamentary action. The Plan of Action calls for the prevention of CAN at all levels, protection of children from all forms of abuse and exploitation, and the recovery and rehabilitation of victims. Although some steps have been taken in that direction, the implementation of the plan is rather weak. The Child Protection Bill calls for the establishment of child protection bureaus, a child protection fund for legal and social support, and the appointment of child protection officers at the community level. Some NGOs are running prevention programs in parts of the country, but their capacity and reach is rather limited.

REFRENCES

[1]   World Health Organization. Guidelines for medico legal care of victims of sexual violence. Geneva: WHO, 2003.
[2]   NCCR-UNICEF. Child abuse and crimes against children in NWFP. Peshawar, Pakistan,1997.
[3]   CRAC-UNICEF. Protection assessment amongst refuges and host communities in major urban areas of Pakistan. Peshawar, Pakistan, 2002.
[4]   WGCSAE-SC. Confronting reality II – Perceptions and incidence of child sexual abuse in Pakistan. Peshawar, Pakistan, 2008.
[5]   CRAC-PPA-UNICEF. Physical abuse of children at homes in NWFP. Peshawar, Pakistan,1998.

In: International Aspects of Child Abuse and Neglect   ISBN: 978-1-60876-703-8
Editors: H. Dubowitz, J. Merrick pp. 29-35   © 2010 Nova Science Publishers, Inc.

Chapter 4

CHILD PROTECTION IN THE PHILIPPINES

Bernadette J Madrid

Child Protection Unit, Philippine General Hospital,
University of the Philippines Manila, Manila, Philippines

The aim of this chapter is to describe how child abuse is defined in the Philippines, its prevalence and the response of the different sectors: Medical, legal, social to a child who is suspected of being abused. It discusses the problems and challenges in the creation of a responsive child protection system in a developing country. It underscores the role of government in bringing up to scale demonstration programs to achieve uniform access nationwide.

INTRODUCTION

The Philippines follows the general definition of violence in the WHO World Report on Violence and Health (1), which states that violence "is the intentional use of physical force or power, threatened or actual, against oneself, another person or against a group or community that either results in or has a high likelihood of resulting in injury, death, psychological harm, maldevelopment or deprivation." The 1999 WHO consultation on Child Abuse Prevention drafted the following definition: "Child abuse or maltreatment constitutes all forms of physical and/or emotional ill-treatment, sexual abuse, neglect or negligent treatment or commercial or other exploitation, resulting in actual or potential harm to the child's health, survival, development or dignity in the context of a relationship of responsibility, trust or power." Also in accordance with Article 19 of the UN Convention on the Rights of the Child of which the Philippines is a signatory since 1990; "violence will include all forms of physical or mental violence, injury and abuse, neglect or negligent treatment, maltreatment or exploitation, including sexual abuse."

After signing the UN CRC, Philippine Congress passed the Child Abuse Law in the Philippines: The Special Protection of Children against Child Abuse, Exploitation and Discrimination Act of 1992 (RA 7610) defines child abuse as "the maltreatment, whether habitual or not, of the child which includes any of the following:

- Psychological and physical abuse, neglect, cruelty, sexual abuse and emotional maltreatment;
- Any act by deeds or words which debases, degrades or demeans the intrinsic worth and dignity of a child as a human being;
- Unreasonable deprivation of his basic needs for survival such as food and shelter; or
- Failure to immediately give medical treatment to an injured child resulting in serious impairment of his growth and development or in his permanent incapacity or death.

The Implementing Rules and Regulations on the Reporting and Investigation of Child Abuse in the enforcement of RA 7610 further defined the following:

- Cruelty refers to any act by word or deed which debases, degrades or demeans the intrinsic worth and dignity of a child as a human being. Discipline administered by a parent or legal guardian does not constitute cruelty provided it is reasonable in manner and moderate in degree and does not constitute physical or psychological injury as defined herein.
- Physical Injury includes but not limited to lacerations, fractured bones, burns, internal injuries, severe injury or serious bodily harm suffered by a child.
- Psychological Injury means harm to a child's psychological or intellectual functioning which may be exhibited by severe anxiety, depression, withdrawal or outward aggressive behavior, or a combination of said behaviors, which may be demonstrated by a change in behavior, emotional response or cognition.
- Neglect means failure to provide, for reasons other than poverty, adequate food, clothing, shelter, basic education or medical care so as to seriously endanger the physical, mental, social and emotional growth and development of the child.
- Sexual abuse includes the employment, use, persuasion, inducement, enticement or coercion of a child to engage in, or assist another person to engage in, sexual intercourse or lascivious conduct or the molestation, prostitution, or incest with children.
- Exploitation means the hiring, employment, persuasion, inducement, or coercion of a child to perform in obscene exhibitions and indecent shows, whether live or in video or film, or to pose or act as a model in obscene publications or pornographic material, or to sell or distribute said materials.

ESTIMATES OF THE BURDEN OF THE PROBLEM

In 2007, the country's population was estimated at 88,706,300; 43% or 38 million were 18 years old and below. Growing annually at 2.35%, the country's population is projected to reach 102.8 million by 2015 (2). There is no centralized nor systemic collection of data on abused children in the Philippines. What is available are reports made to the Department of Social Welfare and Development where duplicative counting of the same case can occur since there is no computerized database. There are also separate reports to non-government organizations based on cases receiving their services. This has resulted in conflicting statistics where a government agency reports a decreasing number of reported abuse cases (figure 1), and an NGO reports (figure 2) increasing cases.

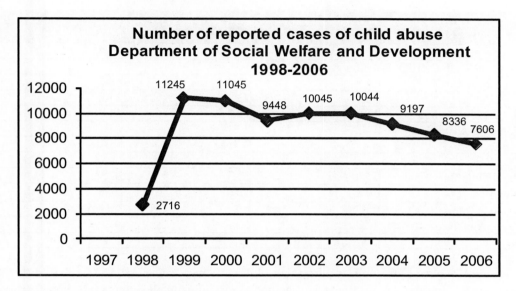

Figure 1. The number of reported cases of child abuse

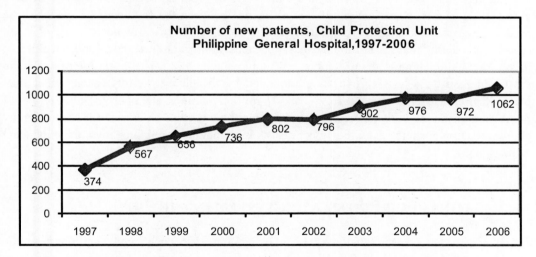

Figure 2. The number of new patients

It is well known that reported cases are simply the tip of the iceberg and do not reflect the true prevalence. The Department of Health in its population-based Baseline Survey for the National Objectives for Health (3) found that the base of the iceberg in the Philippines is indeed huge (see table 1). The survey on child abuse was conducted on 2,704 youth aged 13-24 years in 15 provinces including the National Capital Region as part of other surveys on youth health issues.

Table 1. Percentage of violence, abuse and neglect in adolescence, by gender (from Baseline Surveys for the National Objectives for Health, Philippines, 2000

ADOLESCENTS (n=2704)	TOTAL IN PERCENT	MALE (%) T (n=1348)	FEMALE (%) (n=1356)
Lifetime abuse	85.9	86.6	85.2
HISTORY OF CHILD ABUSE			
Psychological	59.7	65.7	54.5
Physical	82.9	73.7	81.0
Sexual Molestation	11.9	12.8	11.2
Forced Sex/Rape	1.8	3.5	0.2
Neglect	5.4	3.3	7.3
CURRENT ABUSE			
Psychological	35.0	37.3	32.9
Physical	29.8	30.0	29.5
Sexual Molestation	4.0	6.8	1.6
Forced Sex/Rape	1.7	2.8	0.8
Neglect	5.8	9.7	2.4

The high frequency of youth experiencing physical abuse can largely be explained by the acceptance of corporal punishment as a method of discipline in all settings (i.e., home, school, institutions). It is interesting to note that while 98% of reported sexual abuse cases involve girls (4), the survey shows no significant difference between the frequency of sexual abuse reported by male and female youth. The reported number of cases of neglect is low in all reports considering that the Philippines has thousands of street children and 4 million children involved in child labour (Dept of Labour and Employment, 2006). The definition of neglect in the Child Abuse Law (RA 7610) is confounded by the phrase "…for reasons other than poverty". For a country where 26.9% or 4.7 million families are poor (5) and 21.5% of families report moderate to severe hunger (6), poverty is used as an excuse for non-action by child protection agencies in child neglect cases, citing that the solution is beyond the mandate of the agency.

THE CHILD PROTECTION SYSTEM IN THE PHILIPPINES

Any person who suspects that a child is being abused or neglected can report to the Department of Social Welfare (DSWD), the police or any other law enforcement agency or to a local government Council for the Protection of Children. Reporting is mandatory for attending physicians, nurses or heads of any public or private hospital or medical clinic. Failure to report by a physician, nurse or head of a hospital results in a fine. In reality very few report and no one has been penalized for not reporting. The social welfare department and the police have hotlines and an NGO connected to the largest television station also runs a private hotline.

After receipt of a report of possible child abuse, the Dept of Social Welfare is supposed to conduct a home visit within 48 hours to evaluate the situation and to determine the safety of the child. The social workers of DSWD are invested with protective custody powers. Most of the reports go to the hotline run by the NGO which has a high media profile. Reports to the government agencies have not increased through the years, as shown by the statistics of the Dept of Social Welfare and Development, despite increased awareness by the public. This may be explained by the inconsistent response to reports. Only selected hotline reports result in home visits or investigation. There is no centralized repository of reports and more importantly there are no distinct Child Protection Services similar to that of developed countries. Social Welfare agencies run a generic unit that provide services to children, the elderly and migrant families, and offer disaster relief. There is no separate budget for child protection since the Child Protection Law itself (RA 7610) has no budget. Many child-related laws in the Philippines have no budget.

Criminal investigation of a child abuse case begins when a complaint is filed at a Women and Children's Concerns Desk at a police station or any law enforcement agency office by any of the following: 1) a child; 2) parent or legal guardian; 3) relative of the child within the third degree of consanguinity; 4) authorized officer or social worker of DSWD; 5) officer, social worker or representative of a licensed child caring institution; 6) Barangay Chairmen (locally elected officer); 7) at least three concerned responsible citizens of the community, where the abuse took place, who have personal knowledge of the offense committed. The law does not define what is meant by "responsible citizens" and there has never been a case where the complainants have been concerned citizens.

As part of the investigation, the child is brought to a government physician for physical/mental examination and/or medical treatment. If the investigation finds evidence of abuse, the police submit the investigation report together with the results of the physical/mental examination to a prosecutor for filing appropriate charges against the alleged offender. The prosecutor during a preliminary investigation decides whether there is enough prima facie evidence to bring the case to court. There is no jury in the Philippines. The judge alone decides on the case. Depending on the charges filed, penalties range from 6 months to life imprisonment. When the Philippines still had the death penalty (before 2006), incest-rape was punishable by death; now it is up to life imprisonment. In the study by Castillo on the "Legal Outcomes of Sexually Abused Children Evaluated at the Philippine General Hospital Child Protection Unit" (7), 15% of sexual abuse cases reached court. Most (94%) of the perpetrators were known to the child, and 38% involved incest. Almost half the cases (46%) were still unresolved 2 to 5 years after their initiation. The wheels of justice move slowly in the Philippines due to the high volume of cases in family courts; 30% of family courts are in need of a judge. Of the resolved cases, 60% resulted in convictions. The evidence considered in these cases consisted mostly of the victim's testimony and the medical findings. In most cases where the accused is found not guilty, this is due to dismissal on merit based on a child's reluctance to testify following pressure from family members.

Very few physical abuse cases reach court. Those that do, usually involve very serious injuries or death. Most fatal child abuse cases, however, do not reach court. There are many reasons for this: 1) There is no mandatory autopsy for suspicious deaths; 2) Most doctors do not suspect child abuse in cases that they see; child abuse is not part of their training; 3) Most doctors do not want to be involved in the legal system and so do not report cases of child abuse; 4) Investigation of child deaths in the Philippines is still in its infancy and police are not trained in doing death scene investigations; 5) The police require that there be a complainant before investigating a death; in most cases of fatal child abuse there is no complainant; 6) Even in cases reported to DSWD, social workers themselves do not want to be the complainant. Child neglect cases have not reached court at all.

CHILD PROTECTION UNITS

In response to the need to provide abused children and their families comprehensive, coordinated and continuing care by trained professionals, the first Child Protection Unit (CPU) was established in a government tertiary care training hospital in 1997. It was a partnership between the academe, the government and private philanthropy. It cut across the red tape of agencies to put together in one unit - physicians, mental health professionals, social workers, police and lawyers. The goal is to provide immediate and long-term care to abused children and their families for health, safety and optimal development. The investigation and legal protection are done together with rehabilitation and reintegration of the child back to his family and community. Team members work with the community to provide support for families. With scarce resources and minimal political support, initiative, creativity, and perseverance are necessary for success. In areas where CPU's are present, partnerships among health, social welfare, law enforcement, local officials, NGO's, and private philanthropy are crucial. There are 26 CPUs across the country. They are all part of the Child Protection Network that supports the training and continuing development of the member CPU's. The vision is to have one CPU in each of the 81 provinces.

PREVENTION OF CHILD ABUSE

The Philippines can barely provide basic services to children and is far from achieving the millennium development goal of reducing extreme poverty by half. While it seems that the infant mortality rate is steadily decreasing to its present 23 per 1000 live births (5), the rate in the poorest 20% of the population is 42 per 1000 live births (8). The Philippines has problems with poor educational achievement, child labour, a burgeoning population (annual growth rate of 2%) and a high unemployment rate (unemployment rate of 7.4% and underemployment rate of 19%). Much (32%) of the national budget is for debt service-interest payment, while providing insufficient funds for social development and children's programs (9). The share of social services in total government expenditures, including education, health, social security, housing, land distribution, employment, and subsidies to local government is only 28% and has been steadily declining. The budget for health has declined to only 1.7% of the total government budget. It is not surprising that a survey by the Social Weather Station (10) found that only 5% of families needing help received any from the government. The most common source of support for families comes from relatives. A study by Manasan (11), "Financing the Millennium Development Goals," concluded that the Philippine government cannot afford to continue down the current path; rather, it needs to prioritize the necessary resources to achieve the millennium development goals.

Successful initiatives preventing child abuse and neglect, such as home visiting, include helping troubled families, supporting healthy development, keeping children safe by assuring high quality support services, as well as community-based partnerships between child protective agencies and community organizations and cultivating safe neighbourhoods (12). These programs do exist in the Philippines, however, they remain small demonstration programs. The problem is how to sustain and expand them to the scale necessary across the country. There needs to be systematic change brought about by social, political, economic and cultural reform that involves government and all sectors of the society. The Philippines has the talent, ideas, committed and dedicated people, and the model programs to make the country work for children. Leadership and good governance are absolutely necessities.

REFERENCES

[1]   World Health Organization. World report on violence and health. Geneva: WHO, 2002.

[2]   Philippine National Statistics Office. Accessed 2008 Mar 23. URL: http://www.census.gov.ph/CARAGA/Population%20projections%20census%202000-based.htm

[3]   Department of Health. Baseline surveys for the national objectives for health. Manila: Dept Health, 2000.

[4]   Child Protection Unit Network. Manila: Annual report 2007.

[5]   Philippine National Statistical Coordination Board. Accessed 2008 Mar 23. URL: http://www.nscb.gov.ph/stats/mdg/mdg_watch.asp

[6]   Mangahas M. Throwing money at hunger. Philippine Daily Inquirer, 2007 Nov 10.

[7]   Castillo MS. Legal outcomes of sexually abused children evaluated at the Philippine General Hospital Child Protection Unit. Submitted for publication.

[8]   Asian Development Bank. ADB and Philippines 2008 Fact Sheet. Accessed 2008 Mar 23. URL: http:// www.adb.org/Documents/Fact_Sheet/PHI.pdf

[9]   Philippine government report (3rd and 4th periodic report) submitted to the United Nations Committee on the Convention of the Rights of the Child. Manila: September, 2007.

[10]   Social Weather Survey. 38% of Families got help in the past quarter. Manila: Businessworld, 2007 Nov 20.

[11]   Manasan RG. Financing the millenium development goals. Dissertation. Manila: Natl Dev Authority, 2007.

[12]   World Health Organization. Preventing child maltreatment: a guide to taking action and generating evidence. Geneva: WHO, 2006.

In: International Aspects of Child Abuse and Neglect   ISBN: 978-1-60876-703-8
Editors: H. Dubowitz, J. Merrick pp. 37-45   © 2010 Nova Science Publishers, Inc.

Chapter 5

CHILD WELFARE IN EGYPT: INTRODUCING A NEW, RIGHTS-BASED APPROACH TO PROTECT CHILDREN

Ambassador Moushira Khattab [*]
Minister of Family and Population, Cairo, Egypt

Egypt is a developing, middle-income country with a young population—39 percent of Egypt's 74 million citizens are under the age 18 years. Strong macroeconomic performance in recent decades has resulted in considerable improvements in child well-being, but considerable poverty persists, particularly in the rural upper Egypt region. Particular problems, such as children living on the streets, appears to be on the rise. A dearth of national data on child abuse and neglect frustrates attempts to measure the extent of the problem in Egypt or compare it to other countries with a similar background. Recent legal reforms to the Egyptian Child Law initiated and coordinated by the Egyptian National Council for Childhood and Motherhood (NCCM) and passed by parliament in June 2008 have drastically altered the system of child protection in Egypt. Under the new system, and guided by the UN Convention on the Rights of the Child (CRC); children's rights have been recognized and expanded, penalties for particular forms of abuse such child trafficking have been toughened, and new child protection committees have been established in each of Egypt's 29 regions. While many of the laws provisions stirred controversy, they represent a significant improvement in the government's approach to addressing child abuse and neglect and a strong commitment to acting in the best interests in the child. Given the considerable challenges of protecting children in this populous and dynamic country, successful implementation of the new child protection regime will require significant resources and commitment.

INTRODUCTION

Egypt's population of 76.7 million makes it the most populous country in the Arab world and second most populous country in Africa. Despite the great expanse of Egypt's territory (approximately 1 million square kilometers), most of the country is sparsely populated, with

---

[*] *Correspondence:* Ambassador Moushira Khattab, Minister of Family and Population, Cairo, Egypt. E-mail: moushira@e-khattab.com

the vast majority living in densely populated areas along the banks of the Nile River and in the Nile river delta. Just over half (57 percent) of the population lives in rural areas. A predominately young country, Egypt has over 29.5 million children aged 15 or under, representing approximately 31.7% of the population.

Egypt GDP per capita (purchasing power parity) was $5,900 in 2005/06. Over the past few decades, Egypt has seen significant improvements in the economy and strong macroeconomic performance. Between 1995 and 2005, infant mortality and malnutrition among children under five decreased by half. Infant mortality currently stands at 20.5 deaths/1,000 live births. Life expectancy is 71.3 years.

Recent improvements in economic and social indicators have not reached Upper Egypt a predominantly rural region in the south of the country and home to over one third of the population. While poverty has significantly decreased overall since 1995, poverty has increased in Upper Egypt.

The focus of this paper is on child abuse and neglect, a topic that has gained national prominence in Egypt in recent years. In 2008, the government of Egypt passed far reaching amendments to the Egyptian Child Law (Law 126/2008), resulting in a new rights-based and strengthened system of child protection. The legislative process started in 2003 and involved a wide range of stakeholders in an open and inclusive manner. Advocacy efforts, initiated and coordinated by the Egyptian National Council for Childhood and Motherhood (NCCM), convinced decision makers and the general public that children have rights, culminating in parliamentary approval of comprehensive and visionary human rights legislation that safeguards Egypt's children, especially its most vulnerable ones. The law's first articles ensure that Egyptian children receive, at a minimum, all of the rights provided for by the U.N. Convention on the Rights of the Child (CRC), as well as optional protocols on the sale of children, child prostitution and pornography, involvement of children in armed conflict, and other international treaties ratified by Egypt. The law goes on to incorporate the four core values or principles of the CRC: non-discrimination; best interests of the child; right to life, survival, and development within a family empowered to provide protection; and the right of the child to be heard. Taken together, these principles form the foundation of a new, comprehensive approach to ensuring the rights of abused and neglected children.

In the remainder of this paper the central elements of this new child protection system will be discussed.

HOW ARE DIFFERENT TYPES OF CHILD ABUSE AND NEGLECT DEFINED?

The policy framework for child protection is defined at the national level in Egypt. The amended Child Law (126/2008) adopts a rights-based approach to child abuse and neglect as guided by the CRC and other international guidelines and instruments. The law gives children the right to be "protected from all forms of violence, harm, physical, psychological or sexual abuse, neglect, acts of omission, or any other forms of ill-treatment or exploitation."

The law defines child abuse and neglect broadly, including abuse and neglect at home and in public and private institutions (e.g., schools and social care institutions), as well as neglect caused by the denial of rights guaranteed to children under law (e.g., the right to education or healthcare). As such, the amended Child Law adopts a comprehensive approach to the problem, addressing both its manifestation and underlying causes. The forthcoming executive regulations will provide additional definitions of child abuse and neglect, and judges are provided with significant latitude in determining whether a child has been abused either physically, emotionally, or sexually, based on the principle of the best interest of the child and child protection.

The amended Child Law lists instances in which a child is considered at risk or exposed to danger and which would prompt action from child protection authorities (Article 96). These include cases of exposure to violence, in particular physical or sexual abuse; physical neglect (such as the failure to provide adequate food and shelter); exposure to unhealthy or immoral influence (such as exposure to criminal activity, including drugs); inadequate supervision and guidance; denial of access to education; being forced to work in violation of the law; and other areas. Children who are on the street or engaged in dangerous activities such as begging are also identified as "at-risk," allowing government authorities to take action.

The amended Child Law also addresses specific forms of child abuse and neglect that have particular salience in the Egyptian context, including female genital mutilation/cutting, trafficking and sexual exploitation of children using the Internet, child abandonment, and child labor. In each area, definitions have been revised or clarified and penalties strengthened. While corporal punishment by parents is not criminalized, the new Child Law discourages the practice.

Beyond cases of neglect and abuse at home and in institutions, the law provides children with the right to health care and education that, if denied, could be demanded in court. Again, the broad view of child abuse and neglect included in the law's rights-based language forms a comprehensive framework that addresses the issue from both remedial and preventative directions.

WHAT IS KNOWN ABOUT THE EXTENT OF CHILD ABUSE AND NEGLECT?

Scarcity of national data available on different forms of violence and abuse makes it difficult to give an accurate assessment of the problem. The Egyptian Demographic Health Survey (EDHS) of 2005 shows that 90.2% of mothers of children age 3-17 years have yelled or screamed at their children, while 69.1% have hit or slapped their children on his/her body and 50% have hit or slapped their children on the face, head, or ear.

Data available on the extent of the child labor from the National Survey of Child Labour indicates that 2.78 million children are working in Egypt, approximately 21% of children between the ages 6-14 years. However, methodological problems with the survey suggest that it may be undercounting the total number of child laborers. The survey also indicates that 82% of working children are enrolled in schools, though it is likely that many are not actually attending. Though the average age for marriage is rising to over 20 years for the girl child; early marriage is still a problem in some pockets.

Children living on the streets without supervision have become a growing problem in recent years in Egypt but the estimated numbers vary widely. Many of these children are subject to forms of physical, sexual, and emotional abuse and exploitation, in addition to serious health and nutritional hazards. A few incidences of trafficking in the body parts of street children have also been reported.

Finally, the EDHS of 2005 indicates that 96% of ever-married women ages 15 to 49 years reported that they had been circumcised, but the data also suggest the practice is in decline. Data on married women ages 15-17 years indicated that fewer women of this age group (76.5%) had been circumcised. A national survey conducted by the World Health Organization (WHO) and the Egyptian Ministry of Health in 2007 indicates that the prevalence of the practice among girls age 10 to 18 has declined to 50.3% (43% in urban public schools, 62.7% in rural schools, and 9.2% in private urban schools).

WHAT SYSTEMS AND INFRASTRUCTURE EXISTS IN EGYPT TO ADDRESS CHILD ABUSE AND NEGLECT?

With the passage of the amended Child Law (126/ 2008), Egypt strengthened its systems and infrastructure for addressing child abuse and neglect, as well as for the protection of at-risk children in general. The role of the civil society is recognized by the law..

At the policy level, Egypt's child protection efforts are led by the National Council for Childhood and Motherhood (NCCM), is the national body responsible for policy development, coordination, data collection, monitoring and evaluation, public awareness, advocacy, technical assistance, and capacity building for governmental and non-governmental agencies..

The amended law authorizes new protection mechanisms: general child protection committees at the Governorate level, district sub-committees, and the child helpline. NCCM operates a national, toll-free, 24-hour child helpline as a complaint mechanism. The helpline receives calls from parents, children, and others. Solutions are provided through a wide network of government ministries and civil society entities. In its three years of operation, the helpline has handled a wide variety of cases, ranging from child abuse and neglect, to denial of educational or health rights, child labor, and advice to parents and children about child rearing and child development. Street children and other at-risk children, as well as those concerned about their welfare, also regularly use the helpline. The helpline has been instrumental in providing data on violence against children.

General child protection committees are established in each of Egypt's 29 governorates, as well as sub-committees in each local district. These committees will be the front line in developing local child protection policies and recommending actions to help at-risk, abused, and neglected children. In cases requiring the removal or protection of a child, placement of a child in a social welfare institution, or criminal charges, the district child protection committees coordinate with the police, prosecution, and judiciary, each of which maintain specialized personnel for dealing with children.

While child protection committees are expected to handle the majority of cases involving at-risk children, prosecutors and the courts continue to handle criminal matters and cases where protection orders and/or restraining orders are required. Most geographical areas have child courts with prosecutors who specialize in cases involving children. Specialized Family

Courts may also intervene in cases of family disputes involving divorce, alimony, and/or other personal status issues that affect children.

As a last resort, and for the shortest possible duration, a judge can place a child in various child protection facilities managed by the Ministry of Social Solidarity. Children placed in such facilities are separated depending on whether they are in danger, at-risk, or in conflict with the law. They are also divided by age and gender. According to the law, children cannot be placed in detention with adults.

In lieu of placing a child in a child protection facility, children may be placed in foster families registered and monitored by the Ministry of Social Solidarity. The Ministry of Social Solidarity also licenses and oversees a wide range of child protection facilities managed by non-governmental organizations, including a limited number of facilities targeting special groups of at-risk children, such as street children, orphans, and children victims of drug addiction.

Other government ministries and agencies share responsibilities for child protection. For example, the Ministry of Health is responsible for ensuring adequate health care and health insurance coverage, while the Ministry of Education is responsible for ensuring that children are protected from violence while at school and for enforcing the criminalization of corporal punishment in schools. The Ministry of Manpower and Migration is responsible for ensuring through its inspection units that no child is illegally involved in the labor market. Each ministry has a range of administrative penalties on business owners and/or employees at their disposal and can also refer criminal cases to the police and prosecution.

How Does the System Work Regarding Reporting of Possible Child Abuse and Neglect?

Instances of child abuse and neglect can come to the attention of authorities through a number of different pathways. The amended Child Law encourages reporting by anyone who knows of a child in danger and mandates reporting by pubic employees who come into contact with children, for example teachers and healthcare workers. Cases can be reported directly to the police and prosecution or they can be reported to the NCCM child helpline, which will then investigate and refer the case to other agencies for action. In addition, instances of child abuse and neglect can be reported directly to child protection committees. Cases of child abuse and neglect may also be reported through administrative mechanisms in other ministries, as appropriate.

A "Typical" Response by the Responsible Agency(ies)

Upon reporting a case of child abuse or neglect to NCCM child helpline, the case is assessed by the helpline staff, who may (depending on the individual case) dispatch a social worker to rescue the child or to investigate. The system includes social workers placed at NGOs throughout the country. Cases that merit further attention are referred to the appropriate ministry or government agency for action. When a violation of the law is suspected or where immediate action is needed, the helpline team contacts the local or national police or prosecutors directly, who take action as warranted by the case, including further investigation, arrest, prosecution, etc. In emergency circumstances, the prosecutor can order the immediate removal of the child to one of the institutions managed by the Ministry of Social Solidarity (mentioned above) or other safe environment (such as extended family members).

Under the amended law, child protection sub-committees are able to take much of the same actions as the NCCM General Department for Child Helpline, including working with the police and prosecutors to immediately remove a child from danger or ordering corrective actions that serve the best interests of the child. The committees can also fine adults responsible for children (typically parents or guardians) for failure to observe the committee's orders or recommend to the judiciary that the child be removed from home or that additional orders be issued. The committees include representatives of concerned government and non-governmental entities dealing with children, allowing them to deal effectively with a wide variety of cases.

As noted above, the reporting mechanisms of other ministries—such as Education, Social Solidarity, and Manpower—include receiving complaints about specific types of child abuse and neglect. Investigations are conducted to determine the best course of action, whether administrative penalties, such as withdrawing licensing for a social care institution or closing a factory, or referral of the case to the police and prosecution for further investigation and criminal charges.

WHAT ARE THE STRENGTHS OF THE EGYPTIAN APPROACH/SYSTEM?

A completely transformed and decentralized child protection system has been established, enhancing the role and ownership of local community with the child protection committees. Along with protection committees, the NCCM childhelpline network is legally acknowledged as a protection mechanism and give enhanced powers to investigate and take action.

In addition, a new, restorative juvenile justice system inspired by General Comment No. 10 of the Committee on the Rights of the Child recognizes the rights of three categories of children--those at risk, victims and witnesses to crime, and children in conflict with the law. The focus of the reformed system is on preventing child delinquency and the reintegration of children with their families and society. The minimum age of criminal responsibility was raised from 7 to 12 years, in another great achievement, and new corrective measures have been put in place for children in conflict with the law under 15. Deprivation of liberty is now a last resort and for the shortest possible duration with periodic review. Imprisonment during investigation, life imprisonment, and the death penalty for children under 18 are no longer allowed. Specialized child courts and child sensitive court procedures with qualified judges and social workers (including at least one female worker) are being put into place. Since the law was passed in 2008, a capacity building program has been ongoing for all child court professionals according to a preset time bound work plan.

More than the passage of the child law amendments themselves, the ultimate achievement has been convincing increasing numbers of people in government and the general public that children are holders of rights. More salient than ever, many are coming to see gender equality and women's unequal access to citizenship as also effecting children's access to rights.

It has been a very long journey adjusting to the realities on the ground and emerging challenges, such as the Internet and mobile technology. What shocked some people at first has turned into a social movement thanks to the engagement of religious and community leaders, government officials, academics, parliamentarians, media professionals, civil society activists, and children themselves.

WHAT ARE THE WEAKNESSES/CHALLENGES OF EGYPT'S APPROACH/SYSTEM?

Although a momentous achievement, this legal reform only sets the stage for even harder work to come. The law needs to be supported by consistent advocacy to create awareness about its provisions, enforcement, and monitoring mechanisms. Appropriate financial resources need to be dedicated to this fight, educational reform must continue, and all of the entities working with children must coordinate within the framework of the new law.

To continue it success, Egypt also needs to assess the effectiveness of policies and legislation using methods that examine the impact both before and after implementation. These impact assessments should be used to identify gaps and enable potential users to encourage further change. Consolidation of data, better monitoring of law enforcement, and improvements in prosecution are also essential. Finally, there must be collaboration to establish complimentary legislation and enforcement across borders, especially on transnational issues such as trafficking, child pornography, and exploitation using the Internet and other new technologies

Training for professionals working with and for children is also major challenge. A child-centered approach will be instrumental in bringing about the needed change. Targeted groups for continued training include the police, prosecutors, judges, social workers, the media, teachers, NGO professionals, and a wide range of other government officials and the general public. Changing the overall view of children and their rights will continue to require substantial efforts and resources moving forward, making it essential that children and children's issues become more visible in public policy and budget allocations.

Selected areas for further improvements in child protection include changing attitudes toward corporal punishment within the family, continuing to reduce violence in schools, overcoming the traditional silence on sexual abuse and exploitation, continuing to reduce child labor (including addressing its underlying economic causes), continue to combat FGM with the same vigor; and improving services for child victims of abuse and neglect.

Changes will be slow in each of these areas, as they involve changes to societal values and views of children and childhood. The new law is a first step in the introduction of a new culture of respect for the rights of children, but much work needs to be done to instill this culture among the majority of the population.

WHAT ARE THE MAJOR CONTROVERSIES WITH THE EGYPTIAN APPROACH/SYSTEM?

As in most countries, the Egyptian community perceives the rights of children to be detrimental to the authority of adults. A rights-based approach to children victims of abuse and neglect has been met with resistance and generated controversy. The most heated controversies surround the role of the state vis a vis the family, and how and when the state should intervene for the best interests of the child. Heated controversies surrounding the interpretation of religion and the place of traditional practices in a changing world are also major challenges.

In such an environment, the criminalization of female genital mutilation/cutting came as a major achievement. No one, however, can rest assured that the battle is over. Some, though a minority, still argue that the practice accords with religion and/or tradition. That said, many major religious and political leaders have spoken out publicly against FGM/C, and a wide range of public awareness efforts are underway.

Despite strong opposition, the amended law also raises the age of marriage for girls to 18 years (equal to that of boys). Religion was again used to advocate for allowing early marriage. A similar controversy surrounded the right of a woman to register the birth of her child when the father abandons the child, is unknown, or unavailable. Today, Egyptian women can also pass their citizenship to their children, another victory.

Though the silence has been broken, child abuse and neglect in the family is still poorly reported. Debate over the place of corporal punishment has been unleashed, with many supporting its use as a disciplinary measure. Debates area also ongoing about when the state should step in to protect children in cases of violence in the home.

WHAT PREVENTION EFFORTS (PRIMARY, SECONDARY, TERTIARY) ARE IN PLACE AND TO WHAT EXTENT?

Prevention efforts are underdeveloped in Egypt, with government agencies primarily concerned with addressing cases of child abuse and neglect after they occur. That said, each Protection Committee at the governorate-level is charged with developing a child protection policy that includes prevention initiatives. Supporting their efforts, the National Council for Childhood and Motherhood regularly develops prevention plans and leads awareness efforts at the national level in partnership with other government ministries, agencies, and non-governmental organizations. Ongoing campaigns target a wide range of specific issues like deprivation of education; eary marriage; FGM/C, child labor, non-violent resolution of family disputes, and many other areas

On the whole, the provisions of the amended Child Law are designed to reduce factors contributing to child abuse and neglect by ensuring that children and their families receive required health and educational care, social insurance, other needed social and economic services. That said, the implementation of the law will require resources, as will the continuation and expansion of awareness efforts. The recent creation of the Ministry for Family and Population on March 11, 2009 will definitely strengthen national efforts to combat violence against children, including abuse and neglect.

REFERENCES

[1]   El- Zanaty F, Way A. Egypt demographic and health survey 2005, Cairo, Egypt: Min Health Population, 2006.

[2]   Handoussa H. Egypt human development report: Egypt's social contract: The role of civil society. Cairo, Egypt: United Nations Dev Programme, Inst Natl Planning, 2008.

[3]   National Council for Childhood and Motherhood. National Survey on Child Labour in Egypt. Cairo: Author, 2004.

[4]   Social Research Center. Towards policies for child protection: A field study to assess child abuse in deprived communities in Cairo and Alexandria. Cairo: American University Cairo, 2007.

[5]   National Council for Childhood and Motherhood. Street Children Survey: Cairo, Giza, Qalyubiya, and Alexandria Governorates. Cairo: Author, 2007.

[6]   National Council for Childhood and Motherhood. Report on budgeting for children. Cairo: Author, 2007.

[7]   Central Agency for Public Mobilization and Statistics (CAPMAS). Population and establishments census. Cairo: Author, 2006.

In: International Aspects of Child Abuse and Neglect   ISBN: 978-1-60876-703-8
Editors: H. Dubowitz, J. Merrick pp. 47-57   © 2010 Nova Science Publishers, Inc.

Chapter 6

CHILD PROTECTION IN ISRAEL

Rachel Szabo-Lael[1] and Tamar Zemach-Marom[2]
[1]Engelberg Center for Children and Youth
[2]Center for Quality Assurance in the Social Services, Jerusalem, Israel

The aim of this chapter is to summarize some of the main issues related to child protection in Israel. It will discuss the difficulties in defining the term "child abuse and neglect" and measuring the extent of it, describe the mechanisms provided to deal with the phenomenon and their advantages and disadvantages. In Israel, child protection is implemented by the social welfare system, reflecting a belief in social intervention rather than legal action. The main advantage of it is that families have a wide range of services under one roof and do not perceive the agency as a threat. Israel has instituted mandatory reporting of child abuse and neglect. The controversy around this issue, as well as other dilemmas, is discussed.

INTRODUCTION

In recent years, Israeli society has undergone an upheaval in public and professional awareness of the abuse of minors, both in the public and the private domain. This heightened awareness derives, inter alia, from changes in values and from an increased awareness of civil rights, the rights of children and the rights of victims of crimes. These changes are reflected both in the expansion of public protection of children's rights and the provision of new rights, and in a renewed examination of risk situations, including those relating to special groups, such as children who are victims of sexual abuse or children with AIDS. The State's increased commitment to the protection of minors at-risk and in dangerous situations has culminated in legislation, court rulings, and the development of methods of treating both the victims and the perpetrators.

In recent years, much thought has been given to new ways that both the community and the social system can employ in dealing with children at risk: who is responsible for the provision of treatment and solutions?, who has the authority to intervene in the different stages?, and what is the nature of the partnership and the division of responsibility among the relevant parties?.

This paper surveys the child protection system in Israel: the scale of the phenomenon, the mechanisms to deal with it, the advantages and disadvantages of the system and the challenges it faces.

THE DEFINITION OF CHILD ABUSE AND NEGLECT (CAN)

Several laws address the prevention and treatment of child abuse and neglect in Israel, and provide definitions. It is important to note that there is no single definition accepted by all professionals, who work with children. However, these professionals receive tools (indicators) to identify children suffering from abuse and neglect.

The Penal Law of 1977 prohibits acts of physical, emotional or sexual abuse directed at minors (sections 368B, 368C). It also prohibits the neglect of a child and sets penalties for specific breaches of parental obligations, such as failing to provide a child under age 14 with food or clothing (section 362) or leaving a child under six years of age without supervision (section 361). With regard to the criminal offense of abuse of a minor, the Supreme Court defined "physical abuse" as the "direct or indirect use of force or physical means against the body of the victim in a manner and to an extent that may cause physical or emotional harm or both." According to the court, abuse typically involves "cruelty, instilling in the victim considerable fear and terror, degrading or humiliating the victim, or severe risk of (physical and emotional) harm" (1).

Section 2 of the Youth Law (Care and Supervision) 1960 defines seven situations in which a child or youth may be declared by the court as being a "minor in need":

- No one defined as a parent, including a step-parent, adoptive parent or legal guardian, is responsible for the child.
- The adult who is responsible is incapable of caring for the child or neglects to care for him. This refers to parents who suffer from a severe problem that may impair their social functioning (substance abuse or diagnosed mental illness) and their ability to fulfill the child's basic daily needs.
- The child has committed a criminal offense but has not been prosecuted. This refers to a child under 12 who is not criminally liable for an act he committed or a child that committed a criminal offence but there was no solid evidence to prosecute him.
- The child was found loitering, panhandling or peddling. This refers to a child wandering around in the streets without adequate supervision at night or during school hours, or a child being used for panhandling or peddling.
- The child is subject to detrimental influences or lives in a criminal environment. This refers to a child who may be subject to bad influences in his physical environment such as being exposed to drug abuse, prostitution or other criminal activity.
- The child was exposed to drugs in-utero.
- The child's physical or emotional well-being has been or may be impaired. This refers to a child being subjected to physical or emotional abuse, family violence or a child who tries to hurt himself.

Based on these laws, the cases identified and reported by professionals are mostly of children subjected to various forms of neglect: children who are physically neglected – that is, at least one of their basic daily needs is not being met on a regular basis; children who lack adequate supervision, are often left alone, and do not have a daily routine; and children who suffer from educational neglect – that is, their parents do not make sure they attend school regularly. There are also cases of children who suffer from violence directed at them or between their parents, children who suffer from physical or sexual abuse and children involved in criminal activity or who try to commit suicide (1,2).

THE EXTENT OF ABUSE AND NEGLECT

Israel has no single database that contains complete data on the number of children "at risk." It is therefore difficult to obtain accurate figures on children who suffer from abuse or neglect or who are vulnerable to other risk situations. The data on cases reported to the chief child protection officer or the police do not adequately represent the full extent of the phenomenon (1).

According to Tzionit et al (3), 1.9% of all children in Israel in 2006 experienced abuse and/or neglect (those numbers based on cases reported to the chief child protection officer or the police). According to the Report of the Prime Minister's Commission for Disadvantaged and At-risk Children and Youth (4), 6.5% of all children in Israel in 2005 were suffering from neglect and 2% were suffering from abuse; a child can experience both (this is an estimate based on data from different sources).

THE SYSTEM ADDRESSING CAN

In Israel, child protection is implemented by the social welfare system, reflecting a belief in social intervention rather than legal action. This preference is expressed in both the legislation regarding child protection and the organizational structure of the service system. The Social Services Law 1958 obligates local authorities to develop and provide the majority of the welfare services for needy populations, including services for children who are victims of abuse and neglect (1). Child protection services are provided by child protection officers. Child protection officers are social workers with at least a Bachelor's degree in social welfare departments who have undergone specific training and have been appointed by the minister of social affairs.

In most local authorities, they are members of neighborhood teams that also include different kinds of social workers, such as family social workers, or geriatric social workers. The child protection officers are considered experts on children and advise the other professionals on the team. Their role in relation to a child and his or her family varies according to the policy of the local authority and the specific case. A child protection officer may remain "behind the scenes" as a consultant to the family social worker, intervene during a crisis in the family or work in partnership with the family social worker. In some cases, the child protection officer assumes responsibility for intervention and become the case manager for the child and family instead of the family social worker. Occasionally, intervention is carried out under court order. There are thus children who are in the care of child protection officers under court order, others who are not, as well as cases in which child protection officers act as consultants or partners (1,2).

Children who suffer from abuse and neglect are entitled to the same services provided to all children and families by the local social welfare department. A family can be assisted by a family social worker who assesses its needs, counsels, helps with bureaucratic procedures and mediates between the family and other services. The other services can include day care centers; after-school programs that provide children with supervision, hot meals, recreation, informal education and therapeutic services; community-based programs that teach basic life skills such as family budget management, parenting skills and family interaction skills; family counseling services; residential facilities; and foster homes.

At times it is necessary to provide immediate protection for children in an emergency. The way to do so is to provide immediate foster placement as a form of short-term shelter until their situation can be evaluated and a long-term plan devised, or, to place them in emergency centers. Child protection teams in hospitals also provide immediate, emergency placement when the need arises (1,2).

The Penal Law was amended in 1989, introducing mandatory reporting of child abuse or neglect. Section 368D(a) requires an adult to report any case of child abuse or neglect to the police or Child Protection Authority. Failure to do so is a criminal offense that can result in a three-month jail sentence. According to Section 368D(b-c), the law can impose a six-month sentence on professionals (e.g., physicians, nurses, educators, social workers, policemen, psychologists, criminologists and school principals and staff), who fail to do so. According to Section 368D(d), schools and other facilities for children are obligated to report incidents of severe injury, abuse or sexual offenses against a minor committed by caretakers or non-caretakers, including other minors. This mandatory reporting was introduced after the disclosure of several cases of severe abuse and neglect, one of which culminated in the death of a three-year-old girl who had been continuously abused by her uncle, which shocked the public. Teachers, friends and neighbors had been aware of the chronic abuse, but failed to report it to the Child Protection Authority. Despite the passage of this law and an increase in the rate of reporting, it is mostly not being enforced; practically no professionals have been brought to trial for failure to report suspected abuse or neglect (1,2,5). It is important to note that there is no immunity from being sued for reporting: parents can sue professionals including the child protection officers. In addition, the Prevention of Domestic Violence Law 1991 is intended to protect people, including children, from a relative who endangers those living with him or her through physical, sexual or emotional abuse.

In conclusion, the components of the Israeli model include the following: Child protection officers in Israel are an integral part of the system of welfare services; Israel has instituted mandatory reporting, which necessitates a process for screening reports; child protection officers are involved in criminal investigations, although not to gather evidence, but to ensure children's protection; there is no clear division between the therapeutic and legal/protective/authoritative roles of child protection officers; and, there is no clear definition of the division of labor between child protection officers and family social workers.

THE RESPONSE TO A REPORT OF POSSIBLE CAN

Upon receiving a report of a child in need, a child protection officer will investigate the case and gather information with the help of other social workers in the local social welfare department. If there is reason to suspect that a criminal offense has been committed, the child protection officer must report this to the police. Conversely, the police must also consult with a child protection officer. However, if it is the child protection officer's professional opinion that reporting the incident to the police would harm the child, he can seek to refrain from reporting the incident by petitioning a committee made up of representatives of the district attorney's office, a senior police officer and a senior child protection officer. This procedure is rarely used. Once the investigation is complete, intervention begins with or without a court order.

Intervention under court order: A court order may be issued for a "minor in need" if the child protection officer is convinced that the minor is in immediate danger or in need of urgent medical treatment. The child protection officer may take whatever steps deemed necessary to help the child without the consent of the child's guardian for up to one week without court approval. The minor is not required to undergo a psychiatric examination unless so ordered by a regional psychiatrist. Once the court has pronounced the child a "minor in need," the child protection officer may ask that the court take steps required to protect the child. These usually include one of the following:

- A protection order, which places the child in the care of the child protection officer. Although the child continues to live at home, the child and parents are enjoined to cooperate with the treatment plan authorized by the court.
- A custody order, which removes the child from the parents' home and places him or her in the care of the child protection officer until an appropriate out-of-home framework can be found. The court can also order that the child be examined or treated in a psychiatric facility as stipulated by law.

The law also provides for emergency situations. If a child protection officer is convinced that the child is in danger, he is authorized to take all necessary steps – including the child's removal from his home to a safe place – provided the child is not held for more than seven days without the consent of a parent or guardian or court approval (Section 11A). Section 12 of the law states that the court must approve the emergency steps and render an interim decision on the matter before hearing the child or his parents. Its decision is valid for 30 days and may be renewed for up to three months (Section 14).

Intervention without court order: Child protection officers often use their legal authority without actually applying legal procedures. They do so with the knowledge that they can apply such procedures at any stage if the parents fail to cooperate. Once parents agree to a treatment plan, they are asked to sign a contract with the social welfare department that describes the program and mutual expectations (1,2).

THE STRENGTHS OF THE SYSTEM

The main strength of the system is its wide coverage. Very few cases are missed. There are mechanisms to ensure the receipt of extensive and professional assessments that facilitate decision making on the basis of the best interest of the child. The best interest of the child is preserved by, among other things, involving parents and children in decision making when choosing the appropriate intervention. This is stipulated in the guidelines of the decision making committees for children at risk that exist in every local authority (1).

Collaboration by various agencies is another advantage of the system. Hospitals have established special teams (CAN teams) that are on the alert for cases of abuse. If they identify a case in which there is a serious suspicion of abuse, they will notify a child protection officer. Collaboration is embedded not only among various bodies, but also among various professions that provide care for children. As already stated, child protection officers are specially trained social workers who are part of a large, integrated network of social welfare professionals providing services to populations at risk. It should be noted, though, that criticism is sometimes voiced by people in the education and health systems who feel that there is a lack of true collaboration and that child protection officers see them solely as a source of information (6).

The fact that the child protection officer is part of the social services is advantageous in that families have a wide range of services under one roof and do not perceive the agency as a threat (6). In addition, the system is very open to learning and change. The lack of procedures and structure leave the system flexible and adaptable. Many new procedures and a number of new models for providing protective services to children have been developed in recent years (1). One such example is the "Magen" program (which means "protection" in Hebrew). The goal of the program is to reduce risk and improve responses for children at risk. This is achieved by ensuring an immediate response to every report, providing systematic feedback to those in the community who have made reports, collecting information on risk and dangerous situations locally and nationally, as a basis for developing effective responses, ensuring appropriate intervention by defining and upgrading the role of the child protection officer and preventing the recurrence of high risk situations.

Finally, there is a system of checks and balances, and when suspicion arises that the authorities themselves have been remiss, an ad hoc committee is convened by a government minister (e.g., the minister of social affairs and social services) to investigate. Another way to preserve the best interests of the child is through systematic government regulation. A new system of regulation called RAF (Regulation, Assessment and Follow-up) has been implemented in residential facilities for children at risk. The Children and Youth Services under the Ministry of Social Affairs and Social Services is now in the process of expanding the system to all community services for children at risk and interviews with the children for their point of view have been implemented as part of the system (1,7,8).

THE WEAKNESSES AND CHALLENGES OF THE SYSTEM

Services that protect children are still limited and there are significant unmet needs (1,9). The limited scope of available services and their unequal geographic distribution impair the system's ability to both successfully help parents care for their children and adequately protect children. The majority of the services focus on the child rather than on the family as a whole. Innovative best-practice approaches are not broadly disseminated. In out-of-home placements there is a need to improve coordination with the school system and contact with parents (1).

There is little standardization, no clear record of decisions, recommendations or their outcomes, and no dedicated attempt to translate action into legislation. In addition, there is no clear procedure for reporting, a lack of clarity regarding the roles among the various professionals providing care for the child, and no clear guidelines as to the proper caseload for each child protection officer. These professionals often have different approaches and perceptions as to the child's best interests and the preferred method of treatment, and there are no clear guidelines to assist them in the decision making process. The role of the child protection officer may change from one local authority to the next and from one case to the next (1).

The inquiries conducted by the child protection officer are not reviewed on a regular basis. There is no systematic way of determining how a particular decision or recommendation was made and whether it was implemented. There are also delays in obtaining information from agencies and there is no national database on the work of child protection officers. The heavy caseload, stress and inappropriate working conditions of child protection officers (e.g., low salary, inadequate office space, lack of computers, etc.) make it difficult for them to provide sufficient feedback to other professionals.

Child protection officers devote a significant proportion of their time to placement in services for children and their families, leaving little time to fulfill the specific tasks, which require their unique training and knowledge, e.g., legal investigations, working with families resisting care, etc. In addition, child protection officers often lack a clear understanding of the need for their involvement in long-term therapeutic processes, and there is no clear division between their therapeutic roles and legal protection roles (6).

One particular challenge arises from the mandatory reporting law. As a consequence of this law, people can feel that they are responsible for the arrest of a parent and the destruction of a family. The feeling within families that they are being persecuted and that the child protection officer is part of a "police state" have become very harmful to the treatment process and to the families' cooperation. One of the most serious side effects of the law is its misuse in divorce procedures. The law makes it mandatory to investigate each complaint, and the damage to the child who must endure multiple interviews can be enormous. It shifts the focus to the domain of criminal justice rather than treatment and help. The law also puts a great burden on the child protection officer: There has been a large increase in the number of reports of suspicion of abuse or neglect (from 3,000 cases in 1990 to 32,000 in 2002), with about 40% not substantiated (2,5).

THE MAJOR CONTROVERSIES

One controversy pertains to mandatory reporting of child abuse or neglect. On the one hand, it tells the public that the state is serious about the matter. It also deepens both public and professional awareness of the problem, and may lead to reaching more children suffering from abuse or neglect. On the other hand, mandatory reporting increases the number of cases to be investigated. Professionals in particular are quick to report suspicions, which can lead to a waste of resources and sometimes can divert attention from real cases. Children may also hesitate to turn to a social worker if they know it will result in the case being reported to the authorities. It also makes the professional caseworker part of the system that blames and punishes rather than part of the system that provides care. What is more, the duty to report jeopardizes the relationship between the child and the caregiver in that it destroys the confidentiality that is essential for any care process (2). The dilemmas related to mandatory reporting and the abolishment of the law in several countries have raised the issue of possible changes in Israel (2).

Those issues that remain unresolved are the definition and limits of the authority of child protection officers; the balance between their legal and therapeutic roles; the division of responsibility among the various services in the community; and the division of roles and modes of cooperation between child protection officers and other social workers in social welfare departments (6).

The child protection officer experiences an emotional dilemma that can be defined as "compassion vs. control" (10). The parent is perceived, on the one hand, as the victim of a harsh situation, and, on the other, as a criminal responsible for his actions. There are also dilemmas concerning the testimony given by children in court. The decision to seek this testimony has to be based on the child's capacity and sturdiness (11).

There is an ongoing dilemma between the responsibility of the state to prevent child abuse and neglect, and its responsibility to prevent invasions of privacy. As the child protection officer's role is anchored in the criminal code, these responsibilities occasionally contradict one another. Also, when the criminal code does not allow the officer to protect the child in what he considers the best way, he feels distress. Faber (5) suggested that the solution is to change legislation in order to minimize such cases and remove the predominantly criminal component from the relationship between social services and the people. A family in distress is entitled to straightforward care and support without being made to feel – at least initially – like criminals.

ACKNOWLEDGMENTS

We wish to convey our sincere gratitude to Ayal Varshaviak, child protection officer and inter-departmental coordinator for Magen, a nationwide project for upgrading the system of child protection officers in Israel, for sharing with us his knowledge, experience and insights; to Talal Dolev, director of the Engelberg Center for Children and Youth at the Myers-JDC-Brookdale Institute, for her insightful comments; to Dalia Ben-Rabi, senior researcher at the Engelberg Center, for helping us think the issues through; and to Larry Rifkin, Leslie Klineman and Jenny Rosenfeld of the Institute's Publications Department, for their careful editing.

REFERENCES

[1]   Dolev T, Ben-Rabi D, Almog S, Bendor A. Implementation of the convention on the rights of the child (CRC). Jerusalem: Min Justice, Min Foreign Affairs, 2001.

[2]   Faber M, Slutzky H. Between protection and treatment of needy children: the role of the child protection officer. In: Horowitz H, Ben Yehuda Y, Hovav M, eds. Abuse and neglect of children in Israel. Ashalim 2007:951-94. [Hebrew]

[3]   Tzionit Y, Ben Arieh A, Kimche M, eds. The state of the child in Israel - a statistical abstract. Jerusalem: Natl Council Child, 2007. [Hebrew]

[4]   The prime minister's commission for at-risk and disadvantaged children and youth 2006. Jerusalem: Prime Min Office, 2007. [Hebrew]

[5]   Faber M. The obligation to report: Trends and achievements. Lecture for study day on 15 years of mandatory reporting of child abuse. Sha'ari Mishpat College in cooperation with the National Council for the Child, 2005. [Hebrew]

[6]   Szabo-Lael R, Dolev T, Ben-Rabi D. Child protection officers: roles, work methods and challenges. Jerusalem: Myers-JDC Brookdale Inst, 2003. [Hebrew]

[7]   Zemach-Marom T, Fleishman R, Hauslich Z. Improving quality of care in residential settings in Israel through the RAF Method. In: Van den Bergh PM, Knorth EJ, Verheij F, Lane DC, eds. Changing care: enhancing professional quality and client involvement in child and youth care services. Jerusalem: SWP Publ, 2002:30-41.

[8]   Zemach-Marom T. The relationship between research and practice in implementing the RAF Method for Quality Assurance in residential settings for children in Israel. In: Chaskin RJ, Rosenfeld JM, eds. Research for action: cross national perspective on connecting knowledge, policy and practice for children. Oxford: Oxford Univ Press, 2008.

[9]   Dolev T, Rivkin D. Children in the care of child protection officers. Jerusalem: Myers-JDC-Brookdale Inst, 1996. [Hebrew]

[10]   Sela R. Intervening factors in the decision-making process by child protection officers in emergency situations. Dissertation. Haifa: Haifa Univ, 1998. [Hebrew]

[11]   Zur R. Children's court testimonies – dilemmas in permitting their testimony. In: Horowitz H, Ben Yehuda Y, Hovav M, eds. Abuse and neglect of children in Israel. Jerusalem: Ashalim 2007: 309-41. [Hebrew]

In: International Aspects of Child Abuse and Neglect   ISBN: 978-1-60876-703-8
Editors: H. Dubowitz, J. Merrick pp. 57-63   © 2010 Nova Science Publishers, Inc.

Chapter 7

CHILD PROTECTION IN LEBANON SOCIETY AND STRATEGY: MORE THAN ONE?

*Bernard Gerbaka**

Pediatric Intensive Care Unit, Hotel Dieu de France Hospital, Beirut, Lebanon

This chapter reviews the approach and gaps in evaluation and control processes of child abuse and neglect (CAN) in Lebanon. The whole procedure itself is an integrated multileveled approach that incorporates children's rights, professional evidence on maltreatment, relevant social factors and identified intersectoral responsibilities for the control of CAN. Several obstacles hinder the implementation, however, on a national level, including: absence of legislation to provide free child health care under the Constitution, insufficient universal screening for child health problems, and uneven access of children to health care facilities. This report also unveils the means by which the Lebanese strategy for child protection should be developed to comply with the United Nations Convention on the Rights of the Child (CRC), taking into consideration the needs and limitations of a developing, insecure and ill-resourced country like Lebanon.

INTRODUCTION

The prevention of child abuse and neglect (CAN) is a sustained and long-standing process that requires a synchronized, consensual and comprehensive teamwork approach involving universal child rights and cultural processes. Since the regional 2005 United Nations Study on Violence (UNSV) conference in Cairo, the United Nations Convention on the Rights of the Child (CRC) Geneva meeting in 2006 and the UNSV response in 2007, Lebanon has continued to join United Nations efforts to control CAN and violence against children (VAC). Despite many obstacles, a multisectoral team was established within the Higher Council for Childhood, with a common understanding of children's rights. In this strategy, professionals

---

* *Correspondence:* Associate professor Bernard Gerbaka, MD, Pediatric Intensive Care Unit, Hotel Dieu de France Hospital, Beirut, Lebanon. E-mail: Berger@Childoflebanon.org or pedhdf@usj.edu.lb

play a prominent role to develop this framework, in terms of skills, referrals, networking, as well as awareness and advocacy for children's rights on one side and the empowerment of family structures on the other.

WHAT IS THE STATUS OF CHILDREN?

In 2001, the United Nations General Assembly, following recommendations from the CRC, requested that the UN Secretary-General conduct an in-depth study on violence against children. In 2003, Professor Paulo Pinheiro, from Brazil, was appointed as the expert to lead the study. In 2004, World Vision, Human Rights Watch, Save the Children, and the International Society for the Prevention of Child Abuse and Neglect, were appointed as an advisory panel of selected non-governmental organizations to advise on the nature and conduct of the study. The final report was delivered to the UN General Assembly in 2007. The study provided an "in-depth" summary of the extent and burden of the problem of children exposed to violence in their homes, schools, and communities. Representatives from the Arab region participated in the report and provided relevant - yet insufficient - information about the Middle East and North Africa region (MENA) regarding the situation of children and the efforts in this regard. The International Society for the Prevention of Child Abuse and Neglect (ISPCAN) helpled, with the Arab Professionals' Network for the Prevention of Child Abuse and neglect (APNPCAN), in the identification of the procedures that would be more efficient in the respective backgrounds of countries who constitute the arab region, including and interactive approach, taking into consideration the countries' commitments to implement the CRC on tone side and the cultural sensitivities, based either on Religious laws [Muslims (Chiites, Sunnis, Alaouites and Druzes) Christians (Catholics, Protestants and Orthodox) as well as other religious groups, 20 of them existing in Lebanon] or on Regional customs [East Mediterranean, Gulf and North Africa] or on social status [Citizens, Refugees, Displaced, Foreign workers] on the other; ISPCAN has also contributed to increase the knowledge base of those professionals, while reducing the acceptance threshold of CAN, in terms of needs, analysis, procedures, networking, challenges and, mainly, visions for the future.

In this perspective of comparative realizations, Lebanon acknowledges the fact that Child protection strategies have already been set in some countries [Jordan, Morocco, Tunisia, Egypt] and are in the process of development in others [Syria, Bahrain, Yemen] whereas some countries still struggle with safety issues to comfort their child protection policies [Lebanon, Palestine, Sudan, Irak] …again, countries in the Gulf region like the Kingdom of Saudi Arabia [KSA] seem to be in quick motion, in order to install child protection strategies, while less is known about other arab countries, such as Koweit, Emirates, Qatar, Lybia, Algeria and others [ref. the UNSV, 2007 MENA report and recommendations]. ISPCAN has been thoroughly involved in these processes, including the development of national and regional policies in response to the UNSV, mainly –establishing and sustaining of Arab organizations towards the improvement of child protection policies and child friendly processes. In fact, under Law 422, the Lebanese Union for Child Protection [UPEL] is the only institution in Lebanon who has the mandate to ensure proper judicial and social follow-up of maltreated children and juveniles in conflict with law; in case of disclosure, the social worker from UPEL is called by any professional, law enforcement agent and even citizen or NGO in order to offer protection for the child and present with a report to the appropriate judicial reference. Also, UPEL will follow the sequence of the child's file within the Lebanese judicial system until final decision is taken by the judge, including the social protective frame. In that context, professional knowledge about CAN, created by ISPCAN resources, is currently being offered to UPEL and other relevant NGOs in order to increase capacities of professionals working with maltreated children.

WHAT WAS DONE?

Despite ongoing efforts by the government and many organizations to address the multiple social and professional obstacles hindering the implementation of children's rights in Lebanon (Author, Lebanese reports, 2005 and 2006) by reducing violence against children, CAN remains a serious threat to both children - and professionals working with them - in a still deeply unstable Lebanese society. Indeed, initiatives aiming better child protection are also interrupted, disorganized or disoriented by armed conflicts, like the war on Lebanon in July 2006 and the Palestinian Camps war in 2007; they are also challenged by a persistently unstable socio-political situation as well as recurrent riots, the most severe one since the end of the war having just occurred now in 2008.

Furthermore, Lebanon's laws do not yet meet the CRC requirements and there is no specific governmental budget allocated for the strategies and the processes of monitoring child rights, protection and rehabilitation, as well as the prevention of abuse. Instead, children fall under, in terms of civil rights, traditions and the different religious customs in Lebanon. In addition, there are no national independent structures for monitoring children's rights (e.g. National Child Defender), although a university child and youth "observatory" was established in 2007, and a child helpline is being considered.

Currently, many maltreated children still attend - or live in - institutions (schools, local community based foster centers, judicial facilities, and orphanages) that are not adequately sensitive to issues of the CRC, CAN and VAC. In addition, there is a scarcity of therapeutic programs for victims and virtually none for abusers. Furthermore, there is a wide discrepancy in the humanitarian and social situation of refugee children and their Lebanese and non-Lebanese peers living in Lebanon. Since the July 2006 war, children have still been exposed to armed conflict and social insecurity, as well as physical and psychological maltreatment related to their displacement from their homes and villages, as well as to internal reconciliation issues [socio-political turmoil, security and safety concern, economical uncertainty, conflicting youth objectives, and physical and moral confrontations]. These factors increase children's exposure to violence.

Maltreatment concerns are not addressed in the same manner among different social and religious groups, in a hectic political context, where staying alive and peace are the most important issues. For these reasons, children from different communities and diverse settings still suffer from maltreatment, abuse, and neglect of all sorts, without appropriate and comprehensive attention.

What can we do? In such contexts, professionals are expected to pave the way by taking lead roles in terms of diagnostic skills and referral for maltreated children, as well as preventive measures and advocacy. Governmental authorities are expected to invest in child protection - legislation and procedures - as well as social and educational policies.

Realizing the importance of professionals in implementing the CRC requirements in Lebanon, the Higher Council for Childhood selected in 2004 health, law, social and educational professionals for an expert panel - LIBAN-CAN. A code of conduct for professionals working with children is currently required for those working with LIBAN-CAN. Its mission aims at the prevention of maltreatment as well as the identification and management of abused and neglected children. This multidisciplinary task force is in charge for accomplishing that mission. It includes professionals from law enforcement, child welfare and mental health experts, in addition to researchers and health professionals. Since its establishment, LIBAN-CAN has offered its resources to professionals working with children, and those seeking more information about diagnosis, referral and advocacy related to CAN and VAC.

BUILDING THE INFORMATION/KNOWLEDGE BASE

Children subjected to CAN are frequently encountered in health settings; some require urgent medical attention. However, CAN is neither a mandatory reportable nor a regularly disclosed problem. Therefore, measuring the prevalence and incidence of CAN and VAC is not easy, and one cannot rely upon official figures.

In 2005-2006, Child of Lebanon (www.ChildOfLebanon.org) studied the validity of two questionnaires [I-CAST, 4 questionnaires were set: Child home, child institutions, parents, youth retrospective] developed by ISPCAN (www.ISPCAN.org) and APNPCAN (www.APNPCAN.net) for youth and parents (or caregivers) to measure the incidence of CAN in schools, institutions, and the community. In 2007, the youth questionnaire was administered by an NGO dedicated to stopping violence against women and sexual abuse against children [KAFA and Save the children Sweden]to study the prevalence and risk factors of child sexual abuse in selected populations. A "desk review" of institutions and research centers working with injured children and CAN issues, was also performed in 2005-2006 by St Joseph University. This review enabled the compilation of information concerning institutions working with children at risk and exposed to trauma, as well as their capabilities and needs. This review also involved a study of Lebanese laws related to child protection issues, in order to offer a platform to implement the CRC within the Lebanese legislation (www.cusfc@usj.edu.lb).

There is a growing and concerted initiative in Lebanon for the recognition and control of CAN. However, the lack of implementation of the reporting algorithm of children exposed to abuse or neglect calls for an independent, skilled and participatory structure to analyze relevant child-related information. Such a database would enable stakeholders to build child protection initiatives and programs, together with professionals in child related sectors, child and youth associations and NGO's. This is the vision of an inclusive Child and Youth Observatory, capable of presenting data about the situation of children in Lebanon; the growth of such an institution is an ongoing process, growing through a professional network and an intersectoral team competent in the analysis of data collected and the evaluation of society's response. In such an in independent structure, the trained team is enthusiastic to develop a better future for Lebanon's children within the CRC framework. In this perspective, professionals have a major role to play in building the knowledge base, raising the quality of expertise, informing families and stakeholders and modifying their attitudes.

CONCLUSIONS

There are many issues in confronting violence against children in Lebanon. The strategy is the responsibility of the society as a whole, with a special emphasis on the roles, potential and responsibilities of professionals LIBAN-CAN is emerging as a strong national structure, aiming to implement the above goals, where professionals and scientific resources guide its work. Youth participation and children with special needs are directly represented in LIBAN-CAN. We believe that frontline professionals as well as youth can improve the national understanding of children's rights and the definitions of maltreatment. They can also play an important role in the development of focused actions and appropriate policies.

LIBAN-CAN also recommends that teaching institutions in Lebanon include a mandatory course on CAN and VAC in their curricula. This process is underway in other Arab countries to enhance professional education on child protection.

IMPLICATIONS AND FUTURE PERSPECTIVES

Lebanon and other countries in the MENA region are still challenged by the international community but also by dedicated national NGOs to plan child protection systems, to set priorities, to provide frameworks for policies and enhance a social debate on CAN and VAC, in the frame of religious based laws on one side and with the participation of children and youth on the other. We have the following goals:

1. Meet with children and youth, and hear their opinions about CAN and VAC; the I-CAST [child] questionnaire is a useful tool. The main objectives of these meetings are:
    - to agree on definitions of VAC and CAN,
    - to enable children to be informed of the UNSV child version
    - to reach a common understanding about how to confront - and control - violence in children's environments
    - to consider children's responses to the UNSV results and recommendations,
    - to develop procedures children find useful and productive for effective participation and child protection,
    - to include child recommendations in the national Arab strategies for child protection against violence. In this participatory vision, the outreach of children for the child friendly UNSV is actually an ongoing process in Lebanon
2. Meet with parliamentarians and legislators, to:
    - enhance national and local organizations' efforts concerning child protection, while tackling specific needs and priorities, such as refugees camps, areas with limited access for security reasons, crowded slums and displaced populations

- stimulate revision of laws to comply with the provisions of the CRC
- increase knowledge about the UNSV
- and help support appropriate procedures for advocacy and sustainable child protection,

3. Reach a common understanding on how to confront violence and to implement children's rights. This is done annually by many NGOs in Lebanon, with the Lebanese Pediatric Society, many hospitals in Lebanon, the Union for Child Protection in Lebanon (www.UPEL.org), the Lebanese Institute for Child Rights (www.ChildOfLebanon.org), KAFA (www.KAFA.org) , AFEL and others, through posters and leaflets in public spaces, hospitals and schools, with children and community participation. In addition, mass media and opinion leaders are encouraged to publicize the advocacy effort of this new vision. More and more, the private sector and NGOs are invited to participate in this inclusive national Lebanese brainstorming to set a child protection system, as funders and providers

4. Enhance national and local organizations as well as citizens' movements and efforts in child protection, increase child participation in advocacy, raise awareness among youth and educators concerning their rights and opportunities.

5. Stimulate legislative reform to comply with the provisions of the CRC, and the implementation of national laws. ; the modification of prevalence and the reduction of risk factors [based on data collected by the Child and Youth observatory, among other sources of information]. Ultimately, the development of a child protection act and child defender would ensure the CRC implementation; creating a Child Defender institution would indeed offer quick responses to urgent child rights needs by highlighting the gaps within national laws as compared to the CRC, and the difficulties in the implementation of such legislations, thus aiming to reduce inequalities, mainly among vulnerable children

6. Increase professional knowledge about the UNSV and CAN, through the development of curricula in education, health, social work and law schools. Seminars for professionals working with children are useful for the exchanging knowledge and sharing expertise. This process began in December 2007 and will be translated to 3 languages for three categories of professionals: Health, Social and Education, Law. In this chapter, training of professionals with a common tool indeed enhances their efficiency and reduces their vulnerability. ISPCAN and APNPCAN have a major role in such a task, thus increasing local capacities in confronting VAC and CAN

7. Create a child budget, linked to the CRC requirements, recognized national needs and priorities - prioritize - within the national budget.

8. Establish a "Child Helpline" for referrals, as well as social, judicial and emotional support. Differences among religious groups may present obstacles to a common understanding of social conditions or circumstances for controlling CAN and VAC [such as early marriage, multiple spouses, corporal punishment]

9. Upgrade the University Child and Youth Observatory into a national observatory, to build reliable and credible knowledge on child rights and related issues

These perspectives constitute the pillars of knowledge and information on one side, training, and rehabilitation on the other; the prevention and control of VAC and CAN requires education about global child rights and knowledge of local childhood issues.In this arena, professionals working with children are - and should remain - the optimal child defenders.

Of course, this process needs social stability, common vision, and coordinated action by the those in the formal and informal "child" sector, as well as standardized professional intervention and child and youth participation. Of the above, the most challenging element is the last, and also most important. Even Lebanon can top Mount Everest.

REFERENCES

[1] Deeb M, Gerbaka B, Ajouz-Sidani R, Kheir-El-Kadi M. The vulnerable and disadvantaged children in Arab cities. Child and the City Conference, Amman, 2004 [Arabic] www.ChildOfLebanon.org

[2] ISPCAN world perspectives on child abuse, 6th and 7th ed, www.ISPCSAN.org

[3] Gerbaka B. Building a national taskforce in Lebanon for the prevention of child abuse and neglect; Public Health Approaches to Child Maltreatment: Prevention as a Priority; Town and country resort and convention center, San Diego, CA, 2006 Jan 23, www.ChildOfLebanon.org

[4] Gerbaka B. The prevention of child abuse and neglect [CAN] is a long-standing teamwork, relies on a regional expertise and needs an international cooperation; Town and country resort and convention center, San Diego, CA, 2006 Jan 26, www.ChildOfLebanon.org

[5] Gerbaka B, Awada S, Mikhael E. The reply of the Lebanese state on the UN questionnaire on VAC, 2004 [Arabic] www.Atfalouna.gov.lb

[6] The third national report on the situation of children in Lebanon, 1998-2003 [Arabic] www.Atfalouna.gov.lb

[7] The UNGS report on VAC, Paulo Sergio PINHEIRO, 2007

[8] The EU Guidelines on Children and Armed Conflict, 2003.

[9] The four Geneva Conventions of 1949 and its two Additional Protocols of 1977, the Rome Statute of the International Criminal Court (1998) Security Council resolutions devoted to CAAC: 1261 (1999); 1314 (2001); 1379 (2001); 1460 (2003); and 1539 (2004)

[10] The MENA Regional Consultation on Violence against Children, Cairo, June 2005

[11] The International Committee for the Rights of Child meeting with the Lebanese delegation, Geneva, June 2006

[12] Hage G, Gerbaka B. Toward an efficient child protective strategy in Lebanon: A call for pediatricians' true child advocacy. Pediatrica 2007;2:2-3.

In: International Aspects of Child Abuse and Neglect   ISBN: 978-1-60876-703-8
Editors: H. Dubowitz, J. Merrick pp. 65-85   © 2010 Nova Science Publishers, Inc.

Chapter 8

THE ARAB REGION AND THE UNITED NATION STUDY ON VIOLENCE: A GLOBAL MOVEMENT WITH PROFESSIONALS TOWARDS PROTECTING CHILDREN FROM VIOLENCE IN THE MIDDLE EAST AND NORTH AFRICA REGION

Bernard Gerbaka[*]

Pediatric Intensive Care Unit, Hotel Dieu de France Hospital, Beirut, Lebanon

The prevention of child abuse and neglect (CAN) is based on a human rights vision, involving universal child rights and culturally sensitive processes. Since the International Society for the Prevention of Child Abuse and Neglect (ISPCAN) conference in Brisbane and the meeting with the UN special representative for the Study on Violence in 2003, the Arab region was involved in the UNSV (UN Study on Violence) in many tracks:

- Research, with the I-CAST questionnaires - involving academic sectors and NGOs - some endorsed by the UNICEF,
- Advocacy, with the involvement of multiple agencies in the UNSV, including governmental and civil society agencies,
- Training of professionals, with multidisciplinary tools, some of them developed with the WHO, as frameworks and guidelines for an intersectoral approach to the prevention of child abuse,
- Capacity building, by developing multidisciplinary teams within national structures
- Tools for child protection, to be culturally adapted by national teams, in order to set strategies for the prevention of violence against children (VAC)
- Evaluation, integrated within programs, with the purpose of enhancing transparency, sustainability, efficiency and flexibility.

---

[*] *Correspondence:* Associate professor Bernard Gerbaka, MD, Pediatric Intensive Care Unit, Hotel Dieu de France Hospital, Beirut, Lebanon. E-mail: Berger@Childoflebanon.org or pedhdf@usj.edu.lb

INTRODUCTION

The definition of the child is contained in article 1 of the Convention, i.e. "every human being below the age of 18 years unless, under the law applicable to the child, the majority is attained earlier". The definition is adopted by most countries in the Middle East and North Africa regions (MENA).

Violence is defined as presented in the WHO World Report on Violence and Health: "the intentional use of physical force or power, threatened or actual, against oneself, another person, or against a group or community that either results in or has a high likelihood of resulting in injury, death, psychological harm, mal development or deprivation".

The world health organization (WHO) estimates that 40 million children below the age of 15 years suffer from abuse and neglect, and require health and social care. Violence against children is a global problem. Children experience violence in schools, in institutions, on the streets, in the workplace, in prisons, as well as in their own homes. Violence can affect children's physical and mental health, impair their ability to learn and socialize and undermine their development as functional adults and good parents later in life. In the most severe cases, violence against children leads to death.

Violence against children, including physical violence, emotional violence, and neglect, is a violation of children's rights. Article 19 of the convention for the rights of the child (1989) calls for legislative, administrative, social and educational actions to protect children from all forms of violence and abuse.

The UN study on violence against children examined the phenomenon of violence in the Middle East and North Africa Region, its different forms, its causes, and its impact on children, thus identifying the necessary measures for eradicating this phenomenon and the responsible actors, including children themselves, in protecting themselves from exposure to violence [recommendation of the UN General Assembly in its resolution no. 57/190]

The Committee on the Rights of the Child (CRC) has ensured that this study should lead to the development of intervention strategies that aim at protecting children from all forms of violence, with a view to effectively providing the necessary protection and prevention [A/56/488].

The regional 2005 UNSV consultation in Cairo was the first step in the development of regional interaction, followed by the meeting of national teams with the ICRC in Geneva in 2006 and again the Cairo conference in 2007. Those important landmarks allowed stakeholders in a growing number of Arab countries to enhance interaction between ISPCAN and their national representatives, while increasing the networking with Councils for Childhood, National Committees for the prevention of violence, Women and children ministries as well as other official bodies within governmental structures. The purpose of this process is to combat CAN and reduce VAC in the arab region, while installing appropriation structures for efficient programs that would be accepted and developed by diverse cultures in the region.

INTERACTION BETWEEN ISPCAN AND APNCAN

The International Society for Prevention of Child Abuse and Neglect (ISPCAN) is an international organization of professionals working to prevent child abuse and neglect in their countries, regions and internationally. ISPCAN provides education, training, capacity development and research support, information exchange among member professionals and other partners, resources (experts and expertise, little financial support), technical assistance and consultation services. ISPCAN works with regional networks, such as the Arab Professional Network for Prevention of Child Abuse and Neglect (APNPCAN), National Partner Societies, and members to improve their clinical expertise, their community and national capacity in child protection, and increasingly, with governments and international partners - to improve their child abuse and neglect policies, systems, services and internal education to strengthen the efforts of their national professionals to effectively treat abused and at-risk children, and to prevent child abuse and neglect longer term.

PRESENT SITUATION OF ARAB COUNTRIES AND THE UNSV

Child protection strategies have already been set in some countries (Jordan, Morocco, Tunisia, Egypt, Syria) and are in the process of development in others (Saudi Arabia, United Arab Emirates, Yemen, Bahrain), whereas some countries still struggle with safety issues to comfort their child protection policies (Lebanon, Palestine, Irak for example). Less is known about other Arab countries. Since 2003, ISPCAN has been thoroughly involved in different stages of those processes, including the development of national and regional policies in response to the UNSV, mainly in the setting of a sustained support and stable national structures, in order to improve child protection policies as well as child friendly processes. In a significant step to respond to the UN questionnaire on VAC, 9 countries have submitted a report: Egypt, Sudan, Syria, Yemen, Qatar, Kuwait, Morocco, Palestine and Algeria. Lebanon had a catch-up report.

None of the countries, however, provided enough data regarding the situation of violence against children in their respective context. Also, the available studies did not cover all countries in the region. Also, although most Middle Eastern and North African States have endorsed CRC, none of them included in their report their replies to the comments made by the UN regarding the rights of the child. Finally, the voices of children is almost absent from all replies to the questionnaire with the exception of one or two countries, reflecting the absence of children's participation in defining the problem or possible solutions.

Furthermore, although the participation of civil society organizations is mentioned in almost all reports, yet the voice of civil society remains absent in all reports except that of Palestine, where the critical voice of NGOs is represented in discussing the impact of protective measures for children. In more than one location of that report the views of both the executive bodies and those of civil society were highlighted.

A review of the available studies clearly shows that there is a great similarity between countries of the Middle East and North Africa region concerning the causes behind the high prevalence of violence against children in the different areas, including its most common forms. Discrepancies between countries exist regarding certain types of violence such as

FGM (female genital mutilation) or "honor killings" and the size of other phenomena such as street children and child labor. Risk factors may be classified as follows:

- Economic factors: increased rates of poverty and unemployment, which will increase with global economic crisis.
- Social factors: dysfunctional families in multicultural contexts, marital disputes of parents, large size of families, polygamy; social tensions and armed conflicts,
- Prevalent cultural beliefs: attitudes towards raising children (e.g. assumptions that an extent of physical or verbal violence may be useful for child rearing)
- Lack of awareness: regarding appropriate child rearing practices and the harm that some might provoke (e.g. shaking babies)
- Role of the media and programs which sometimes encourage violence (e.g. scenes of violence and child participation in armed conflicts)
- Legislation: lacks provisions that target the protection of children. In cases where those laws are present they may not be adequately enforced.

Also, reporting of violence against children is not compulsory in most of the countries in the MENA region

SITUATIONAL ANALYSIS

Most studies refer the scarcity of data on violence against children to a number of reasons, such as the sensitivity of the issue especially when it happens in certain contexts such as the family, the tendency to under report on violence against children, the lack of awareness of its negative consequences, etc. finally the issue did not attract enough attention from researchers and investigators except recently, despite the abundance of studies addressing violence in the community in general in the last decade. Some of the country reports have mentioned that such data are not available because of lack of field studies and epidemiological research on part of relevant bodies.

THE MIDDLE-EAST REGION

In Egypt and Lebanon, for example no periodic reports are available regarding child deaths due to violence, because such crimes usually happen as individual cases and do not represent a phenomenon; moreover, they are often attributed to accidental injuries. Thus, there are no government reports on child deaths suspected to be secondary to violence. In 2009 however, a child deaths review team was created in Lebanon, between a university hospital-based group and the child protection services, in accordance with the Ministry of Justice. In this perspective, a child protection unit was also installed in the same premises.

In Syria the reply to the UNSV admits the widespread prevalence of violence against children, whether in the home, at school, on the street or at the work place. The reported cases of violence do not represent however the whole reality due to lack of accurate monitoring mechanisms. Also there is lack of media coverage of the issue.

Palestine does not report an estimate of the size of the problem, and refers to the absence of such statistics. Also there is no monitoring of crimes committed against children nor of the complaints associated with that violence.

THE GULF REGION

"The Meeting of Experts in the Region of Gulf Cooperation Council" on the maltreatment of children, held in the Kingdom of Saudi Arabia in 2004, agreed on the presence of cases of child maltreatment in all countries of the region.

In Yemen, although the government of did not undertake any national surveys during the last decade addressing the issue of violence against children in particular, still there are some studies which address family violence in general. Also, there is a public system that officially investigates causes of death, including deaths of children. A periodic monthly report is published, describing a summarized statistical review of deaths which are known or suspected to be as a result of violence.

In Qatar, no previous surveys have been made regarding the prevalence of violence against children; there is, however, a report that shows the total number of cases of violence against children as given by relevant state bodies.

Kuwait stated that violence does not constitute a phenomenon in the country; therefore there are no available statistics on that matter. Also there are no governmental bodies specialized in addressing violence against children in particular. There are, however, administrations and bodies within state ministries which are concerned with all human rights issues who undertake the follow up of all human rights issues and the defense against any violation of those rights, including children's rights and any form of violence that children might face.

NORTH AFRICA

Sudan indicates that some research and surveys have been done concerning the market children, domestic laborers, child labor and juvenile justice, but did not report the findings of those surveys.

Algeria has s system of fact finding and research which allows official investigation of cases of child deaths by the security authorities and the police once the issue is addressed in a legal investigation and reports statistics regarding child deaths due to violence. A forensic death certificate is needed for such an investigation. The legal security authorities and the police have to periodically submit a statistical report on deaths and send it to relevant bodies and ministries.

THE WHOLE REGION

Several reports on violence against children in different countries of the MENA and Gulf regions (Iran , Jordan, Lebanon, Yemen and North Africa) have indicated the prevalence of different forms of violence (physical, verbal, sexual, neglect) at the home or at school. However, the size of the problem is yet not clarified in most of the countries. Useful tools in this perspective include:

- The I-CAST questionnaires (Lebanon, 2006, 2007, 2008; Egypt, 2006)
- Definitions of CAN, that need to be integrated within the provisions of law (Lebanon, KSA, 2009) as being in accordance with:
- The provisions of the CRC
- The professionals' descriptions, mainly in the health sector
- The societies' culture and awareness.

ISPCAN AND THE UNSV IN THE ARAB WORLD

ISPCAN has contributed, with the Arab professionals network for the prevention of child abuse and neglect (www.APNPCAN.net) in the identification of the procedures that would be more efficient in the respective backgrounds, including cultural sensitivities; Arab and international networks have also increased the knowledge base - while reducing the acceptance threshold of CAN - in terms of needs, analysis, procedures, networking, challenges - thus enhancing the quality of national visions in terms of efficient child oriented policies. In some areas of the Arab world, these initiatives were hindered by armed conflicts, like the war in Lebanon July 2006 and the Nahr-el-Bared camp war in 2007, the everlasting Palestinian struggle and the Iraq situation; they are also challenged by unstable socio-political situations in many counties of the MENA region.

However, despite many obstacles, the perspective of child protection is strongly developing within national systems and regional networks, in the presence of increasing levels of common values and universal understanding of child rights. In reality, child dedicated structures are grass rooting initiatives; they rely on political decisions, local and national human resources, regional expertise and international cooperation; they seek for strategies at the countries levels in order to implant child protection systems, and recently expanded the network in order to learn from experiences in other arab countries:

- 1st ISPCAN Arab regional conference on CAN, Amman, Jordan, 2005: "Breaking the silence"
- 2nd ISPCAN arab regional conference on CAN, Sana'a, Yemen, 2007: "Towards a strategy for child protection"
- 3rd ISPCAN arab regional conference on CAN, Riyadh, KSA, 2009: "Working together towards safer childhood".
- Also, in between those dates, professionals' training seminars were held in: Syria, Lebanon, Egypt, Bahrain, KSA, etc.

On those diverse occasions, the Arab initiative - then the UNSV - presented a setting-based framework for the description of child abuse in countries and the efforts developed to stop violence. The International Society for the Prevention of Child Abuse and Neglect was also partner within the advisory panel to advice on the nature and definitions of VAC on one side, and conduct the UNSV on the other.

Based on an expanding knowledge base, the UNSV intends to highlight on the status of children confronted with violence in their different environments, to increase the national - as well as informal capacities to build systems that focus on the integration of protection and prevention - as well as child participation - in the human rights commitments and implementation processes. All procedures would be based on a CRC matrix that incorporates children's rights, professional evidence, relevant social factors and intersectoral responsibilities for the prevention of VAC and the control of CAN, as a priority in Governmental programs.

The final report from the study was delivered to the UN General Assembly in the beginning of 2007. The study provided an "in-depth" summary of the extent of violence against children, where children are exposed to violence in their homes, their communities and in the schools. Representatives from the arab region and APNPCAN participated in the UNSV and in the "World perspectives" ISPCAN document and provided therefore relevant - yet insufficient - information about the MENA situation of children and the efforts undertaken in this regard to relieve their conditions.

Obviously, the scarcity of child specific health and social support services are obstacles to child protection, and should then be made available to families and accessible to children. In reality, the capacities of those services are sometimes overwhelmed, especially during armed conflicts and social instability, when children are involved in violent situations and at increased risk of different types of abuse and violence. In such contexts, free childcare, universal health screening and universal access to free medical care become even more critical, as is, in general, the universal access to free health care for all citizens.

National strategies for child protection would indeed comply with the United Nations Convention on the Rights of the Child, with attention to the needs and possibilities of some developing, insecure and ill-resourced countries. The potential challenges and impacts of the CRC implementation should also be explored for future landmarks of democracies and freedom of opinions, mainly in terms of:

- Independent structures: child observatories, at local and national levels, are actually available in Morocco, Tunis and Lebanon. There are still no child defenders or child ombudsman, though a proposition of law was presented in this regard in Lebanon, 2004.
- Child protection acts or child-friendly and environment-centered legislations, actually available in Egypt, Jordan, Syria, pending in Lebanon
- Budgets for Child protection and child oriented projects, not distinctively available
- Helpline for children and professionals, for the reporting of child maltreatment and for psychosocial support to victims of violence, available in Egypt, pending in Lebanon
- Training of pilot and decentralized multisectoral teams and building of professional curricula, actually in expanding process in Syria, Lebanon, Jordan and Egypt
- Study the extent of VAC, based on three I-CAST questionnaires (Child, Retrospective and parents) tested and implemented in Egypt and Lebanon.

- Participation of children and youth in the evaluation of problems, analysis of situations, setting of reports, implementation of processes and re-evaluation of actions, present in many country reports, where few evidence of efficiency is however available
- Support of child-friendly media: auto-censorship on aggressive viewings, to reduce violence and enhance educative programs - with children - on screens; in this regards, workshops for child friendly media have been held in many countries in the region, with two main outcomes: abused children are rarely visualized on media, and more child friendly programs are developed
- Code of conduct for professionals working with children: Lebanon is considering the implementation of the code with professionals working for/with children, within the provisions of the coming modification of relevant law.

Despite ongoing efforts by Arab governments and many NGOs to address the multiple social, cultural and professional pitfalls, CAN remains a serious threat to child rights implementation. There is still no child budget and no child protection acts in many counties. There are few independent structures for child rights monitoring (National child defender, national child observatory) and scarce child helplines. Children are still present in high numbers in institutions. Therapy programs are limited for victims - yet increasing - and most often virtual for perpetrators. Legislations are subject to national consultations to meet the CRC requirements. The human and social situation of refugees is sometimes dramatic or still waiting for the settlement of the Arab-Israeli conflict. Internally and regionally displaced children are repeatedly exposed to extreme types of violence and abuse.

In some countries, children are viewed as - and submitted to - their religious references, in terms - and place - of civil rights. In such countries, children are exposed to problems that alter their growth, development, social interaction, safety, education and health.

It is therefore important for Arab professionals to rely on - and encourage - the governments who show intention to build child protection systems, but also to contribute in drawing a sharing platform of knowledge and knowhow, from observations and findings of professionals, experts and NGOs who work closely with children; in this regard, cooperation with ISPCAN may increase the capacities of stakeholders in confronting violence with peaceful stands, based on firm and clear evidence of efficient programs.

The mission of the professionals' network - at academic or informal levels - aims at the prevention of maltreatment as well as the identification and management of abused and neglected children. Established in taskforces, they accomplish this mission within multidisciplinary teams, formed of law enforcement personnel, child welfare and mental health specialists in addition to research resources and health professionals. However, and unless controlled by reliable monitoring systems, professional training and societal implication, further increase of violence against children is expected in many countries of the Arab region - in view of the alarming rates of associated risk factors.

VIOLENCE IN DIFFERENT SETTINGS

Four settings of violence against children have been identified. Those are the family, the school, institutions and the local community. The family harbors several forms of gender based violence such as female genital mutilation (FGM), early marriage and honor killings.

Violence against children in the home and family

Family does not refer only to the small nuclear family, but also involves the extended family and other forms of relationships that define family life and relations.

Punishment and violence within families as disciplinary methods is widespread and still culturally and legally tolerated (Lebanon, Tunisia, Yemen, Kuwait) while measures taken to address that violence are inadequate (Egypt, Jordan, Kuwait, Saudi Arabia, and Algeria). In Morocco all forms of violence and mutilation, such as FGM, are criminalized by law.

In countries where Islamic Sharia'a laws regarding personal affairs are not standardized yet, there is more likelihood of random application of laws which may differ from one local community to the other.

Prevalent beliefs and concepts of honor and the association of family honor with women's sexual conduct outside of marriage frequently lead to what is called honor crimes, which constitute the severest form of family violence against young women.

In reality, corporal punishment is a mainly visible and common means of discipline to children in most arab countries - not excluding many others in the world. Severe physical abuse is often easily recognized; however, cases of fatal or severe shaken babies and alleged or factitious disorders (Münchausen by proxy) as well as unidentified sudden infant deaths are reasons of concern; on the other hand, allegations of CAN have been raised in situations of family dislocation and cause important disruption in the child well-being and deviations in court decisions, when bribing and corruption may induce false certificates. In the mainstream, it is not exaggerated to stipulate that 95% of children with problems in behavior are subject to physical means of discipline, which leaves a broad grey band to be interpreted by individuals, based on their knowledge on one side, and cultural background and beliefs on the other. Risk factors for child maltreatment also include: poverty, scattered families and poor skills in conflict management. In some countries, political violence and politicization of children are fertile fields for VAC and child violence.

Arab professionals have stimulated some responses to violence against children in the home and family; some of those are ongoing:

- Organizing campaigns for stopping corporal punishment, with participation of media and education stakeholders in the process; those campaigns targeted to increase child and family awareness about CAN, advocate for child protection and encourage the participation of children. (Syria, Lebanon, Jordan, KSA)
- Setting workshops, in the perspective of child helplines on one side and alternatives to corporal punishment on the other (Egypt, Lebanon)
- Support of individual child and family mental health rehabilitation and promoting home visitation for families at risk (Lebanon, 2009)

- Modification of relevant legislations (ongoing in most countries who have reported to the UNSV)
- Development of multisectoral curriculae and training of health oriented professionals (One of the main projects for the APNPVAC (New denomination of the APNPCAN) in recent years; however, curricula have only been implemented in few countries: Lebanon, Syria, Jordan)

Violence against children in schools and educational settings

This includes corporal punishment at schools or threat to use any form of physical violence in addition to humiliation, ridicule, verbal abuse or neglect. Physical punishment continues to be widespread in schools, even in states which have legislated against such violence (e.g. Egypt, Morocco, Algeria) and states which have not provided clear legal provisions that ban physical punishments at school such as Iraq, Kuwait, Lebanon and Yemen, where such measures are accepted as disciplinary tools, in spite of a strong professional and NGOs movement towards banning permissive relevant laws.

In school settings, corporal punishment is a common means of discipline to children. Severe physical abuse is rare in such environments; anecdotal cases are, however, reported.

Corporal punishment is a classical tool to control discipline of children in schools: more than 50% of children - as opposed to 95% of children with behavioral problems - are subject to physical violence; nearly 50% of teachers and administrators use these physical means for education and discipline. The WR/VAC/2007/Chap 4/Page 125 indicates that between 30% (females) and 40% (males) of children aged 13 to 15 years have been bullied at least once within the 30 last days, less than Jordan, as much as Oman, more than the UAE. Also, 30% of females and 65% of males aged 11, 13 and 15 years have been involved in a physical fight within the last 12 months, less than Jordan, more than Greece, UAE and Oman. Other consequences of violence include: Bullying, violence against teachers, deterioration of school performance, school drop-out, drug dealing, peer stimulation or alcohol abuse.

The treatment of children in care institutions ranges between cruel and moderately violent when children make a mistake. Parties using violence with children are teachers, supervisors, guards and social workers. A number of factors contribute to those practices, among which are lack of qualification of staff entrusted with the supervision and care of children, lack of accountability mechanisms in most institutions, lack of reporting mechanisms which the children can use to complain and also lack of effective penalties in the case of submitting a complaint.

There have been, with Arab professionals and other resources, some responses to violence against children in the schools, nurseries and other educational settings:

- As in home violence, workshops on alternative measures for discipline were organized. Also, peaceful conflict resolution is an original experience undertaken in schools settings; results are promising, but need adequate environments and appropriate advocacy
- Legislation, customs and educative procedures were also identified and alternative plans set in order to stop corporal punishment in schools.

- Also, elected parents councils and child representatives induce safer environments for children, as well as efficient means of disclosure

Violence against children in care and justice institutions

Most children in those institutions are victims of sexual abuse, usually by guards and teachers, or by older children. Children may also be transferred with adult criminals who in turn inflict violence or sexual abuse on the children.

Ages of penal responsibility vary between arab countries, from 7 to 14 years, increasing under the pressure of evidence, showing the incompatibility of low ranges of age with the CRC. Eventually, the UNSV consultation has also tackled the issue of children in institutions, where diverse and additive types of abuse and neglect are inflicted to children. Regional meetings, organized with ISPCAN and APNPCAN, provided tools and given exposure to new ideas for lobbying in favor of de-institutionalization and child protection in the judiciary systems.

In many countries of the MENA region, too many children are still in institutional care-and-stay, sometimes mixed with adults. Given the predicted difficulties that children encounter in such settings, only hazy figures are available about the extent and nature of the phenomenon. Also, the situation of children in institutions is hardly described in the absence of evaluative and disclosure procedures, requiring:

1. Training for professionals working with children
2. Alternative care of child in foster family

In institutional care the WR/VAC/2007/Chap 5/Page 183/children in institutions [1999-2000] shows the numbers of children who live in institutional care; given the critical child-rights aspect of the problem, studies about children in institutions need to be performed in arab countries, with a timetable, including:

- Gathering resources and increasing knowledge,
- Train professionals working with children,
- Promote alternative education processes
- Provide consensual and comprehensive terms of understanding with institutions of care, including codes of conduct
- and perform relevant modifications in law

Some experiences deserve however replication (SOS children's village case study, the WR/VAC/2007/Chap 5/Page 208) as some institutions help families to care for children at home, with micro credit strategies, partial institutionalization, local networking as well as support and thorough social follow-up. Such support may provide possibilities for self-reliability for woman-headed, multi-children families, with eventually absent or incapacitated fathers.

In custody and detention most children, who are in conflict with law and placed for institutional rehabilitation are in child environments. In such situations, children beneficiate from judicial assistance, educational and job learning programs, as well as leisure possibilities, outdoor activities and playtime. The number of children held in prisons is difficult to publish and always on the move; they are subject to surveillance - daytime - by diversely competent personnel and benefit from job training opportunities.

The issue of violence in care and justice institutions has been the center of many debates, with Arab professionals and other resources; some of the responses include:

- Modification of relevant laws, to make their provisions more child-friendly and to offer better protection to the minors in conflict with law and threatened children who need protection.
- Alternative measures to imprisonment of children in conflict with law, towards rehabilitation and reparation procedures in communities; currently and since 2006, alternative measures to imprisonment is a judicial strategy adopted by a growing number of judges in juvenile settings in Lebanon
- In some countries, in the presence of allegations of CAN, ad hoc or institutional committees - constituted of professionals in child health, mental health, social workers, judges and law institutions - meet to study the files of children in need of protection, with respect to laws. Child protection units have also been instituted in hospital (Lebanon, KSA) and social settings (Syria)
- In cases of severe CAN, cases are also submitted, in some countries, to child fatality and severe abuse teams, in order to present an accurate diagnosis to court. Ref: WR/VAC/2007/Chap3/page91. For example, in 2009, a child fatality review team has been instituted in a university hospital-based setting in Lebanon.
- Arab professionals have been leaders in editing, since 2003, relevant algorithms and guidelines to help in the diagnosis and management of CAN cases, and co-organized training sessions with ISPCAN, to multisectoral first liners [law, social, health, education] in order to increase the efficiency of system response to disclosures of CAN. The medical certification and child abuse curriculum is ongoing in some arab countries and remains to be developed in others
- Lately, there has been an emerging movement to increase the age of penal responsibility. Main concern is aggravated exposure of the child to conflict with law, leading some countries to discuss an incremental increase of the age of penal responsibility. (e.g., honor crimes)

Violence against children in places of work

In most Arab countries, rural life and street environments are places, where children work. Sexual and commercial exploitation of children and organs is also a significant concern, with insufficient data on these common appearances; in such context, some children work in extreme and dangerous conditions.

Because of poverty and ignorance, as well as exploitation networks, working at a young age may be considered as a positive, where children contribute to the family budget.

The phenomenon of child labor is prevalent in many countries of the Middle East and North Africa; the extent varies according to the definition and methodology used in each country in assessing the nature and size of the problem. In most countries it is difficult to specific the size of the phenomenon since children usually work in the informal sector and in small workshop and take up marginal jobs. Available research on child labor in the different countries such as Egypt, Lebanon, Morocco and Jordan indicates that children work under extremely difficult circumstances and may be subject to violence, an be either verbal or physical, mostly in the form of beating. Also, they are deprived of any health care and many of them work in dangerous jobs that threaten their health and distort their growth and development. In all those countries there are laws for the protection of children. Lack of supervision and inspection especially in the agricultural sector and in family institutions (Egypt and Morocco) expresses concern regarding he involvement of extremely young girls in domestic labor and their exposure to violence and the cruel working conditions.

The report of countries of Gulf Council cooperation mentions the issue of children Jockeys used in camel races, especially in United Arab Emirates. The respective governments (Emirates, Qatar, Oman) launched a campaign against smuggling of children, banned the use of children in such dangerous jobs and prohibited the employment of children.

To make things worse, children are not beneficiaries of health and injury protection, and cost therefore even less to the workplace than adults.

Such commercial abuse boosts the street children problem, and mixes in some countries with the problem of refugees. In home settings, the working girl issue is predominant, whereas boys may dominate in rural areas, in the streets and factories.

A network of professionals working with children can advocate to stakeholders for more awareness about the effects of child labor on the predicament of children in places of work:

- Countries are entitled to comply with optional protocols to confront child labor, reduce the phenomenon of child labor, with incremental procedures and stop the worst forms of child exploitation
- The project of child protection in the streets is a huge enterprise, too big for one country alone; the Arab council for childhood and development proposes the following steps:
  o Execute field studies, with the cooperation of local resources and NGOs
  o Set training sessions for capacity building of first liners working with street children
  o Review relevant laws with regard to protection of children in the streets
  o Organize local networks and enhance cooperation with arab experiences
  o Promote family oriented programs (micro credit, education sponsoring)
  o Stimulate coordination between formal and informal sectors to control child labor in the streets

Other directions need also to be explored, such as work on a MENA platform to control street children phenomenon and improve with ILO the Law referential on child labor and street children.

Violence against children in the community - Street violence

Children are subject to violence on the street as a result of disputes between them and their neighbors or age peers or as a result of street car accidents or due to the dangerous games played by children on the street. The most group of children exposed various forms of violence on the street are the "street children". This phenomenon is prevalent in many countries in the Middle East and North Africa region.

The definition of who is a street child differs from one country to the other. But the general definition involves living on the street most of the time and earning one's living from the street.

Available research concerning this category of children reveals the different types of violence of which they may be victims. Those range between physical harm, sexual abuse, risk of addiction and crime and may reach up to murder.

Violence in armed conflicts

The Israel-Arab conflict, as well as social conflicts in Lebanon, Iraq, Somalia and Sudan have had a significant impact on children. Many crimes have added to the forms of violence which are suffered by the rest of the children in the Arab region and the world. Since the structural violence exercised directly influence and lead to an escalation of violence within Palestinian society resulting in even more poverty and frustration and a need to ventilate that frustration against whoever is available among the family members. Accordingly women and children become the immediate target.

The definition of a child is a concern: for example, it is applied according to the convention on Israeli children, while Palestinian children are subject to military laws. Such definitional issues are also a concern in Sudan and Darfur.

The refugees' related problems concern millions of people in the MENA region and provoke religious and demographic instability; it also creates hot areas of armed violence, uncontrolled by some states. The humanitarian conditions inside the camps and slumps affect important numbers of children, exposed to community violence, customs and discrimination that may even be irrelevant with legislation.

Qualitatively, the situation of children is also highly concerning. Some reports - shadow reports - bring information about the condition of children in such housings and social settings, where commercial and sexual exploitation are current, adding violence over violence to poverty, clan violence, discrimination and religious confrontations. The situation of children also addresses the insufficiency of the international community in carrying out Article 1 obligation to "ensure respect" for the Geneva Conventions and the protection of civilians during armed conflicts throughout the Arab region, ...to pass a resolution denouncing the deteriorating respect for international humanitarian law in the Arab region, including in Iraq, the OPTs, Darfur and Yemen.

SEXUAL EXPLOITATION AND TRAFFICKING IN CHILDREN

Children may be subject to sexual abuse in the family or school or in the different institutions. However, the term sexual exploitation is used to refer to childhood prostitution and their use in pornographic activities. The same applies to trafficking in children where the child is transferred from one person to another in exchange for money. This is usually done in order to use those children in different forms of domestic labor, agricultural labor and also in sex tourism.

Laws in all countries of the Middle East and North Africa region prohibit sexual exploitation of children and the production of pornographic material in the context of prohibiting prostitution and sexual exploitation in general.

As for sexual abuse, many countries do not have specific laws that protect children subject to rape. The penalty is usually a severe one in case the victim is under age. The rapist may be spared the penalty, if he agrees to marry the victim and in many cases the girls are forced to marry their rapists.

In the regional conference on Commercial Sexual Exploitation of Children in North Africa (ECPAT), organized in Rabat, Morocco in June 2003, the five participating countries submitted a report regarding the situation of sexual exploitation of children and suggested recommendations to address this phenomenon. Lebanon is also, by nature, a place for sexual tourism, where legislation is not tackling directly internet crimes, sexual exploitation, extra-territoriality, aggravating conditions for sexual abuse, etc. On the same subject, an International Conference on Effective Strategies for the Prevention of Child Online Pornography Trafficking and Abuse was held in Bahrain, March 2009.

Reports from Arab countries agree that it is difficult to obtain accurate data and information regarding the prevalence of sexual exploitation. Police records also do not provide an estimate of the size of the problem.

The prevalent form of sexual exploitation in the North Africa region is child prostitution; child trafficking is associated more with economic exploitation than with sexual exploitation since it is associated with child labor in areas such as domestic labor.

The sectors most at risk are street children beggars and domestic laborers. Forced early marriage, especially in Egypt, Mauritania and Chad are considered a form of sexual exploitation, as are the child trafficking in Iraq and the problem of smuggling children inside the state of Libya for the purpose of prostitution and slave trade.

Responses to violence against children in the community: Arab professionals provide expertise to decision makers about the condition of children in such settings, where problems are too big for one arab country, including living conditions and social challenges, sexual and commercial exploitation of humans and organs, humanitarian assistance and support, as well as access to education and control of frontiers, arm smuggling and corruption.

ARAB PROFESSIONALS HAVE OBJECTIVES, TOOLS AND EXPERTISE

Organized in networks, professionals integrate institutions and enrich human resources in contact with children ; based on an interdisciplinary team approach, they develop skills and knowledge, encourage collaboration within local and governmental institutions, call on academic and research organizations, stimulate funding from private sectors, interact with families and informal sector and - last but not least - innovate opportunities for youth participation. Some of the objectives of Arab professionals are:

- To identify valuable resources and key persons working with children
- To develop and improve models for detection and management
- To increase public awareness in the definition, recognition and prevention of CAN.
- To design and facilitate educational and training materials, and provide a sustainable educational support for professionals and NGOs working in the area of CAN.
- To support local and governmental cooperation, and encourage the Arab region (MENA) and global efforts in child protection, mainly with ISPCAN expertise.
- To help launch specialized centers for research and others for the management of maltreated children
- To ensure that adequate and independent surveillance systems are available and that monitoring of extent and pattern of child maltreatment is studied

An important aspect of the mission includes comprehensive reporting on CAN and involves the efforts to improve child protection. In this vision, the major objectives are as follows:

- Provide professional expertise and technical support to gather information from resources and professionals
- Establish a core group of trained and committed multidisciplinary professionals, to report on cases involving CAN, and monitor actions to comply with CRC provisions.
- Increase the quality of practice in terms of intersectoral and intra professional work, in the areas of health, law, education and welfare services.

In the UNSV perspective, professionals integrate subcommittees or working groups, dealing with: the legal framework, the training needs, the research resources… in all types of CAN. As actors in addressing violence, professionals also tackle policies and programs to address violence against children: data collection and research, analysis and evaluation, awareness and advocacy curricula and training.

In reality, despite the professionals pressing demands and the consequent efforts deployed by governments from the levels of policies and legislations to those of implementation and practice, violence against children is still a challenge for several reasons, which can be summarized as follows:

- Examples of cultural beliefs: Some types of CAN, such as corporal punishment, female genital mutilation, early marriage and violence against girls still are diversely perceived by stakeholders and citizens; they remain sometimes in arab societies as private matter or cultural specificities. Modifications are expected in the provisions of national legislations.
- Challenges in education: Lack of awareness about child rights among families, educators and child caregivers, remain a challenge. School-based initiatives are needed in that regard, like "ambassadors of peace", "One World 2011".

- Types of structural obstacles to the CRC implementation: The lack of monitoring systems relating to violence is still a gap in the evaluation and control of violence against children. Child observatories exist in some arab countries and need to be replicated with more independence. Also, the Child Defender project would help national child protection strategies reach rapid, adapted, legalized and socially acceptable interventions toward the implementation of the CRC. Furthermore, the Child helpline, available in some countries, is warming up in some others. "Child Friendly Budgeting" is an emerging concept in Jordan, involving Governmental and Nongovernmental sectors. The Child Friendly Budget initiative aims at increasing the attention of policy makers and legislators on public spending that best responds to children's matters and priorities, ensuring its integration into governmental planning in the fields of health, education and social development.

- Legislation discrepancies and pitfalls: All countries of the Middle East and North Africa region have endorsed the CRC. Some countries did not make any reservations, while others have made reservations regarding provisions that were taken to be incompatible with Islamic jurisprudence. Seven countries (Egypt, Lebanon, Jordan, Yemen, Qatar and Tunisia) have equally endorsed the optional protocol regarding child trafficking, child prostitution and child pornography.

The definition of a child varies however from one country to another, with subsequent variation in the definition of the age of criminal responsibility. In many countries that age is very young, and is therefore not compatible with CRC (e.g. 7 years in Lebanon…to be increased to 10; Libya, Qatar, Saudi Arabia, Emirates, Yemen and Egypt). Subsequently a child that young could be convicted. In some countries which have no definite age of adulthood, children may receive the death penalty, life imprisonment or flogging (especially in Qatar, Saudi Arabia and Emirates).

Maltreatment of juveniles and their detention in difficult circumstances stress the violence they might be subject to by officials and their deprivation of the right to contact their families such as is the case in Lebanon, Libya, Morocco, Syria and Tunisia. In some countries such as Syria and Egypt beggars and street children are treated like criminals.

Weaknesses in enforcement of legal provisions included in the CRC, as well as some discrepancies within national legislations, are congruent problems. There are still, however, important efforts produced towards child friendly laws. This issue is particularly important in the Juvenile Justice and children at risk. Alternative measures for juveniles in conflict with law are on the track, with compensation, reintegration and restoring justice. Legislation and capacity building also appear as critical requirements in the street children problem in the Arab world.

- Training and capacity building, gaps to fill: Professional capacities and institutional frames are critical points in the efficiency of initiative aiming to provide control of violence and protection of victims. In fact, Arab professionals offer expertise to the institutional settings to increase the level and quality of knowledge on the science of intersectoral cooperation and /or the usefulness of such a coordinative process, to optimize the development of child protection systems, thus encouraging the participatory process and increasing the capacities of the informal sector to build networks for interventions and collaboration.

- Monitoring and reporting. Reporting cases of violence against children is still very limited. There is lack of popular awareness regarding mechanisms of filing complaints or reporting. Also, the available mechanisms of complaints assume that the child is capable of dealing with the complicated judicial authorities. They also assume that the custodian of the child will complain on his or her behalf. There is generally no mechanism that allows the child to complain if it is against the will of the parent or custodian - or against them if they are the source of violence. Law 422/2002 in Lebanon has allowed children or civil society to report and file complaints on one side, while reporting is mandatory for physicians and recommended for other professionals working with children on the other.
- Role of civil society in combating violence against children. Reports from different countries have highlighted civil society organizations to different degrees as active parties in addressing violence against children. Also, in some countries, civil society plays a major role in designing policies, palpating the pulse of community in term of compliance to law, and changing societies' understanding of child protection. NGOs seem however to lack up-to-date skills in data collection, documentation and reporting etc. The majority of NGO activities focus on training and awareness raising as well as carrying out studies and research. In this perspective, most training seminars are multidisciplinary and include professionals working with children as well as front liners from NGOs delivering services to children.
- Participation of children: The participation of children is still very limited in addressing the issue of violence against them, whether in the design of the activities and programs or in their implementation and monitoring or even as regards expressing what they think about the issue, what it means to them and how it affects them.

Children have no idea of the legal measures or otherwise which target their protection from violence. In this regard, the child -friendly version of the UNSV has been the subject of consultations in some countries of the region (Jordan, Lebanon). In order to interview children and communicate legal procedures and social values, it is important to be aware that they can identify the following forms of violence:

- Physical and verbal violence by teachers.
- Lack of any school response regarding that violence.
- Laws prohibiting violence in school are not enforced.
- Poor students are more subject to violence.
- Children also propose solutions to problems concerning them:
- A system of accountability and punishment of teachers who practice violence.
- Training social workers and teachers to be able to address violence.
- Involvement of parents' councils in addressing the problem and suggesting solutions.
- Establishment of activity clubs (painting, music) in schools to divert violence into creative activities.
- Organization of media campaigns on the issue.

The regional endeavor focuses on the legal aspect of VAC, targeting a solid legal framework to be effectively used. The law of the child is considered a first and essential step in that direction and has been issued in Syria and Egypt; the process is ongoing in Lebanon, Jordan, KSA and other countries. Children can also collaborate in other legal procedures, such as the reporting and monitoring, evaluation and follow up; they can also contribute in lobbying and advocacy, in non-governmental organizations and local capacities, in cooperative tools and capacities of national and local committees. As an example of child empowerment, the first UNICEF Regional Awards for Media on Child Rights were handed out in Amman by the Queen. Special awards also went to two determined 16-year-olds from Jordan and the Palestinian territories that produced media projects without financial support from any governmental or private entity.

CONCLUSIONS

Addressing violence against children in the Middle East and North Africa region is the responsibility of the whole society including the state. The state bears an essential responsibility in that respect since it is the party that drafts policies, draws legislations that serve those policies, follows up their implementation, in addition to providing the necessary resources for the implementation of those programs, ensuring that they are not based on short term projects - scope and duration - but rather on a nationwide sustainable strategy. In this perspective, it is critical that the child victim of violence in all Arab programs and policies is not addressed as an object for charity or protection alone, but rather as a present non-voting citizen, entitled to all human rights and a life free of violence.

Recently, it is noticed that the issue of violence against children is not marginalized in a growing number of countries in Middle East and North Africa. Many of them have established councils and national organizations concerned with human rights in general or even with the human rights of children in particular. Violence against children is now addressed in a way that includes more socially sensitive areas, such as violence inflicted by parents on children in the context of the family, or early marriage or traditions and norms that lead to violent practices against children, like FGM and honor crimes. The theoretical model needs however implementation, evaluation and sustainability.

The right perspective in addressing any form of violence is an essential perspective and entry point to enable interventions and legal amendments to protect that right in the face of violations. This perspective also requires that children be an essential actor in the design of intervention policies, their evaluation, monitoring of implementation and their amendment or development leading to a sustainable protection of that right.

The Arab professionals gave birth to the APNPCAN, in 2004, and changed the name to APNPVAC in order to comply with the UNSV. Both ISPCAN and the arab network played an active role in the 2005 MENA regional UNSV consultation context, the 2006 ICRC critics in Geneva and the 2007 UNSV report and meeting in Cairo. The network contributed to widen the platform of interventions and deepen their efficiency in confronting violence against children, as this problem appears to be more and more accepted as the responsibility of the society as a whole. The inclusion of the informal sectors in the State prerogatives remains however a challenge in many countries. The emerging child protection movement is presently in a continuously growing, expanding, and hopefully inclusive and participative design. The result of this social congruence and intersectoral teamwork, led by professionals, with children with whom they work, will be a mixture of cultures, values, beliefs and challenges.

IMPLICATIONS AND FUTURE PERSPECTIVES

Arab countries live, now more than ever, with identity crises and armed conflicts. They are, however, challenged to plan systems, set priorities and provide a basis for political and social debate on the present and the future condition of children, with the participation of children. In this perspective, the APNPCAN/VAC can plan the following activities:

- Meet with children and youth, to discuss their opinions about CAN and VAC; the I-CAST [child] questionnaire developed by ISPCAN and supported by UNICEF is indeed a useful tool in such a task. The main objectives of those meetings are:
  - o to agree on definitions of VAC and CAN
  - o to enable more children to outreach the UNSV child version
  - o to reach a common understanding about the way to confront violence in child environments
  - o to exchange with children their outputs on the UNSV results and recommendations
  - o to develop procedures children find useful and productive for child effective participation and child protection,
  - o to include, in an effective process, child recommendations within national Arab strategies for child protection
- Lobby with parliamentarians and legislators, to:
  - o enhance already existing national and local movements towards child protection, while tackling specific needs and priorities
  - o stimulate legislative revision of laws, to comply with the provisions of the CRC and optional protocols
  - o increase local and national knowledge about the UNSV
  - o and contribute in finding appropriate procedures to initiate advocacy and sustainable child protection.
- Work with other professionals to:
  - o Increase common knowledge and develop training tools
  - o Upgrade the informal knowledge to a comprehensive curriculum
  - o Base their interventions on evidence of qualitative assessment and efficient actions
  - o Carry out comprehensive national surveys. It is essential that children participate in the survey
  - o Support research and study centers
  - o Develop mechanisms that enable violated children to make their complaints
  - o Provide psychological and physical rehabilitation services

- o Prepare periodic reports and meetings
- o Develop training programs for personnel working with children regarding best practices
- o Set up counseling centers that receive reports and complaints
- o Embody the reform of child protection by being candidates in city councils, parliaments and governments, in order to set up parliamentary committees, amend existing legislation (rights of the child, criminalization of violence and enforce the provisions of CRC)
- o Reduce gender discrimination

Countries in the Arab region are urged to launch CRC compliant and socially accepted - child protection systems that would be comprehensive melting pots of existing and developing programs. Success stories and reports on obstacles are most welcome, to improve MENA knowledge about the status of children, in a dynamic and proactive way. In this perspective it is important to note that there was an Arab League meeting in 2009 to amend Arab chapter on Child Rights.

In different – and sometimes conflicting - contexts of security and safety, the arab efforts to integrate children's rights within global human rights matrix - and child health and well-being requirements - need, in fact, strong social links and individual stands towards child protection acts. Child helplines, child defenders and child observatories are the pivots of knowledge base, data collection and training, rehabilitation and prevention, global child rights and local childhood requisites.

In each step, the APNPCAN/VAC can demonstrate the efficiency of professionals in promoting children's globally recognized rights within their liveplaces. Such initiatives work best when social stability, common vision, effective interaction between formal and informal sector, and child efficient participation...are available. Indeed, such initiatives towards child protection are most needed when those conditions are not yet available. Most challenging options are in most difficult - yet enriching - environments! Where the most vulnerable is not the slowest!

ACKNOWLEDGMENTS

Jamila Bia, Barbara Bonner, Howard Dubowitz, Majid Eissa, Adib Essali, Danya Glaser, Aida Gorbel, Hani Jahshan, Hassan Kassim, Abdelouadoud Kharbouch, Fadheela Mahroos, Marcellina Mian, Elie Mikhael, Maha Muneef, Kim Oates, Desmond Runyan and Randa Yousef.

In: International Aspects of Child Abuse and Neglect   ISBN: 978-1-60876-703-8
Editors: H. Dubowitz, J. Merrick pp. 87-96   © 2010 Nova Science Publishers, Inc.

Chapter 9

CHILD PROTECTION SYSTEMS IN TURKEY

Figen Sahin, MD and Ufuk Beyazova[*]

Department of Social Pediatrics, Gazi University Faculty of Medicine and
Gazi University Child Protection Center, Ankara, Turkey

The aim of this chapter is to discuss the current situation of child abuse and neglect in Turkey and to provide information about child protection system in this country. Definitions and extent of the problem of child abuse and neglect are given followed by information about the structure and functioning of the child protection system in Turkey. There are three main parts in this system: social services and child protection agency, medical and legal systems. By reporting how a sexual abuse case was managed, the authors discuss the mechanism of child protection system, and the gaps and problems within this system. In the final part of the article, preventive efforts of governmental and non-governmental organizations to combat child abuse and neglect in Turkey are mentioned.

INTRODUCTION

The concept of child abuse and neglect is gradually developing in Turkey. This development has led to more studies on the subject and increased sensitivity of the media to abused children, helping raise public awareness and influencing the definitions of abuse and neglect.

DEFINITIONS OF CHILD MALTREATMENT

Although there are universal definitions about child abuse and neglect, the perceptions of each society may differ regarding the acts considered as abuse. Corporal punishment, for example, may be acceptable in some populations as a way of disciplining a child. In Turkey,

---

[*] Correspondence: Figen Sahin, MD, Associate Professor of Pediatrics, Gazi University Faculty of Medicine, Department of Social Pediatrics, Besevler, Ankara, Turkey. E-mail: figens2001@yahoo.com or fsahin@gazi.edu.tr

although the cultural norms change with increasing educational level, the traditional approach to corporal punishment still exists in many regions. In a thesis entitled "Physical abuse and neglect of the child by the parents," conducted in 1995, the author surveyed 317 families from three different sociocultural levels. The results revealed that at three socioeconomic levels, children were beaten approximately once every week, mostly by their mothers, and that slapping was the most common form. In the lower sociocultural level beating, locking inside the house or throwing out of the house were more common (1).

A more recent study, which investigated views of "acceptable" disciplinary methods in a group of pediatricians and medical school students in Ankara, the capital, demonstrated that almost half thought that beating a child was acceptable (2). This traditional view also reveals itself in proverbs, such as "beating comes from heaven, if you don't beat your daughter, you beat your knees later on, (you feel regret), and, a rose blooms from the spot where the teacher slaps." In another study from Izmir, on the western coast and one of the most developed parts of Turkey, 15% of participants believed that the family had the right to severely beat a child for discipline - described as "beating that causes a physical mark or injury" (3).

In contrast to the tolerance of some milder forms of physical abuse such as corporal punishment, sexual abuse of a child is considered highly immoral. Love and affection are expressed by hugging, kissing and touching more commonly than in western societies, especially towards young children, but sexual forms of touch are clearly unacceptable. In fact, sexuality itself is taboo and not talked about within the family. Families don't usually educate their children about sexual subjects. Although boys are encouraged to engage in sexual relations, sexual intercourse for a girl and losing "one's virginity" before marriage, is considered as ruining the family honor; it may even be a reason for murder by shamed family members in some regions (4).

Legal definitions of child abuse and neglect exist in the Turkish Penal Code (5). Although no provisions specifically exist for physical child abuse, all articles about causing physical harm to individuals intentionally (article 86), torturing (article 94) and murdering (article 82) also apply to child abuse. For child sexual abuse on the other hand, there are special articles (articles 103-105). According to these, sexual behaviour towards a child younger than 15 years is subject to punishment, even if nobody files a complaint. For children between 15-18 years, the sexual act is considered a crime only if a complaint is filed but in this case if the perpetrator is 5 or more years older than the victim, the act is considered a crime anyway. If the perpetrator is a relative or somebody responsible for taking care of the victimized child, it is considered as aggravated assault and the penalty is increased by half.

Neglect is defined in the Turkish Penal Code as failure by parents to provide care, support or educational needs of the child, and is subject to punishment if reported. The Turkish Law of Education says that it is mandatory to send a child 6-14 years of age to school; 8 years of primary school education are compulsory. It is forbidden to make children under 15 years of age work. Children between 15-18 can work in "suitable" areas like food and textile industries, provided that they do not interrupt their education, and they still attend school. Hard and unsafe labor in which children between 15 and 18 should not work is defined by the Ministry of Labor and Social Security (5).

According to the Social Services and Child Protection Agency's definition, "a child in need of protection" is a child whose physical, spiritual and moral development or personal safety is endangered, and who does not have a mother/father or both, and information regarding his/her parents' whereabouts is unknown or has been abandoned by them, and who is neglected and abused (6).

EXTENT OF THE PROBLEM

Turkey is a one of the 20 most populous countries in the world with a population of around 70 million; almost one third are under 18 years. Family ties are generally very strong; even when the family lives as a nuclear family, grandparents often help take care of young children while parents work (7). Children are valued in both rural and urban areas. Families from less developed regions prefer to have more children (more help working in the fields) and they prefer boys (females are considered to belong to the husband's family once married). Children living in the villages and children of poor families are expected to work and contribute to the family budget from an early age (8).

Geographically the country is divided into 7 regions and social, economical and cultural differences exist among these regions. Therefore, it is difficult to obtain data about the frequency of child abuse. While there is no single study of the whole country, regional studies help understand the extent of the problem in Turkey.

For example, a retrospective adult study from Turkey reported childhood sexual abuse in 2.5%, physical abuse in 8.9%, emotional abuse in 8.9%, and neglect in 33.9% of the group (9). In other studies, childhood sexual abuse was reported to have 13.4% and 28% prevalence rates in two school-based populations (10,11) and physical abuse was found to have a 35% prevalence in a broad population-based study (12). Konanç et al (13) analysed 48,165 court cases in three cities in Turkey in 1985-86. They found that 701 cases (1.5%) were related to child abuse, 68.3% involved sexual abuse with almost half (46%) involving males. Fifty-five percent of sexual abuse victims were younger than 12 years and 1.4% were mentally retarded. Of all the sexual abuse cases, one-third were committed by adolescents. In only 14% of cases were the perpetrators the victims' parents. The authors speculated that incest cases are generally not referred to the courts (13).

A study was conducted in an Apprentice Education Center in a city in eastern Turkey. Of 476 apprentices (mean age 17 years), 82% stated that they had been exposed to violence at some time in their lives. Within the last year, 5.5% and 8.4% of the apprentices had been exposed to violence in the family and at work respectively (14).

Violence in schools is also a problem in Turkey. The Ministry of Education collected the studies on violence in schools and peer abuse in a book. They reported that 44%, 30% and 9% of high school students were exposed to emotional, physical and sexual abuse respectively, with a peak at 15-16 years of age (15).

Child labor is another problem. According to a 2006 survey on child labor, 22.3% of 6-17 year-old children work and 15.3% of them do not attend school (i.e., approximately 4% of Turkish children). Forty percent of working children are engaged in agriculture (16).

Children working or living on the street in a city on the Mediterranean coast of Turkey were investigated in a study which included 916 teenagers. It revealed that 64% of them had been exposed to physical or sexual abuse (17).

Most of the children working and/or living on the street in Turkey do have a family and return home at night. They are usually in poor families who have migrated to large cities from rural regions, and they usually have problematic family relations (8). They are often engaged in work that does not demand physical strength, such as shoe polishing, and selling bottled water, bagels, and paper tissues.

The situation of street children in Diyarbakir and Gaziantep was reported by a commission of the Turkish Parliament. This revealed that 96% and 54% of the mothers and fathers of these children respectively were illiterate. Ninety-four percent of the mothers and 58% of the fathers were unemployed, 73% of the families lived in a shanty, 78% of the families needed the children's income, and 42% said they would force their children to work even if they did not want to. Half of the parents also said that the child deserves to be beaten if he or she spends the money earned without permission of the parents (18).

INFRASTRUCTURE

Social Services and Child Protection Agency (SSCPA)

SSCPA is a nation-wide web with directorates in all 81 provinces of Turkey (6). It serves children and adults who need financial and/or social support and it coordinates adoption and foster care procedures. It is also the coordinating agency for implementation of the UN Convention on the Rights of the Child (CRC) in Turkey.

As the number of foster parents is very limited in Turkey, children in need of protection usually live in SSCPA institutions. Institutional care is designed separately for children 0-12 and 13-18 years. According to 2006 data, there are 220 residential institutions with almost 20,000 children and adolescents. They may remain there until age 20 years, if they attend high school and until 25 years, if in college. The government provides jobs for those children after they have completed their institutional care.

There are also 42 "youth institutions" serving street children, working on their rehabilitation. These institutions have an "open door" policy, allowing adolescents to decide whether to stay.

A disadvantage of large institutions is that they create a feeling of "not having a family." Therefore, another system of "home" institutions, has arisen recently. In these homes, 4-5 children live with caregivers, employees of Social Services. There are 810 such homes in eight provinces.

SSCPA provides institutional care for disabled children whose parents cannot or will not take care of their children. National and international adoptions are coordinated by SSCPA. Social workers make the necessary evaluations about the suitability of the applicant families. They also follow up on the children in foster care or who have been adopted.

Medical system

Medical services in Turkey consist of primary health care services which are outpatient clinics. For secondary and tertiary health care, there are state and university hospitals respectively. There is no single unit dealing with abused children and there is no specialty on this subject. Pediatricians, pediatric surgeons, forensic medicine doctors and child psychiatrists most commonly see abused and/or neglected children. Recently, multi-disciplinary teams have been being developed in the university and state hospitals of the big cities such as Ankara, Izmir, Istanbul, Kayseri and Adana. In 1998, one of the first teams was established in a state teaching hospital in Izmir (19,20). Two reports on child abuse cases in the two university hospitals in Ankara have been published. (21,22). Gazi University Hospital's child protection center, established in 2001, was the first officially recognized center (22).

Child abuse and neglect is a relatively new area for Turkish medicine. There is a need to educate primary care physicians and other health care personnel working with children to increase their knowledge and skills in detection, assessment, reporting, treatment, and prevention of child abuse and neglect (23,24). Recently, the Ministry of Health and Turkish Medical Association organized several courses on child abuse and neglect for practicing physicians, in collaboration with the Turkish Society for Prevention of Child Abuse and Neglect.

Reporting to legal authorities is mandatory for health care personnel when they see an abused child in the course of their professional practice (Penal Code article 280) (5). Filing a report to social services can also be done, but is not mandatory.

Legal system

a. Law enforcement is the first point of contact when an offense is committed or suspected against a child. They provide a nation-wide service. They have specialized units, "juvenile police," which deal with victimized children and children in conflict with the law. A total of 3,050 personnel, 1,700 of which are specially trained juvenile police officers serve throughout the country (25).

b. The Council of Forensic Medicine is the official organ of the Ministry of Justice which reports on forensic cases. Approximately 85,000 reports each year are written about technical and scientific subjects required by the courts and district attorneys (26). This institution also offers specialty training in forensic medicine.

c. Legal Framework: The main laws about child abuse in the Turkish legal system are the Turkish Civil Code, the Penal Code, the Criminal Procedure Code and the Code of Protection of Family. The Civil Code includes issues like protection orders for children, custody right, and compensation. The Code of Family Protection includes removing offenders from the home in domestic violence cases and measures like alimony. The Turkish Penal Code includes penalties for all offenses and has changed extensively in 2005 (see definitions). Articles concerning the protection of victimized children were included for the first time in the Turkish legal system: the victimized child will be provided an attorney - free of charge; the child's testimony will be obtained only once and will be videotaped; and, a professional, experienced in child interviews, such as a psychologist or social worker will be present while the child testifies (5).

d. Courts: There are three different types of courts in the Turkish legal system regarding children: juvenile court, family court and criminal court.

    i. Juvenile court is established for juvenile offenders (children <18 years) and for children in need of protection. In the law concerning juvenile courts, it is stated

   that if a child was younger than 12 years when he/she committed a crime, he/she
   is not criminally responsible, and protective and supportive measures can be
   ordered by the court. If a crime is committed when he/she was between 12-18
   years old, he/she can be held criminally responsible. Children can be sentenced
   to prison, or, supportive measures (counseling, education, care, health measures)
   and observation by probation officers.

ii. Family court deals with family issues (divorce, guardianship, custody, etc). The
     Turkish Civil Code Article 272 states that a judge can set aside a family's right
     to custody and issue a protection order for a child whose family does not provide
     adequate care, or abuses the right of custody by abusing the child physically,
     sexually, emotionally or economically (e.g., making him/her beg on the street). If
     the violation of the custody right is not serious, a court can limit the custody
     right while ordering services for the family (guidance, counselling, treatment).

iii. Criminal court is for adult perpetrators. There are 3 different types according to
     the severity of crime: Peace Criminal Court, Basic Criminal Court, High
     Criminal Court.

The legal system starts with law enforcement when a crime is thought to have been
committed against a child. This crime may be brought to attention by anyone who witnessed
the event, or by the health care personnel who found the medical evidence of an abuse, or, by
the victim. The law enforcement officer is responsible for reporting the case to the prosecuter.
Prosecuters interrogate suspects and decide whether to file a case, if there is enough evidence.
In this phase, he/she usually asks for a report from the Council of Forensic Medicine or from
other authorities that can file a forensic report (eg, forensic medicine specialists or the
recently established child protection centers in university or state hospitals) Depending on the
findings obtained from the first investigation, the prosecuter may decide not to file a suit. If
there is a decision to prosecute, the trial usually lasts long, sometimes for several years.
During this time, the accused may or may not be in custody.

CASE REPORT

A 14-year old girl was brought by her mother to the Child Protection Center (CPC) of Gazi
University together with her 4-year old brother. She related a history of sexual abuse by her
father since she was seven years old. She said she at first did not understand what her father
was doing. When she reached puberty, she realized that it was wrong and told her mother.
The mother who is an uneducated woman preferred not to tell anybody, thinking that it would
ruin her daughter's honor. She did not talk to her husband about this, because she was scared
of him. He could be violent, especially when he drank. She could not leave him, because she
did not have any income and did not know where to go. So, she tried to protect her daughter
at home, sleeping with her at night.

One night when she was sleeping with her daughter, her young son who was sleeping in a
bed with his father called her to the bathroom saying his anus hurt. She was horrified to see
that his anus was bleeding. The boy said he did not know what had happened. She took him
to the nearest primary health care center early in the morning. The general practitioner

working there said he might have been sexually abused, but did not file a report and said that they must go to the forensic medicine department of a hospital. As the mother did not have enough money for transportation and did not know how to go to the hospital, they returned home. Two weeks later a neighbor asked her why she was so sad and she shared the family's secret with her. She said she knew a CPC in a university hospital and helped her get there.

When they arrived at the CPC, both the 14-year old girl and her brother were interviewed by the social worker. The boy could not divulge what had happened to him, but his sister told clearly of her abuse, over years. She said her father abused her sexually, but to protect her virginity did not penetrate her vagina. Her genital examination was normal. Anal examination of the little boy was also normal. It was thought that during the two weeks since the last incident, evidence of trauma had healed. The report filed by the multidisciplinary team included a psychological evaluation of the girl. The comment of the physicians was: "Although no physical evidence was found, we concluded from her interview that the girl was sexually abused." A forensic report was filed and sent to the police.

The father was arrested and a trial has been continuing for two years. The Bar provided them with an attorney free of charge. The girl, the CPC pediatrician, and the general practitioner all testified. The mother applied for divorce. The Social Services gave financial support to the mother. The children received therapy in the CPC.

DISCUSSION

This is a typical case of sexual abuse in Turkey. It reflects the influence of society's values. The daughter's silence for so many years is very common, as elsewhere in the world. The cultural context, and the mother's lack of education, poverty and helplessness complicate the issue. She tried to hide the abuse, fearing it would harm her daughter's reputation. This is a very common response among families of sexually abused children. Even when they apply for medical help, they ask the physicians not to report (27). This case reveals the gaps in our child protection system, too. Physicians' knowledge of the legal and social management of these cases is limited; therefore, even if they suspect and diagnose abuse, they may fail to report to the police and/or social services (22). In this case, the general practitioner who should have filed a report thought that the forensic medicine doctors should do so, and sent the boy to such a unit. He did not follow up to ensure this occurred. The mother could not reach there, but later – somewhat by chance - she did reach a CPC. If she had not been able to do so, the abuse would probably have continued. Victims in Turkey usually enter the child protection system via medical facilities by seeking medical help; therefore, coordination of medical services with the legal and social systems is very important. If not, the child may have to tell his/her story more than once at each unit in which the child is seen, and physical examinations may be repeated.

Another option for the mother would have been to apply directly to a law enforcement agency. The police would have sent the file to a prosecuter, who would have asked for the opinion of the Council of Forensic Medicine. The caseload of the Council of Forensic Medicine is immense; cases are evaluated within minutes. Until recently, cases were usually evaluated based only on the physical findings, disregarding the psychosocial evidence. This approach is gradually changing. There was no physical finding in these two patients. Thus, if the prosecuter received such a report without the psychosocial evidence, he would probably not have filed a suit. During the process, the girl had to tell her story of abuse several times in different places, the hospital, police department, prosecuter's office and court. Since the amendments in the criminal code in 2005, it is required that the child testifies only once. During this interview, a specialist must be present and the interview must be videotaped.

Although the designated agency for mandatory reporting is the social services agency in many countries, in Turkey physicians must report child abuse to the police or prosecutor. The legal system approaches child abuse cases from the standpoint of evidence collection, not from the perspective of child protection. The Social Services Agency which is supposed to be the cornerstone of child protection has inadequate resources in Turkey. The foster care system is underdeveloped, so a court-ordered protection order mostly means sending a child to an institution, which is not ideal for child development. In this case, the mother could have had better support from the social services; only financial support was provided

Challenges in the legal system are mainly due to the huge caseloads. Court cases are protracted, lasting years. The offender may be imprisoned, but not rehabilitated, and may be a danger to society after release.

In spite of these challenges, the existence of a social service system, amendments to the legal system, and the establishment of hospital-based child protection teams are strengths of the child protection system in Turkey. The increasing awareness of the population about child abuse and neglect is also important.

PREVENTIVE EFFORTS

In addition to the government's efforts to eliminate poverty, to increase educational and occupational facilities, to decrease social and financial inequalities, numerous non-governmental organizations (NGO) contribute to education with reading and writing courses)especially for women), parenting classes, and building campaigns for schooling young girls. There are some NGO's which directly deal with children's rights and prevention of child abuse and neglect (28-30). They also collaborate in networks.

The SSCPA has 59 "Public Centers" in 31 of 81 provinces offering courses in vocational training, parenting programs and reading and writing classes, and 22 "Family Counseling Centers" in 21 provinces. SSCPA also has centers for preventive services for street children (6).

The Ministry of Labor and Social Security, a partner of the International Labor Organization (ILO) in the "International Program on the Elimination of Child Labor (IPEC), works to combat child labor (31).

The Ministry of Health has a wide web of services reaching even small villages. The health care personel working in primary health care centers follow up infants and children starting prenatally. They give anticipatory guidance (i.e., advice on anticipated child rearing issues, such as feeding and behavior) during these visits, and identify families at risk of abusing their children. There are treatment centers, affiliated with the Ministry of Health, for children with the problem of substance abuse (32).

The Ministry of National Education: The school guidance and counseling system is working well. There are counselors in many schools whose roles include "supporting students to help prevent them from having social, personal and academic problems." They identify and report children at risk as well (33). This Ministry also organizes parenting programs in their "Public Education Centers." There are projects conducted by this Ministry to prevent violence in schools.

UNICEF Turkey: Together with governmental and non-governmental partners, UNICEF is working with and for children and their families to ensure the effective implementation of social and economic policies to reduce poverty and inequality in Turkey by 2010. The main projects being carried out by UNICEF involve child survival, girls' education, adolescent development, effective parenting, child development and child protection (34).

In-service training programs are conducted in most of the sectors whose personnel work with children, such as law enforcement, lawyers, teachers and physicians. Child protection teams within university and state hospitals and other improvements in the system are promising for children's rights and protection in Turkey.

REFERENCES

[1]   Tercan M. Çocuklarin anne babalari tarafindan fiziksel istismari ve ihmali. [Physical abuse and neglect of the child by the parents.] Dissertation. Ankara: Ankara Univ, 1995.

[2]   Orhon FS, Ulukol B, Bingoler B, Gulnar SB. Attitudes of Turkish parents, pediatric residents, and medical students toward child disciplinary practices. Child Abuse Negl 2006;30:1081-92.

[3]   Zeytinoglu S, Kozcu S. A study of physical child abuse in Turkey. Paper presented at the first European Congress of Child Abuse and Neglect, Rhodes, Greece, 1987.

[4]   Tezcan M. Ulkemizde Aile içi tore ya da namus cinayetleri [Intrafamilial honor murders in our country] In: Honor Murders. Republic of Turkey, Prime Ministry Publications, Ankara., 1999.

[5]   Agir ve tehlikeli isler cizelgesi [Chart of hard and unsafe labor] Accessed 2008 August. URL: http://www.mevzuat.adalet.gov.tr/html/21902.html

[6]   Korunmaya muhtac cocuk [Child in need of protection] Accessed 2008 March. URL: http://www.shcek.gov.tr

[7]   Zeytinoglu S. Country context Turkey In: Mapping the number and characteristics of children under three in institutions across Europe at risk of harm. European Commission Daphne Programme. Copenhagen: WHO Regional Office Eur, 2005:96-102.

[8]   Zeytinoglu S. Türkiye'de sokakta çalisan ve/veya yasayan çocuklar. [Children working and/or living on street] In: Çalisan çocuklarin istismari ve ihmali [Abuse and neglect of working children], Izmir, Ege University press , 2001:151-86.

[9]   Akyuz G, Sar V, Kugu N, Dogan O. Reported childhood trauma, attempted suicide and self-mutilative behavior among women in the general population. Eur Psychiatry 2005;20:268-73.

[10]   Alikasifoglu M, Erginoz E, Ercan O, Albayrak-Kaymak D, Uysal O, Ilter O. Sexual abuse among female high school students in Istanbul, Turkey. Child Abuse Negl 2006;30:247-55.

[11]   Eskin M, Kaynak-Demir H, Demir S. Same-sex sexual orientation, childhood sexual abuse, and suicidal behavior in university students in Turkey. Arch Sex Behav 2005;34:185-95.

[12]   Bilir S, Ari M, Donmez NB. 4-12 yaslari arasinda 16000 cocukta orselenme durumlari ile ilgili inceleme. [A review about child abuse in 16000 children aged 4-12] Cocuk Gelisimi ve Egitimi Dergisi [Journal of Child Development and Education] 1986;1:7-14.

[13]   Konanc E, Zeytinoglu S, Kozcu S. Analysis of child abuse and neglect court cases in three cities in Turkey. In: Viano EC, ed. Critical issues in victimology. International perspectives. New York: Springer, 1987:101-9.

[14]   Deveci S.E, Acik Y, Oral R, Polat S.A. Elazig ciraklik egitim merkezi ogrencilerinin yasamlarinin herhangi bir doneminde fiziksel siddete maruz kalma durumlari ve siddete yaklasimlari [The status of

Elazig Apprentice Educational Center students to physical violence exposure in any time in their lives and their attitudes toward violence] Saglik ve Toplum [Health and Population], 2004;14:95-102.

[15]   Kiliç R. Okullarda siddetin onlenmesi ve azaltilmasi. [Prevention of violence in schools] In: Gelbal S, ed. Okullarda siddetin onlenmesi, mevcut uygulamalar ve sonuçlari [Prevention of violence in schools, current interventions and results], Ankara TED Press, 2007:25-48.

[16]   Child Labor. Accessed 2008 March. URL: http://www.tuik.gov.tr/prehaberbultenleri.do?id=482

[17]   Kurt AO, Bugdayci R, Sasmaz T, Oner S, Ugurhan F, Tezcan H. Mersin il merkezinde sokakta calisan ya da yasayan cocuklarda istismarin boyutlari ve etkileyen faktorler. [Extent of abuse for children working or living on streets in the city center of Mersin and affecting factors.] Saglik ve Toplum [Health and Population], 2005;15:41-8

[18]   Sokakta_Yasayan_Calisan_Cocuklar [Children living or working on the streets]. Accessed 2008 March. URL: http://www.shcek.gov.tr/ hizmetler/Sokakta_Yasayan_Calisan_Cocuklar/

[19]   Oral R, Can D, Hanci H, Miral S, Ersahin Y, Tepeli N, et al. A multicenter child maltreatment study: twenty-eight cases followed-up on a multidisciplinary basis. Turk J Pediatr 1998;40:515-23.

[20]   Oral R, Can D, Kaplan S, Polat S, Ates N, Cetin G, et al. Child abuse in Turkey: An experience in overcoming denial and a description of 50 cases. Child Abuse Negl 2001;25:279-90.

[21]   Cengel-Kültür E, Cuhadaroglu-Cetin F, Gökler B. Demographic and clinical features of child abuse and neglect cases. Turk J Pediatr 2007;49:256-62.

[22]   Sahin F, Kuruoglu AC, Demirel B, Akar T, Camurdan AD, Iseri E, et al. Six year experience of a hospital based child protection team in Turkey. Turk J Pediatr, in press.

[23]   Canbaz S, Turla A, Aker S, Peksen Y. Samsun merkez saglik ocaklarinda görev yapan pratisyen hekimlerin çocuk istismari ve ihmali konusunda bilgi ve tutumlari [Knowledge and attitude of general practitioners working in primary health-care centers in Samsun -city center about child abuse and neglect] Surekli Tip Egitimi Dergisi [Journal of Continuing Medical Education] 2005;14:241-6.

[24]   Tamer A, Sahin F, Ilhan MN, Camurdan AD, Yoney A. Ankara'daki hastanelerde cocuk istismari ve ihmali olgularina takim yaklasimi [Team approach to the child abuse and neglect cases in the hospitals of Ankara]. Surekli Tip Egitimi Dergisi [J Continuing Med Educ] 2008;17: 49-56.

[25]   Çocuk   polisi   [juvenile   police].   Accessed   2008   March.   URL: http:// www.emniyet.gov.tr/cocuk.polisi.asp

[26]   Adli   Tip   Kurumu   [Council   of   Forensic   Medicine].   Accessed   2008   March.   URL: www.atk.gov.tr/0english.swf

[27]   Sahin F, Beyazova U. Çocugun cinsel istismarinda adli bildirim: Hekimin ikilemi. [Reporting child sexual abuse: The dilemma of the physician] Adli Tip Dergisi [J Forensic Med] 2003;17:47-51.

[28]   Cocuk Istismarini ve Ihmalini Onleme Dernegi [Turkish Society for Prevention of Child Abuse and Neglect]. Accessed 2008 March. URL: http://www.tspcan.org

[29]   Uluslararasi Cocuk Merkezi [International Children's Center]. Accessed 2008 March. URL: http://www.icc.org.tr

[30]   Cocuk Haklari Ulusal Iletisim Agi [National Network on Child Rights]. Accessed 2008 March. URL: http://www.0-18.org

[31]   International Program on the Elimination of Child Labor (IPEC). Accessed 2008 March. URL:http:// ww.ilo.org/public/english/region/eurpro/ankara/programme/ipec/support.pdf

[32]   Treatment and education center for alcohol and substance dependency Accessed 2008 March. URL: http://www.amatem.gov.tr/index.htm

[33]   Turkish Ministry of Health, Directorate of school guidance and counseling Accessed 2008 March. URL: http://www.orgm.meb.gov.tr/Mevzuat/genelgeler/

[34]   UNICEF Turkey Accessed 2008 March. URL: http://www.unicef.org/turkey

In: International Aspects of Child Abuse and Neglect   ISBN: 978-1-60876-703-8
Editors: H. Dubowitz, J. Merrick pp. 97-110   © 2010 Nova Science Publishers, Inc.

Chapter 10

FROM PROTECTED OBJECT TO LAWFUL SUBJECT. PRACTICAL APPLICATIONS OF THE BELGIAN MODEL OF CHILD PROTECTION

Peter Adriaenssens[*]

University Hospital Gasthuisberg, Catholic University, Leuven, Belgium

Most European countries endorsed the United Nations Convention of the Rights of the Child at the end of the eighties, thus unmistakably influencing the evolution of national legislation. As a result, several European countries, including Belgium, reorganized their child protection system in the early 1990s. Until 1987, only the Department of Justice was authorized to respond to reports of physical and sexual violence towards children. After child protection was transferred to the communities, the role of the Justice Department was limited to juvenile judges and prosecutors who both can be informed after meeting all conditions of the subsidiary principle. Child protection services consist of two organizations focussed on voluntary aid: the Special Childcare and the Confidential Centres for Child Abuse and Neglect. The Confidential Centres fill a societal need by being a place of justice for children. The social debate that drew attention to the need for their existence can only have a positive effect on the rights of the individual. In this paper the process is described, epidemiology, presentation of a case and comparison of our system with other countries in Europe. The Confidential Centres have a broad view of child abuse, not limiting their work to children with visible or documentable harm. We aim to shift the focus to early indicators of family violence. Rather than being primarily concerned with what is punishable, we prioritize the assistance that can and must be offered to troubled families.

INTRODUCTION

Thirty years ago, an important part of the jurisdiction with regard to child protection and child abuse was withdrawn from the Belgian judicial system. Hence, the subsidiary principle

---
[*] *Correspondence:* Professor Peter Adriaenssens, Confidential Centre Vertrouwenscentrum Kindermishandeling, Justus Lipsiusstraat 71, 3000 Leuven, Belgium. E-mail: peter.adriaenssens@uzleuven.be

became a priority. This decision was based on the view that all children have the right to be treated respectfully in our society. The starting point for the authorities is the human equivalence, regardless of age, implying that human rights are applicable to children as well. This was the start of a new way of thinking about children. In the past, emphasis was put on protecting children "for their own sake." Nowadays, the input of children is highly appreciated in such a way that they increasingly become active partners in protecting their own rights. Children have evolved from protected objects into lawful subjects. This paper describes how this evolution has lead to the organisation of child protection to achieve its role from a more educational perspective. Mandatory reporting of child abuse and neglect does not exist. Instead, Confidential Centres are recognised as centres for child abuse, providing assessment and intervention, without informing the Department of Justice. We focus on the approach of these Centres, their strengths and weakness.

The relatively small Belgian population (10 million) may contribute to a high level of public agreement regarding serious threats to children's safety and integrity. This is manifested in the general approval of the Confidential Centres' model, which now exists for twenty years. On the other hand, there is an unmistakable protection from the European social model of which Belgium is part. This is a vision of society that combines sustainable economic growth with ever-improving living and working conditions. This involves full employment, safe and healthy jobs, equal opportunity, social protection for all, social inclusion, and involving citizens in the decisions that affect them. Belgian social security legislation minimizes the risks linked to certain socio-economic factors. Social security payments are provided either to those who have or had a professional activity (pensions, unemployment benefit, sickness and disability benefits, industrial accident, occupational diseases), and are extended to all the members of the family (family allowance, sickness insurance). The vaccination level is 98%, there is free medical care, primary school reaches 98% of children, poverty affects around 8%, unemployment is around 5%, only 2% of adults used drugs in the last 12 months, which is less than in several surrounding countries. This and several other social measures help protect our population in part from serious and prevalent family violence. When comparing models for child protection - prevention and intervention with child abuse in particular - it is very important to consider these contextual circumstances. In our opinion, the existence of different models to approach child abuse functions as a protection for children. The consequent discussions contribute to a continuous critical analysis of the quality of the clinical and judicial approach. The exchange of collaborators between countries with a different approach should be encouraged in order to stimulate this process.

Although the term child protection is an international concept, its practical interpretation is very diverse. Most European countries endorsed the United Nations Convention of the Rights of the Child at the end of the eighties, thus unmistakably influencing the evolution of national legislation. As a result, several European countries, including Belgium, reorganized their child protection system in the early 1990s (1).

At the same time, Belgium evolved into an efficient federal structure. Belgium has a federal government with important national responsibilities such as the Department of Justice. The population of 10 million persons consists of three communities, the Flemish (5.8 million), French (4 million) and German (80.000) speaking communities. Each community has a regional government with autonomy at different levels, such as child protection.

In 1991, the communities fundamentally reformed child protection. A key element of this rearrangement is the "subsidiary" principle, meaning that priority is always given to the intervention that most adequately meets the families' needs, that is most accessible to them, and that least compromises their liberty. The communities set up non-profit organizations with government grants to offer a variety of services in the best interests of children and parents. These services include nurseries, babysitters, education shops (where every parent can explain his/her educational problem concerning children (up to age 18 years) to an educational specialist), educational support, counselling, day care centres, family centres, evaluation centres, and treatment centres. Most of these services are free.

The national importance of the subsidiary principle explains the limited role of the justice system in the protection of minors in cases of child abuse, involving physical, emotional or sexual abuse and neglect within the family. This change in policy represents the intention to evolve from a punitive strategy to a supportive one, encouraging every individual to take responsibility at their level, and to encourage everyone to take initiative when there is any early signal that a child's health or development might be in danger. This resulted in the following policy developments (2):

- The government agrees that the priority for any care must be the rights of the child. The fulfilment of this task should be the prime concern in future development of health care sector and judicial procedures.
- Violence towards children is clearly divided into intra-familial and extra-familial.
- Intra-familial violence is best reported to a multidisciplinary team, called Confidential Centres in Flanders or SOS Child Teams in the French speaking region. The centres provide assessment and intervention without any obligation to report to the judicial authorities, except when the child's safety cannot be guaranteed.
- In the case of child victims of extra-familial offenders, the judicial authorities are brought in, and their investigation takes priority. The investigation includes only a forensic team, without clinicians.

WHAT ARE THE DEFINITIONS OF THE DIFFERENT TYPES OF CHILD ABUSE AND NEGLECT? THE JUDICIAL FRAMEWORK

Although it is not mandatory to report child abuse and neglect (CAN) to the Department of Justice, every citizen is free to do so. The definition of child abuse is laid down in criminal law. The criminal code primarily deals with the deliberate infliction of injury, such as punches and wounds, malnutrition and endangering health (3). Sexual abuse is covered under indecent assault and rape (4). Since 1989, rape has been regarded as "any act of sexual penetration of whatever nature and using whatever means, committed against a person who does not give his or her consent." Sexual penetration of a child under the age of fourteen is always regarded as rape, irrespective of whether coercion was involved.

While it is not mandatory to report child abuse, every citizen is obligated by civil law to provide help to a person in need. He/she can inform local police or any professional to seek help. For these professionals, including medical doctors, criminal law implies that, if their own efforts of voluntary help fail and the safety of a young person is clearly still in jeopardy, they should refer the family for specialist help, such as at a Confidential Centre or a department of child psychiatry, or, report this to the Justice Department if the child's life is threatened.

THE NON-JUDICIAL FRAMEWORK

The definition of child abuse used in child protection should first of all contribute to a growing alertness for any warning signal from children. The aim is to teach adults to think about child abuse as a possible contributor to many symptoms in children. Most victims show very general symptoms including learning problems, bed-wetting, biting or lying. Child abuse and neglect is any situation in which the child is the victim of physical, psychological or sexual violence, whether passively or actively. This broad definition invites all persons to contact professionals if any suspicion of child abuse is present.

WHAT IS KNOWN ABOUT THE EXTENT OF THE PROBLEM?

Child abuse data are being registered centrally only in Flanders. In 2006, 47.1 out of 10,000 minors were reported to the Confidential Centres (8,172). For 74.2% of them, the diagnosis was: 41.1% physical abuse, 32.8% sexual abuse, 26.7% emotional and physical neglect and for 0.4% Munchausen by Proxy. Thirteen percent were evaluated as being "risk situations." The situation remained unclear in 5.7% and the problem was related to recovery of previous abuse in 2.1% of cases. Finally, in 4.4% of reports, no child abuse was found (5). In the same time period, 6,321 youngsters were reported to the Department of Justice for the whole country (Flanders and Wallonia)(5). In the Flemish Confidential Centres, 40% of reports originated from the child's extended family, and 20% were reported by schools (6). A further 20% of the reports originated in the healthcare sector. The fear that this model would encourage fake reporting seems to be groundless. Manipulation and abuse of the report is shown only in 4% of the files.

THE INFRASTRUCTURE TO ADDRESS CAN

Until 1987, only the Department of Justice was authorized to respond to reports of physical and sexual violence towards children. After child protection was transferred to the communities, the role of the Justice Department was limited to juvenile judges and prosecutors who both can be informed after meeting all conditions of the subsidiary principle. This means that all possible efforts have been undertaken to make parents accept the voluntary help, but they did not work or did not adequately protect the child (7). The first question when child abuse is reported is whether the alleged perpetrators are family members or not. For extra-familial perpetrators, only the Justice Department is responsible. The reports, including from the Confidential Centres, are referred to them. For intra-familial violence, the subsidiary principle guides the approach; voluntary help is most important. The role of the Justice Department is restricted, only becoming involved after exhaustive efforts of the

Confidential Centres (physical and sexual abuse) and Special Childcare (neglect and education failure) (1).

CHILD PROTECTION SERVICES

Child protection services consist of two organizations focussed on voluntary aid: the Special Childcare and the Confidential Centres for Child Abuse and Neglect. They work independently.

Special child care

Most concerns regarding youngsters and families in need are handled by this organization, which is led by a committee of representatives of the community who are informed by social workers/counsellors, and especially deals with reports of neglect and high risk families with serious psychosocial difficulties. In consultation with parents, Special Childcare evaluates the parents' demand for help. The subsidiary principle is followed here as the family's own demand has the highest acceptance rate. The offer consists of many free services such as home counseling, day and night nurseries, and mental health consultation. These services use risk taxation instruments and treatment protocols to evaluate and adjust their assessments. When parents refuse voluntary care and when the child protection service considers the situation as harmful to the child, the course of events depends upon the specific region in Belgium. In the French-speaking community, the file can be forwarded to a juvenile prosecutor. In Flanders, additional efforts are required to make voluntary assistance successful by submitting the file to a mediation commission. This commission, active in every judicial district since 1991, focuses on parents and children as well as other caretakers familiar with the situation. The mediation commission is flexible in working with families. For example, evening meetings are very common. When an agreement is reached, work is coordinated by the Special Childcare on a voluntary basis. If no agreement is reached with the parents and if the commission confirms the dangerous situation of the minor, the commission transfers the file to a juvenile judge.

The Confidential Centres for child abuse and neglect

The government also developed special teams to receive child abuse reports, assess concerns, and to offer assistance when needed. The teams were modelled after the Dutch Confidential Doctor Centres, founded in 1972. The confidential doctor is entrusted with confidential information about abuse or neglect. This information can be given without risk of prosecution, for violation of professional confidentiality or for avoiding reporting to them. Experimental teams were founded in Flanders and French-speaking Belgium. These teams agreed that the duty to report child abuse to the Justice Department led to avoidance of child abuse recognition and belated notifications by professionals. The judicial inquiry encouraged parents to deny and avoid problems rather than face them and accept assistance. Parents did not learn to change their parenting behaviour. The Confidential Centres worked in a discordant context between the judicial authorities and the communities. This situation ended in 1987, when the roles of Confidential Centres were regulated by law. The Regional Executive stipulates that the Centres are specialised in the following tasks:

- provision of expert support to professionals confronted with child abuse in their work environment, and assistance to families and others involved
- assessment, coordination, intervention and, if necessary, psychotherapy for families and other persons involved in a case
- Raising awareness of health care providers, teachers and the general public regarding child abuse and neglect, in order to optimise detection.

The legislation also requires the Centres to be multidisciplinary (the cooperation of a medical doctor, a psychologist and a social worker form the minimum requirement) and to be accessible day and night (8). Each province has its own centre, providing free services.

A simple concern can be sufficient for reporting. The help procedure is started as soon as possible, followed by an assessment. The initial help can then be adjusted progressively after the assessment. This order of sequences is a specific characteristic of these Centres. Thee team's tasks include a number of initial phases in the therapeutic process: assessment, confrontation, conclusion, motivation for therapy, and the transfer to an external child welfare or mental health service. If there are no referral options, the centre may offer psychotherapy.

This model has been similarly developed by the six Confidential Centres in Flanders and their counterpart in the French-speaking part of the country, the SOS Child Teams. In the Netherlands, where the concept of Confidential Centres was first developed, there have been changes. The original Confidential Doctors are now integrated into the Advice and Reporting Centres for Child Abuse. In these Centres, reports are received and orientated to social, therapeutic or judicial authorities, depending on the content. Unlike the Flemish Confidential Centres, these Centres do not provide treatment. The aspect of confidentiality remains important in encouraging citizens to report their concerns at an early stage. In Belgium as well as in the Netherlands, there is no obligation to report child abuse to the Justice Department, but Confidential Centres employees must take responsibility for children's safety based on the principle of shared vulnerability. It is a legal obligation to help a person in need, implying that the employees are responsible by criminal law for not reporting to Justice when they know a child's life is threatened and they do not adequately protect the child. In 2007, the death of two children in Flanders was considered by the government as a consequence of child abuse. Therefore, the evaluation of possible danger seems to be clearly established.

THE JUDICIAL COMPONENT

Belgium is divided into judicial districts, where child abuse can be reported to a prosecutor, who can bring the case before a juvenile judge. This latter decides which intervention is the least intrusive, will try to mediate, and can enforce a decision if necessary. On the one hand, social services will report to the judge. On the other hand, the judge will meet with the youngster, the parents and, if applicable, the previously involved caretakers. From the age of 12 years, every child has the right to be heard by the juvenile judge and get advice from his or her own lawyer. A juvenile judge can remove the youngster from the parents' environment and put him/her into protective care if his/her physical or psychological integrity is in immediate and serious danger. The judge's decision has to be reviewed at least yearly and has to be confirmed or finalized on the basis of follow-up information from social services. During the conclusion, a child and family can be referred to voluntary Special Childcare.

HOW DOES THE SYSTEM WORK REGARDING REPORTING OF POSSIBLE CAN?

Unlike in many countries, in Belgium it is not mandatory to report child abuse to the judicial authorities, except in cases where protection is not possible. In the first place, child abuse is considered to be a health and welfare problem for the child and family. Only if initial responses fail, does legal intervention become necessary. This vision is translated by the call to the public to report any suspicion of child abuse. Every parent that reports a problem from his or her own family or agrees to cooperate with the Confidential Centre when abuse is suspected will get help, and will not be reported to the judicial authorities. If a report proves to be malicious (e.g. in divorce matters), both parents are informed about this decision. Different media convey the message that at least 10% of children are confronted with child abuse, that this problem is a fact in our society. We should not be ashamed to seek help for this problem, but, we are responsible if no help is sought. In this framework, parents are invited to acknowledge that child abuse took place in the family.

What does this mean in practice? Suppose a fifteen-month old baby is admitted to hospital, showing clear injuries indicative of Shaken Infant Syndrome. He has bleeding around the brain and in the retinas. During the conversation with the medical doctor, the mother describes severe tension recently between the couple, and that she was beaten by her husband on several occasions. Over the past 48 hours, this happened twice while she was holding the baby. The second time the baby fell from her arms and bumped into a closet. The baby cried, but could not be soothed. Father was in a panic, and shook him to quiet him. The father acknowledges the problem. The parents regret that these events occurred and wish for their child to receive the best possible care. They are willing to enter a counselling programme.

In these circumstances, there is no need to report the incident to the judicial authorities. The events have been clearly identified as signs of child abuse. The parents responded well to this by acknowledging the events and by immediately coming forward with a story that is consistent with the child's injuries. The parents immediately sought appropriate care for the child. They agreed to leave their child in the hospital until he had fully recovered and until counselling had been initiated. And finally, the aim of counselling the parents was to better understand the history and risk factors that contributed to this violence. The primary conditions of lawmakers have been met: assistance is rendered to a child in distress, safety is guaranteed because the child is hospitalised, the child has been admitted, and there is the prospect of working together with the parents. What if the child is ready for discharge in a few days? Anger management may have just begun, and there's the risk of dad losing his cool again? Naturally, promises to behave better are a good start, but just a start. If the child goes home soon, the father is asked to temporarily stay elsewhere in order to ensure the child's safety. In this case, the advantage for the child is to be home soon with the safe parent. If the father refuses, the child can stay with a foster family for a short period or can go to crisis centre for children. In some cases, the father is allowed to stay at home on the condition of home counseling. In other situations, the mother prefers to leave her husband so she can go on with the baby. In that case, a child guidance clinic is called in. The core principle remains achieving maximum cooperation between the parents, the child and the available social services. By exploring diverse forms of help, the agreements are more faithfully followed.

There are alternative scenarios. The same child could have been admitted by the parents, with the story that they found the child in this condition in bed. They add that the child went quietly to sleep the night before, that they awoke in the middle of the night because the child was groaning in bed, that they found the child convulsing, and that they rushed him to the hospital. The parents are faced with the findings that the injuries sustained by their child point to Shaken Infant Syndrome. The parents are outraged; they say that nothing ever happened in their home, and that the baby has not been with any other adult in the past 48 hours. The physical findings are sufficient for the neuropediatrician to give a guideline: as the parents do not want to answer questions about their functioning as a family and couple and want to avoid the possibility of child abuse from the investigation, we inform them that we will notify the judicial authorities. We are unable to protect the child, as we do not know who he should be protected from.

A "TYPICAL" RESPONSE BY THE RESPONSIBLE AGENCY(IES)

A professional making a report to a Confidential Centre admits he is powerless to provide safety and recovery for a child in need. This is an act of courage. "Reporting to a Confidential Centre is not betrayal: it is a request for help." With this pithy saying, Pieterse (8) clearly sums up how the Confidential Centres should approach the process of reporting. Obviously, "Who reported me?" is the first reaction of most parents, because they experience this as a betrayal. It is up to the team of the Confidential Centre to change this reaction into: "Whoever calls our Centre does not want to harm you, because this person knows we are not a judicial service. Help is recommended and together with you, we want to evaluate the concern, together with you, as well as what the next steps should be."

FROM SUSPICION TO CARE

A mere suspicion is sufficient to launch the process. It provides a Confidential Centre with an opportunity to talk to the child or young person and his or her parents. We clearly explain the concerns. We explain why we want to help. Consequently, we explain how the child's problem may be due to child abuse. The assessment by the Confidential Centre should clarify the situation. We use a protocol that consists of three parts: 1) the genogram of the family (to investigate boundaries, feedback mechanisms, hierarchies, coalitions, and transgenerational processes); 2) The Child Abuse Observation Chart (to collect all observations and findings regarding behaviour, emotion, physical examination and body language, play/drawings/narrative information) and 3) The Resilience Chart (to focus on competence and resources of individuals, the family system and the context). The Centre is responsible for setting standards: "your child is being sexually abused, this cannot be permitted." Reference is made to a child's unjust situation and the abuse of power. Once this aspect has been investigated, the Centre can begin to look into the parents' history and the elements causing this type of behaviour. It is important to avoid a one-sided portrayal of the case: either by treating one or both of the parents as criminals, or, by minimising the offence in view of the parents' history. A quarter of the cases are reported to the judicial authorities if cooperation with the family is impossible and/or if the child's safety cannot be guaranteed (9).

CONFRONTATION

Confrontation is a key feature in the work of Confidential Centres (8,10). In the first place, referral is made to the mandate the Centre has been given by the Parliament, included in Belgian law, to examine suspicions of child abuse and to offer help to families. The second reference is to the United Nations Convention on the Rights of the Child (UNCRC). The third is the knowledge about the impact of physical and sexual abuse on children's development. Together they justify the emphatic, supportive and confrontational style. In contrast to what occurs in many countries after an extensive assessment, we have a meeting with parents very early, based on first impressions. We confront parents with our hypothesis, even though we have limited data to support this hypothesis at that time, and we invite them to become our partners. This is the opportunity for them to be real parents, by helping us telling their story of the facts. The most valuable information we may obtain is a parent telling us "that he/she is beating his/her child for years, but that this is the first time it resulted in fractures, but the child is to blame as he resisted." Although every testimony is likely to be only a part of the truth, the breakthrough is that the secret of family violence is broken by the parents. From this moment on, discussions can take place and specific enquiries of which parents and children knowing the final aim, can start. Breaking this cycle of violence and secrecy is the ultimate goal, giving us a better and faster insight into the violence within this family, the chronicity of the problems, and co-morbidity. For the offender, it is important to acknowledge the facts very clearly and unambiguously. This needs to be named within the family. The way the family deals with this is evaluated by the team. Once physical or sexual abuse are named and acknowledged, therapeutic work with the youngster, the offender and other members of the family can begin. When abuse has occurred, the offender must present himself to a special team for offender counselling. At the Confidential Centre, the victim and the non-abusive parent are mostly involved in systemic family therapy, with or without cognitive behavioural therapy (CBT) or Parent-Child Interaction therapy (PCIT).

A CASE STORY

Jirka is 21 years old and calls the Confidential Centre. Her 14-year old sister told her that her father touches her genitals. The Confidential Centre requests that Jirka visit the Centre. She only wants to do so if her anonymity is guaranteed; the Centre agrees. We give her a false name under which she can register.

Jirka visits the Confidential Centre and talks about her family. It consists of four children, Jirka being the eldest. Her younger sister Laura told her "strange things happened" with their father. Jirka is not surprised; she was also sexually abused by her father. If confidentiality is assured, she is willing to come to the Centre with her sister. We contact the girl's school, so she can come during school time. Both sisters come together. Laura is very quiet. She says she doesn't want her father to leave their home, and that she does not want to leave either. She tells that she fainted a few times at school. Once she was taken to hospital, but the examination was normal and her parents took her home.

We suggest to Laura that she be admitted to hospital, to ensure her safety and take her into our care. She agrees, she says "I cannot take it any longer, what my father is doing!" We explain to her that hospital admission means that her parents will be invited to the Confidential Centre. Laura agrees.

A few days later, the school doctor admits Laura into the hospital, as planned. For social control, Laura's room is in front of the nurses' station. An employee of the Confidential Centre calls the mother and invites her to come to the Centre together with her husband. During this conversation they are told that Laura was admitted to hospital, because of her fainting, that the physical examination was normal, but that the multidisciplinary evaluation was worrying from another point of view: there are symptoms and signals that sexual abuse is involved. The functioning of the Confidential Centre is explained to the parents and they are told that the majority of offenders are family members. The father remains very calm and clearly indicates that he has had nothing to do with it; the reaction of the mother is less clear. She says the facts are not known to her, she has no clue about what is going on. The couple is split up and they talk separately with a staff member. The father keeps denying abuse, while admitting "trivial touches", he accidentally touched his daughter's breast, that he likes to tickle and that she probably confuses this with touching her genitals. It is explained to him that the examples he is giving point in the right direction, that he clearly understands that we are talking about sexual abuse, but that the facts we are talking about are much more serious. We ask the father to consider this and to come again for discussion the next day and to agree that Laura stays in hospital on a voluntary basis.

When talking to the mother, she is asked to carefully think about her daughter's development over the last few years as well as about the other children in the family. Mother will also come back the next day. Both parents agree that Laura can stay in the hospital on a voluntary basis and that it is up to her to decide whether she wants her mother to visit her.

The next day, the second daughter of the family, 20 years of age, calls for an appointment. She visits the hospital that same day and explains that the Centre has got the whole thing wrong. The father is a good family man and nothing suspicious is going on. She is listened to very carefully and it is explained to her by the team-workers that there are serious reasons for concern, because symptoms of the impact of sexual abuse are present, such as post-traumatic stress disorder (PTSD) and trauma related psychosomatic complaints. Does she think Laura should be told that her sisters are convinced that she is safe? Gradually, the sister starts to hesitate, she tells small fragments of the things she seems to recognize, and finally confirms that Laura also told her about the abuse.

Through subsequent conversations, the parents get to know the true story. Father says he had to learn not to think about painful or difficult things in life and that we don't have to ask him what had happened. We try to understand where this proposition comes from. When he was 12 years old, he was raped by his father; he talked about this to a teacher, who told him to forget it and to look forward in life. Father tells what happened with his two daughters, but minimizes the impact of it. Mother did not believe the story of her daughters until hearing confirmation by her husband. She reacted numbly, and stated that she wanted to stay with her husband; she did not want to be alone, because that would drive her crazy. This is what she was taught by her mother. She tells that she grew up without a father, her parents split up, when she was very young. Throughout her childhood she heard the bitter stories of her mother, about the absent father. Eventually psychiatric symptoms became evident and her mother had to be hospitalized. As a child she was put into foster care, where she was abused by a cousin of that family, somebody her own age. Losing her husband would be losing a father figure for the second time. She says: "One can only be a good mother when there is a father at one's side."

The Confidential Centre develops a treatment contract. Father has to leave the house immediately, until the Centre says he can move back in. He is referred to the Centre for Sex Offender Management. They perform their own assessment, and decide independently whether this perpetrator is eligible for offender therapy or whether they consider him to be too dangerous and think treatment under judicial auspices is appropriate. In the latter case, the Confidential Centre refers the perpetrator to the Department of Justice. Mother and daughters receive individual and family therapy at the Confidential Centre. Laura will only return home, when we are sure the contract is signed and executed. The contract also states that in case of violation of one of the agreements or threats to Laura's safety, the file will be transferred to the Justice Department (12).

THE STRENGTHS IN THE BELGIAN APPROACH/SYSTEM

Models approaching child abuse seem to move on a continuum between control and voluntariness. The control model is expressed by interventions that are strictly regulated by the government, stating what should be reported. In duty-to-report models, the legislator decides what is in the child's best interest. The other extreme are models based on voluntariness - as existed 40 years ago. Doctors and other professionals had to decide to the best of their ability what needed to be done. It seems to be a 'laissez-faire' approach where parents are supposed to know what is best for them. The strength of the Confidential Centre Model is that it seeks to integrate both extremes and find a reasonable middle ground. On the one hand, a child in distress needs protection, requiring elements of control. At the same time, we want to acknowledge and respect the parents' and children's expertise about the possibilities within their family. This allows them to help find realistic solutions including shelter at friends, possible therapy, and people they can trust to ensure their safety. The model introduces a system of "positive sanctioning" that, on one hand, encourages everybody to cooperate and, on the other clearly aims to end the abuse. In this model, "controlled voluntariness" is the key element.

An argument favouring a decriminalizing approach to child abuse and neglect is its high prevalence. If at least 1 out of 10 children is maltreated, a breakthrough will not obtained by judicial interventions based on sufficient evidence. Rather, there is need to change the style of parenting, primarily a task of welfare and mental health care. Secondly, in most cases of sexual abuse there is little or no physical evidence. We will not rely exclusively on children's testimony, but on all the systematically collected observational data. Finally, recovery from traumatic experiences is rooted in the respect of the victim's perception, the recognition of his feelings, and the opportunity to work at it together. We encourage this recognition as it contributes to the child's recovery and safety.

The effectiveness of the approach by the Confidential Centres is indicated by the increased self-reports over the past 20 years, from 7% of all reports in 1987 to 46% in 2006. The number of unjustified reports remained stable around 4.4% (5,6). Throughout the years, the model has been supported by broad public opinion. In the 1990s, the relationship with the Justice Department evolved from distrust to mutual respect. Both parties realized that the phenomenon of family violence is so prevalent that no organization can handle it alone. The number of reports of physical and sexual abuse to the Justice Department did not change over the last ten years (5). Over the past 20 years, none of the Confidential Centres has been found guilty of malpractice, suggesting a high level of professional competence.

WEAKNESSES/CHALLENGES IN THE BELGIAN APPROACH/SYSTEM

The improved relationship between the Confidential Centres and the Justice Department is reflected in the number of shared cases. The number of youngsters reported by the Centres to the Justice Department increased from 5% (1990) to 25% currently (10). There is increased conviction that child abuse assistance should always start at the level of the child and that all partners should integrate their knowledge to achieve an optimal approach.

In the current model, the family is interviewed several times by staff of the Confidential Centre before it may be concluded that some families do not want to cooperate, or, that an offender is dangerous to society. A report to the Justice Department may complicate the independence of the judicial inquiry. Often a child does not want to repeat to a police officer what she or he has already told at a Confidential Centre, stating "they should ask the Centre." Then the forensic interview may be stuck. The model of the Confidential Centre works well among families that accept voluntary help, but it can cause problems in others.

The surveillance of child abuse and neglect is weak in Belgium, because of the lack of uniformity within different communities. Even within Flanders, no uniform system exists. For example, Special Childcare, Confidential Centres and the Justice Department use separate registries. If it is difficult to maintain a uniform registration system within one country, it makes it especially difficult to compare the approaches of different countries. We think that more effort is needed at the international level is develop a uniform approach to surveillance.

CONTROVERSIES IN OUR APPROACH/SYSTEM

In order to study juvenile protection in a country, it is not sufficient to describe its organization and to listen to the practice. Descriptions of interventions are generally similar, while differing in practice (10). Most describe assessment and intervention including trauma therapy. But, when visiting teams in different countries, it seems that the specific methods vary greatly. For some, the assessment procedure is emphasized and is required to get to the helping stage. In our model help starts as soon a child tells something and diagnostics are built throughout the contacts. In some countries, the confrontational conversations we perform are only conducted during forensic interviews. We have come to conclude that parents often expressing a paranoid attitude towards adults are supported by a clear conversation and hypothesizing child abuse without an aggressive tone. There they see what a good parent should be like: strong, clear, but just and open-minded in order to find solutions together.

The decision to remove a child from a family depends upon the way a child's interest is regarded, and, how the balance between voluntary assistance and mandatory steps is required by law (8). The manner that juvenile protection is applied in a community can be considered the result of a dynamic interaction among the ways roles and responsibilities are authorized, the ways social care and justice are organized, and the cultural features of the population. If professionals are trained to always report to a justice department, a generation is fostered with a 'logic' that might no longer be questioned. This is the same in our country. The 'logic of reporting to a Confidential Centre' is leading to assumptions and complacency that can impede improving the model. The has resulted in the interest existing in our Centre in Leuven for models in the USA and UK. By observing the clinical practice of child abuse in Child Advocacy Centres and reviewing the vast research in these countries, we come to the conclusion that a mutual approach by professionals as well as justice can be very supportive for certain children, acknowledging their victimization. We want to learn from this, and we are currently investigating how to implement this approach in our practice. Therefore we should not regret the ongoing discussions on the different approaches of child abuse. It is important to understand a country's culture(s) to understand the possibilities and the limitations of different approaches (12). It inspires us and encourages ongoing questioning of our approach. This should be the mission of all child abuse teams: children are subjected to the way help is organized, hence we our obliged to be questioned by others, colleagues as well as justice and victim groups.

CONCLUSIONS

The Confidential Centres fill a societal need by being a place of justice for children. The social debate that drew attention to the need for their existence can only have a positive effect on the rights of the individual. The Confidential Centres have a broad view of child abuse, not limiting their work to children with visible or documentable harm. We aim to shift the focus to early indicators of family violence. Rather than being primarily concerned with what is punishable, we prioritize the assistance that can and must be offered to troubled families.

ACKNOWLEDGMENTS

This paper includes the cumulated inputs and suggestions of my colleagues at the Leuven Confidential Centre. They are all acknowledged for their feedback and constructive criticism.

REFERENCES

[1]   Ang F, Berghmans E, Cattrijsse L. Participation rights of children. Mortsel: Intersentia, 2006:82-93.

[2]   Cappelaere G, Adriaenssens P. National Commission against sexual exploitation of children. Brussels: Fgov, 1998:22-62.

[3]   Belgian Code of Criminal Law. Article 398, Article 401bis. Brussels: Belgisch Strafwetboek, 2006:Titel VIII Afdeling II.

[4]   Belgian Code of Criminal Law. Article 372. Brussels: Belgisch Strafwetboek, 2006:Titel VIII Afdeling II.

[5]   Kenniscentrum Statistiek Vlaanderen. Annual reports, www.flanders.be, 2007.

[6]   Kind and Gezin. Annual reports, http://www.kindengezin.be/KG/English_pages/, 2007.

[7]   Put J. The Juvenile Justice System in Belgium. In: Giostra G, Patané V, eds. European Juvenile Justice Systems. Milano: Giuffrè Editore, 2007:3-37.

[8]   Adriaenssens P, Smeyers L, Ivens C, Vanbekkevoort B. In vertrouwen genomen. (The Leuven approach of child abuse & neglect). Tielt: Lannoo, 2000:82-90.

[9]   Adriaenssens P. Vertrouwenscentrum Kindermishandeling Leuven Annual Report. Leuven : UZLeuven, 2006:3-6.

[10]   Grevot A. Voyage en protection de l'enfance. Vaucresson: CNFE-PJJ, 2001:111-23.

[11]   Smeyers L, Ivens C. La protection de la jeunesse en Belgique. In : Grevot A. Voyage en protection de l'enfance. Vaucresson : CNFE-PJJ, 2001:118-20.

[12]   Gilbert N. Combating child abuse: International perspectives and trends. New York: Oxford Univ Press, 1997:168-70.

In: International Aspects of Child Abuse and Neglect
Editors: H. Dubowitz, J. Merrick pp. 111-121

ISBN: 978-1-60876-703-8
© 2010 Nova Science Publishers, Inc.

Chapter 11

PROTECTING CHILDREN FROM ABUSE AND NEGLECT IN ENGLAND

Jenny Gray, Dip Social Work

Department for Children, Schools and Families, Safeguarding Children Policy Unit,
Sanctuary Buildings, London, England

The aim of this chapter is to describe the system for protecting children from abuse and neglect in England. The government sets the statutory framework through legislation, regulations and guidance. Organisations and people have a statutory responsibility to implement these at a local level, and for ensuring that staff access continuing professional development. The framework has been judged to be sound but there are ongoing challenges to ensure that the quality of practice is consistently high across the country. At the time of writing the government had commissioned a review of the child protection system which was intended to inform future developments in both policy and practice.

INTRODUCTION

The current statutory system for protecting children from child abuse and neglect has been evolving in England for over half a century (1). It continues to be underpinned by legislation, regulations and detailed statutory guidance. The principle of effective multi-agency, multi-disciplinary working to ensure that children are safe, their developmental needs are met and families are supported wherever possible to bring up their children is embedded in both the legislation and associated guidance. The United Nations Convention on the Rights of the Child was enshrined in the Children Act 1989 (2). This Act places a general duty on local authorities to safeguard and promote the welfare of children in their area. Descriptions of different types of child abuse and neglect are set out in the government's statutory guidance, Working Together to Safeguard Children (3). This guidance also describes how agencies and professionals should work together at a local level to safeguard and promote the welfare of children. In England, the legislative framework for protecting children has been found to be sound (4): the challenge is to implement it in ways which ensure that all children are safe and achieving their optimal outcomes.

DESCRIPTION OF CHILD ABUSE AND NEGLECT

In England, all professionals work to the same descriptions of abuse or neglect which are set out in government guidance. These relate to the State's responsibility to intervene, where necessary, to safeguard and promote the welfare of children. The descriptions are revised from time to time when the guidance is updated. Four types of abuse are described in the Government's statutory guidance Working Together to Safeguard Children (3) (paragraphs 1.30 – 1.33). These are as follows:

Physical abuse

Physical abuse may involve hitting, shaking, throwing, poisoning, burning or scalding, drowning, suffocating or otherwise causing physical harm to a child. Physical harm may be also caused when a parent or carer fabricates the symptoms of or deliberately induces illness in a child.

Emotional abuse

Emotional abuse is the persistent emotional maltreatment of a child such as to cause severe and persistent adverse effects on a child's emotional development. It may involve conveying to children that they are worthless or unloved, inadequate or valued only insofar as they meet the needs of another person. It may feature age or developmentally inappropriate expectations being imposed on children.

Sexual abuse

Sexual abuse involves forcing or enticing a child or young person to take part in sexual activities, including prostitution, whether or not the child is aware of what is happening. The activities may involve physical contact, including penetrative (for example rape, buggery or oral sex) or non-penetrative acts. They may include non-contact activities, such as involving children in looking at, or in the production of, sexual on-line images, watching sexual activities, or encouraging children to behave in sexually inappropriate ways.

Neglect

Neglect is the persistent failure to meet a child's basic physical and/or psychological needs, likely to result in the serious impairment of a child's health or development. Neglect may occur during pregnancy as a result of maternal substance abuse.

THE INCIDENCE AND PREVALENCE OF CHILD ABUSE AND NEGLECT

The Government publishes annual statistics on the number of children about whom people have concerns that they may be suffering or at risk of suffering harm (4). This includes children who are the subject of a child protection plan: recent government statistics indicated that, at 31 March 2008, there were 29,200 such children – a rate of 27 children per 10,000 of the population aged under 18. (In England, the total child population is 11 million). The official figures clearly do not represent the full extent of child abuse or neglect. They are the children known to public agencies, and who following enquiries led by Local Authority children's social care are determined to be at continuing risk of significant harm. These children are deemed to be in need of a multi-agency child protection plan. In each year some 538,500 children are referred to children's social care, of whom 319,900 go on to be assessed by the Local Authority as to whether they children in need (this figure included those who may be suffering or likely to suffer harm).

The Government does not, however, routinely collect information on the prevalence of child abuse and neglect. In the most recent study in the United Kingdom (5), researchers rated 7% of the sample as experiencing serious physical abuse in their families, 6% experiencing a serious absence of care and 6% experiencing serious emotional maltreatment. Six percent of the total sample assessed themselves as having been sexually abused. The NSPCC is in the process of repeating this study.

INFRASTRUCTURE

The Government's guidance Working Together to Safeguard Children (3) sets out the processes to be followed by all professionals and agencies, when there are concerns about possible child abuse or neglect. It also describes the roles and responsibilities of those professionals and agencies most likely to be in contact or working with children. At a local level, each local authority (of which there are 150 in England) is required by the Children Act 2004 (4) to set up a Local Safeguarding Children Board (LSCB). The core objectives of the LSCB are:

- to co-ordinate work done by board members to safeguard and promote the welfare of children and
- to ensure the effectiveness of what is done.

The core functions of LSCBs are set out in the Local Safeguarding Children Board Regulations (7). These cover the following areas in relation to safeguarding and promoting the welfare of children:

- policies and procedures;
- communicating and raising awareness;
- monitoring and evaluation;
- participating in planning and commissioning services;
- collecting and analysing information about child deaths;

- reviewing serious cases; and
- other activities compatible with their functions.

LSCBs are made up of both statutory and non-statutory members. Statutory members include the local authority, police, health bodies and probation. Non-statutory agencies include schools and further education colleges, domestic violence forums, drug and alcohol services, and housing providers. The chair of the LSCB is accountable to the Director of Children's Services in a local authority all the way up to the Minister for Children and Young People in the responsible government department i.e. the Department for Children, Schools and Families.

CHILD WELFARE LEGISLATION

The primary legislation governing child abuse and neglect in England is the Children Act 1989 (2). Under section 17(1) of the Children Act 1989, the local authority has a general duty to safeguard and promote the welfare of children in need in its area. Children in need are defined as those children whose vulnerability is such that they are unlikely to reach or maintain a satisfactory level of health or development, or whose health and development will be significantly impaired without the provision of services (Section 17(10) of the Children Act 1989).

Working Together to Safeguard Children (3) (pg 34) defines safeguarding and promoting the welfare of children as follows:

- 'protecting children from maltreatment;
- preventing impairment of children's health or development;
- ensuring that children are growing up in circumstances with the provision of safe and effective care; and
- undertaking that role so as to enable those children to have optimal life chances and to enter adulthood successfully.'

The Children Act 1989 also places on local authorities a statutory duty to make enquiries when there are concerns about possible significant harm to a child. In addition, the Children Act 2004 places a responsibility on a range of people and organisations to make arrangements to ensure that their functions, and any services provided by contractors on their behalf, safeguard and promote the welfare of children. The 2004 Act represents an important milestone in England's legislative provision to protect children from harm. For the first time, direct responsibility is placed on all those core agencies and people responsible for managing agencies who work with children to safeguard and promote their welfare. These responsibilities are set out in detail in statutory guidance (8).

RESPONDING TO CONCERN ABOUT CHILD WELFARE

The legislation provides the broad statutory framework for safeguarding and promoting the welfare of children. Chapter 5 of Working Together (3) sets out in detail how agencies and their staff should respond to concerns about the welfare of a child or children, in particular where abuse or neglect is suspected. The guidance covers both children who are living with their own families and those living away from home. In England, professionals are not under a mandatory duty to report suspected cases of child abuse and neglect, however, all are expected to follow the guidance set out in Working Together. This guidance is statutory and if, therefore, agencies or staff deviate from it they need to be able to justify their decisions, if necessary, in court of law. In general, this responsibility to comply with statutory guidance is well understood in the professional community and by members of the public.

The statutory guidance (8) sets out that everybody who works, or has contact, with children should be able to recognise and respond to concerns that a child's health or development is or may be impaired. This applies especially when they are concerned that a child may be suffering or, is at risk of, suffering significant harm. It is, however, the statutory responsibility of the local authority to intervene in relation to the child's welfare. The police may also be involved if criminal investigations are being undertaken. Other professionals employed, for example, in health bodies, nurseries or schools may also be involved with these enquiries if they know the particular child or children in the family.

The guidance (3,8) makes clear that all key agencies involved with the child and family prior to concerns being raised, together with those agencies which will provide specific services as part of a multi-agency plan, should work together in a coordinated, multi-agency way. There is also an expectation that agencies should work, wherever possible, in partnership with children and family members involving them in the assessment, planning and reviewing processes and, in particular, in carrying out the plan. The legislation (6) also requires that, in undertaking its functions, the local authority children's social care services should consider the child's wishes and feelings when planning interventions.

There are four key processes which underpin work with children and families: assessing, planning, intervening and reviewing. Each has to be carried out effectively in order to achieve optimal outcomes for children. The inter-agency processes set out in Working Together (3) cover the following five key areas:

- referral of concerns about a child to a statutory organisation (local authority children's social care or police) with responsibility to safeguard and promote the welfare of children;
- followed by the undertaking of an initial assessment of the child's situation, led by a local authority social worker;
- where necessary, using statutory powers to take emergency action to protect a child from immediate harm;
- when there are concerns about a child's safety, holding a discussion, led by a manager in children's social care, and involving all key agencies; this may lead to the initiation of statutory enquiries which require a more in depth core assessment to be completed, and if there are concerns about harm, a multi-agency child protection conference to be convened and
- finally, at a child protection conference deciding whether the child is at continuing risk of significant harm. If so, the child will become the subject of a child protection plan. This plan is implemented by a core group of key agencies working together

with the child and family. The plan is regularly reviewed at set intervals in line with statutory guidance.

DEVELOPMENTAL NEEDS OF CHILDREN

When following the above processes, statutory assessments of children in need, including where there are concerns about possible significant harm, follow the government's guidance set out in The Framework for the Assessment of Children in Need and their Families (9). During an assessment, information is gathered in the three domains of the Assessment Framework, namely the:

- child's developmental needs;
- parents' or carers' capacity to respond appropriately to these needs; and
- wider family and environmental factors.

Following a referral to children's social care and the initial assessment, the practitioners should be able to answer the following questions:

- What are the developmental needs of the child?
- Are the parents able to respond appropriately to the child's identified needs?
- Is the child being adequately safeguarded from significant harm, and are the parents able to promote the child's health and development?
- What impact are family functioning and history, the wider family and environmental factors having on the parents' capacity to respond to their child's needs and the child's developmental progress?
- Is action required to safeguard and promote the welfare of the child? (3, paragraph 5.38)

Where enquiries are being undertaken in response to concerns about possible significant harm, an in-depth core assessment, building on the initial assessment, is required to understand the child's and family's needs more fully. This information will inform decisions about whether the child should be the subject of a child protection plan and what services are necessary to achieve the planned outcomes for the child. This plan will be reviewed at regular intervals and updated as appropriate.

In order to support LSCBs in their work, the government produced statutory guidance and other materials. In particular, it developed the practice guidance What to do if you're worried a child is being abused (10) which is directed at all practitioners and managers whose work brings them into contact with children. This publication has helped them be clear about their roles and responsibilities. The government has also commissioned multi-agency training materials, including Safeguarding Children – a shared responsibility (11) to help LSCBs and agencies train their staff.

STRENGTHS IN THE SYSTEM

The multi-agency, multi-disciplinary approach to child protection described in this paper has been evolving in England over the last fifty years. This means that professionals and agencies are familiar with the overall processes even if some may not have a detailed understanding of each stage. The process of holding multi-agency child protection conferences in response to concerns about a child suffering harm has been in place since the early 1980s. They have succeeded in bringing together professionals from all agencies to discuss and plan, together with the child and family, how the child might be protected from subsequent harm. A proportion of these cases will, however, go on to be considered by the family courts.

One of the new responsibilities of the LSCB is to ensure the effectiveness of the work done by partner agencies. This requires LSCBs to develop ways of monitoring the effectiveness of all the different organisations, both statutory and independent, who work with children. They, then, need to ensure the findings are implemented. Another key issue for LSCBs is ensuring that all relevant staff receive appropriate training. This is an ongoing process, and requires organisations to take seriously their responsibilities to ensure that all staff, including those working primarily with adults, receive such training.

Although, in general, all agencies working together have a clear understanding about who from which agency, has lead responsibility for what, for example, the police lead on criminal investigations and children's social care services lead on child welfare, there are examples of cases where collaborative working between professionals has not been effective. A statutory Inquiry (12) into the death of an eight year old child Victoria Climbié concluded that the English legislation and statutory processes were sound and the focus of future policy needed to be on their successful implementation. In the words of the Inquiry's chair, Lord Laming, "the answer lies in doing relatively straightforward things well". More recent events in England have continued to highlight the difficulties in working together to protect children from harm (13). At the time of writing the government has asked Lord Laming to review the system to identify what more needs to be done to improve its functioning.

WEAKNESS AND CHALLENGES

Making safeguarding everyone's business - the government's vision for safeguarding children (14-16) - is one of the major challenges facing both central and local government. This means ensuring that all those who either work or have contact with children or parents, or adults in contact with children, understand their roles and responsibilities and are competent to carry them out. Those employed in housing and the fire service have as important a role to play in safeguarding children as doctors, social workers and the police: those working in small organisations are as important as those in large statutory agencies. This message is clear in all the government's guidance (3,8) and related training materials (11). A key priority in the government's Children's Plan (15) is the safety of children. The Staying Safe: Action Plan (14) is the first ever cross-government strategy for improving children's and young people's safety. This strategy is underpinned by a Public Service Agreement on child safety which has four indicators to be worked towards over the next three years (17).

LSCBs, in place since 2006, drew on the experiences of their predecessors Area Child Protection Committees (ACPCs) which had been in place under various names since 1974. Their responsibilities, however, have been widened from a focus on protecting children from abuse or neglect to also preventing them from for example, being bullied or suffering injury or death from accidents. It is a major undertaking to engage agencies and organisations at all levels, as well as to engage members of the community in safeguarding the welfare of all children.

In England, since 2008, LSCBs have been required to review the deaths of all children in their area, and to use the information collected to decide which deaths could have been prevented (3). This new statutory provision also means that local agencies and professionals are expected to work together collaboratively, according to an agreed plan, when a child dies unexpectedly. LSCBs are required to put in place their own local policies and practices and to ensure that all relevant staff are trained in these new processes. These are major tasks to achieve. In the early stages of implementation, particular concerns were raised about the resources – human and financial – to undertake these new processes. Government funding has since been made available to support the child death review processes, as have training resources (18,19). As with any new policy initiative, there is a need to continue to monitor its implementation and to use the lessons learnt to refine both policy and practice (20).

CONTROVERSIES

The current child protection system has been evolving since the 1950s when the first government circular was issued on joint agency working to protect children from abuse and neglect (1). Indeed, the first local area child protection committees came into being in 1974 following the tragic death of a foster child, Maria Colwell: she was the subject of a major public Inquiry (21). As stated earlier, the Inquiry chaired by Lord Laming was very clear that the child protection system in England did not require change. Despite everyone's best efforts, however, a number of children continue to suffer abuse or neglect. Each year, some 80 to 90 serious case reviews are undertaken when a child has died (22,23). These cases involve possible abuse or neglect as well as concerns about the way in which professionals and services worked together. Some cases receive high profile coverage in the media: inevitably questions are asked about what professionals should or could have done better to prevent a particular child from dying or suffering serious abuse or neglect. It is because of such concerns that Lord Laming has been recently asked to review the child protection systems in England, including those systems for reviewing serious case reviews and learning the lessons from them.

Recently the government published two overviews of serious case reviews highlighting the complexity of situations in which some children live (22,23). These reports demonstrated the very difficult task that professionals have in ensuring that each and every child remains safe. Many of the key issues identified are well known from previous studies, inquiries or research (12,24,25). For example, problems include poor or no communication about the child between professionals, lack of relevant training, and a focus on the adults to the extent that some children become lost to the system and hence almost invisible to the professionals who have a responsibility to protect them. Particular concerns have been raised about older children who seem to have been neglected not only by their families, but also by the system. Another long-standing issue highlighted again and by other research into domestic violence and mental health in child protection cases (26) is the difficulty professionals often experience collaborating across the children's and adult services boundaries. In particular, this involves those working in the substance misuse, domestic violence or mental health fields. Although these concerns are not new (24,25), and despite the wide dissemination of these findings and the development of government commissioned training materials (27-29) as well as clear guidance for both adult and children's services staff, knowledge about these areas is still not widely implemented. It seems that each new generation of staff need to relearn the same lessons, rather than there being a progression in our use of knowledge.

Evidence based decision making requires quality assessments based on child welfare knowledge. Concerns about the quality of assessments and the ability of staff to undertake interventions in relation to child protection led to the government developing and implementing the Framework for the Assessment of Children in Need and their Families (9) and the Integrated Children's System (30) as well as the major Safeguarding Children research programme. Social work training was reformed in 2000 to improve its quality; further work is being undertaken to reform the children's work force to support the government's programme to ensure that all children achieve their developmental potential (33,31). The quality of service provision not only depends on the calibre of staff, but also the availability of appropriate services for children and families. To ensure that these services are available, the local authority has a statutory responsibility to plan at a strategic level what resources should and will be available (32). This should mean that, in response to assessed needs, individual children, parents and families receive services in accordance with the agreed plan.

PREVENTION EFFORTS

Following the Inquiry into the death of Victoria Climbié, the government announced a major programme for children's services - Every Child Matters (33). This programme is guided by five key outcomes which children and young people themselves said are important to their wellbeing. Keeping children safe is one. The other four are 'being healthy, enjoying and achieving, making a positive contribution, and achieving economic wellbeing'. The government's Green Paper, Every Child Matters and the subsequent Children Act 2004 set out plans for the integration of services around the needs of children through the creation of children's trusts. In addition, it includes a requirement that local authorities set up inter-agency local safeguarding children boards and that all agencies which work or are in contact with children safeguard and promote their welfare. A key aim of the government's policy is both early intervention to prevent problems developing and reaching a serious level and intervening early in children's lives to give them the best possible start. This early intervention strategy led to the setting up of 125,000 children's centres across England by 2008 to ensure that children and their families are provided with a comprehensive range of child and family services based around a school and that they can access these services early on when they want additional help. More recently, the government has announced that it will legislate to set up children's trust boards to ensure that local services - including schools, health, social services and the police - work together to improve outcomes for children and young people (16).

The Staying Safe: action plan (14) sets out an extensive programme to keep children safe. It includes ensuring that children have opportunities for play and are able to undertake activities which may contain an element of risk in as safe a way as possible as well as the prevention of accidents, educating parents on how their children can use IT safely and intervening effectively when children are harmed. The government's aim is that all children have the opportunity to grow up and enter adulthood successfully, and achieve their potential in relation to the five outcomes. This means that the more narrowly defined concept of child protection has been superseded by focusing on the broader safeguarding children agenda and improving the wellbeing of all children in our community.

CONCLUSIONS

A key achievement of the Every Child Matters programme has been to place safeguarding and promoting the welfare of children and improving children's wellbeing on the national agenda and to make the programme something that all individuals in England, i.e. children, parents, communities and professionals feel a part of. Safeguarding children from harm has never had a higher government profile. The big challenge now is to translate the legislation and policy together with the policy aspirations of government into reality by delivering services on the ground that will truly improve the wellbeing of all children in our community.

REFERENCES

[1]   Home Office, Ministry of Health, Ministry of Education. Joint Circular from the Home Office, Ministry of Health and Ministry of Education. Children neglected or ill-treated in their homes. London: Home Office, 1950.

[2]   Children Act 1989. London: HMSO, 1989.

[3]   HM Government. Working together to safeguard children. London: Stationery Office, 2006.

[4]   Department for Children, Schools and Families. Referrals, assessments and children and young people who are subject to a child protection plan, England. Year ending 31 March 2008 (Statistical volume). London: Stationery Office, 2008.

[5]   Cawson P, Wattam C, Brooker S, Kelly G. Child maltreatment in the family. A study of the prevalence of child abuse and neglect. London: NSPCC, 2000.

[6]   Children Act 2004. London: HMSO, 2004.

[7]   The Local Safeguarding Children Board Regulations. SI 2006/90. London: HMSO, 2006.

[8]   HM Government. Statutory guidance on making arrangements to safeguard and promote the welfare of children under the Children Act 2004. London: Dept Children Schools Fam, 2007.

[9]   Department of Health, Department for Education and Employment and Home Office. Framework for the assessment of children in need and their families. London: Stationery Office, 2000.

[10]   HM Government. What to do if you're worried a child is being abused. London: Dept Children Schools Fam, 2006.

[11]   The Department for Children, Schools and Families, the NSPCC, Royal Holloway University. Safeguarding children - a shared responsibility. London: Dept Children Schools Fam, 2007.

[12]   Cm 5730. The Victoria Climbié inquiry report. London: HMSO, 2003.

[13] Ofsted, Healthcare Commision and Her Majesty's Inspectorate of Constabulary. Joint area review. Haringey children's services authority area review of services for children and young people, with particular reference to safeguarding. London: Ofsted, 2008.

[14] HM Government. Staying safe: action plan. London: Dept Children Schools Fam, 2008.

[15] The Department for Children, Schools and Families. The children's plan. London: Dept Children Schools Fam, 2007.

[16] The Department for Children, Schools and Families. The children's plan one year on. London: Dept Children Schools Fam, 2008.

[17] HM Government. PSA Delivery Agreement 13: Improve children and young people's safety. London: HM Treasury, 2008.

[18] The Department for Children, Schools and Families. Why Jason died. London: Dept Children Schools Fam, 2007.

[19] The Department for Children, Schools and Families. Responding when a child dies. A training resource to support Local Safeguarding Children Boards in implementing the child death review processes in Working Together to Safeguard Children. London: Dept Children Schools Fam, 2008.

[20] Sidebotham P, Fox J, Horwath J, Powell C, Perwez S. Preventing childhood deaths. A study of 'early starter' child death overview panels in England. London: Dept Children Schools Fam, 2008.

[21] Department of Health and Social Security. Child abuse. A study of inquiry reports 1973-1981. London: Stationery Office, 1982.

[22] Rose W, Barnes J. Improving safeguarding practice. Study of serious case reviews 2001 – 2003. London: Dept Children Schools Fam, 2008.

[23] Brandon M, Belderson P, Warren C, Howe D, Gardner R, Dodsworth J, et al. Analysing child deaths and serious injury through child abuse and neglect: what can we learn? A biennial analysis of serious case reviews 2003 – 2005. London: Dept Children Schools Fam 2008.

[24] Department of Health. Child protection: messages from research. London: HM Stationery Office, 1995.

[25] Falkov A. A study of working together "Part 8" reports: fatal child abuse and parental psychiatric disorder. London: Dept Health, 1996.

[26] Cleaver H, Nicholson D, Tarr S, Cleaver D. Child protection, domestic violence and parental substance misuse. London: Jessica Kingsley, 2007.

[27] Cleaver H, Unell I, Aldgate J. Children's needs – parenting capacity: The impact of parental mental illness, problem alcohol and drug use, and domestic violence on children's development. London: Stationery Office, 1999.

[28] Falkov A, Mayes K, Diggins M, Silverdale N. Cox A. Crossing bridges – training resources for working with mentally ill parents and their children. Brighton: Pavilion Publ, 1998.

[29] Department of Health, University of Bristol, the NSPCC and Barnardos. Making an impact: children and domestic violence. Training resource. London: Barnardos, 1998.

[30] Department of Health. The integrated children's system. Working with children in need and their families. Consultation document. London: Dept Health, 2003.

[31] Department for Children, Schools and Families. 2020 children and young people's workforce strategy. London: Dept Children Schools Fam,2008.

[32] Children and Young People's Plan (England) Regulations 2005. SI 2005 No 2149. London: Stationery Office, 2005.

[33] Cm 5860. Every child matters. London: Stationery Office, 2003.

In: International Aspects of Child Abuse and Neglect   ISBN: 978-1-60876-703-8
Editors: H. Dubowitz, J. Merrick pp. 123-129   © 2010 Nova Science Publishers, Inc.

Chapter 12

CHILD PROTECTION IN FRANCE

Gaby Taub

Territorial Correspondent for Paris, Children's Ombudsman of France, Paris, France

The child protection system in France is a two-tiered system: administrative and judiciary. Despite its complexity, the system allows for great flexibility in protecting children from abuse and neglect. The French child protection system is characterized by the ease with which it is possible to pass from the administrative framework to the judicial framework and back, in the interest of children and their families. This chapter will attempt to examine some of the philosophical underpinnings of the French system that account for its flexibility. It will also briefly examine the positive and negative aspects of a system which opens the way to intensive public intervention in the private family sphere.

INTRODUCTION

The child protection system in France is a two-tiered system: administrative and judiciary. Its legitimacy rests on the jurisdictions of the "départements" – 99 French territorial sub-divisions – and the state. Despite its complexity, the system allows for great flexibility in protecting children from child abuse and neglect.

France sees itself as an indivisible, secular, democratic, and social Republic that applies the same policy and law to its entire territory and entire population. The French state consists of the sum of its legislative, executive and national administrative institutions. It is both a political and an administrative entity. The state is comprised of three types of territorial collectivities: 22 regions (such as Normandy, Burgundy, and Provence), 99 Departments (such as the Loire, Dordogne, or Martinique), and 36,757 communes (such as Paris, Dijon, or Bordeaux). These territorial collectivities are respectively governed by elected assemblies known as regional councils, general councils and municipal councils, each with their own sphere of power as defined by the law of the State.

The current child protection system is based on policies dating back to 1945, with regard to juvenile offenders, and to 1958 and 1959, with regard to the protection of children and adolescents. As a result of the decentralization laws of 1983 and 1986, authority over social welfare was largely transferred from the State to the Departments, causing significant developments in the child protection system.

The Prevention of Child Abuse and Neglect Law passed in 1989 holds the President of the General Council ultimately responsible for child protection in each Department. It also provides for mandatory reporting, a child abuse hot line, a register of victims, multidisciplinary assessments, and training programs for professionals at the Departmental level.

Nevertheless, the State still has basic responsibilities. The state (or national government) has sole legislative authority and develops the national policies that greatly influence the conditions of social welfare. The Minister of Justice, also at the State level, is ultimately responsible for ensuring that judges' decisions get carried out, notably with respect to child protection.

HOW IS CHILD MALTREATMENT DEFINED IN FRANCE?

According to the Decentralized Observatory of Social Action, a mistreated child is a child victim of physical abuse, sexual abuse, psychological abuse, and/or neglect having grave consequences for his/her physical and psychological development. A child at risk is a child whose living conditions pose a risk to his/her health, security, education or physical well-being, even though he/she is not mistreated.

WHAT IS KNOWN ABOUT THE INCIDENCE OF CHILD MALTREATMENT?

The following statistics were provided by the Decentralized Observatory of Social Action based on cases reported by child protection services: In 2005, there were 20,000 mistreated children and 77,000 children at risk. Of the 20,000 mistreated children, 6,400 were victims of physical abuse, 4,700 of sexual abuse, 5,100 of neglect and 3,800 were victims of psychological abuse.

THE PHILOSOPHICAL UNDERPINNINGS OF THE FRENCH SYSTEM

Four major principles govern French policy with regard to child protection:

- Respect for birthrights and filial relationships
- Consideration for children's identity
- Consideration for parents' identity and cultural background
- Recognition of parents' responsibility

France attributes great importance to birthrights and filial relationships. A child is considered to be, first and foremost, a member of a family. Child protection services emphasize maintaining the child within the family. When it is necessary to separate children from their families, placement is always a temporary measure with the child's return to the family as its ultimate goal. Recent reforms reaffirm the notion of parental authority, even going back several generations in the same family (preference, for example, is usually given to grandparents in decisions regarding placement). The law establishes equal parental responsibility between the mother and father and stipulates that children must have access to both parents, even in cases of severe conflict, separation, and divorce. Furthermore, family mediation and shared custody are written into the Civil Code. Whether their parents are married or not, all children have equal rights in the eyes of the law. Distinctions between legitimate and illegitimate children with regard to inheritance laws have recently been abolished.

Great importance is also accorded to children's identity. In France, the strong Republican and secular traditions contribute to individuals being considered as citizens with equal rights, regardless of religion or ethnic origin. If for example, a child needs to be taken into state custody, psychological considerations bear greater weight in the choice of a placement facility than the child's language and culture. Nevertheless, though it may not be uncommon to select a French Catholic foster family for an African Moslem child, care is taken to respect the child's background and identity.

High value is also placed on parents' cultural background. Both the Child Welfare Department and the Children's Court are required by the law to take religious and cultural preferences of families into consideration when making decisions concerning their children.

Most striking, perhaps, is the importance attributed to parental authority. The French child protection system is characterized by a strong alliance between State and parents for the purpose of raising children under the best possible conditions. It is commonly accepted that families and public powers share a stake in raising the future citizens of the Republic. Thus, for example, the Child Welfare Department and the Children's Court are bound by law to enlist the cooperation of families when making decisions concerning their children. The obligation to seek common ground when providing assistance in raising children is a feature of the French child protection system. Under this system, the government progressively compensates for parents' shortcomings and limitations.

In summary, French child protection policies are less centered on the child than on the family as a whole. All child protection laws in France are guided by the principle that public intervention in the private sphere aims primarily to support families and to assure that the child remains bound to his/her family.

A TWO-TIERED SYSTEM OF CHILD PROTECTION

The French child protection system is organized around two separate sectors:

- Judicial protection, created in 1958
- Administrative protection, created in 1959

JUDICIAL PROTECTION

Judicial protection is controlled by the state, with the aid of the departments and the voluntary sector. It includes all social intervention based on decisions made by a Children's Judge. Article 375 of the Civil Code states that protective measures ordered by a Children's Judge can be initiated at the request of the parents or caregivers, of the child, or of the Public Prosecutor "if the health, safety, or moral development of a non-emancipated minor is in danger or if the conditions of his/her upbringing are seriously compromised."

In the French legal system, Children's Judges have a dual jurisdiction: penal with regard to juvenile offenders and civil with regard to child protection - in cases of clear and present danger due to inadequate parental authority or child abuse and neglect. These Judges are independent and their role is to administer justice.

The function of Children's Judges was created in 1945 to deal with juvenile delinquency, thus granting a specific status to minors charged with crimes or misdemeanors. In 1958, the jurisdiction of Children's Judges was expanded to include the protection of children in physical or psychological danger. While the Judge has broad powers to intervene in private family affairs, it is incumbent upon him/her to specify the nature of the danger motivating his/her decisions. Matters of parental conflict over child custody in cases of separation or divorce and questions of parental authority remain within the jurisdiction of Family Judges. Children's Judges intervene only in cases of abusive or deficient parental authority.

Reports of children in danger, usually emanating from the Child Welfare Department, are transmitted by a Public Prosecutor to a Children's Judge. Police brigades specializing in children and adolescents are part of the judicial police and, although they are not present in all communes, they are present in all regions and "départements." They play an important role in investigating allegations of child abuse and neglect at the request of a Public Prosecutor or a Children's Judge.

As a result of mandatory reporting, children's courts in France are faced with ever-increasing numbers of cases involving suspected child abuse and neglect. Court-mandated assessment is a procedure that has been developed in France to facilitate the optimal professional response to humane and efficient handling of these cases in the judicial system.

To obtain help in making an informed decision, the judge can designate a child protection services agency to conduct an in-depth evaluation. The aim of the court-mandated assessment, as defined by the law, is to do an evaluation of the child's psychological functioning personality and to broaden the scope of the evaluation to include the child's family and social environment. Ultimately, the goal of the court-mandated assessment is two-fold: to help the judge make an informed decision and to help the family develop a feasible treatment plan.

Faced with a complex family situation that poses a grave threat to the child's well being, the judge is empowered to make a rapid and clear decision. Yet, if there is persisting doubt or uncertainty concerning the parents' ability to protect their child, the judge may choose to temporarily suspend judgment and allow time for a court-mandated assessment of the family situation. This measure is not subject to appeal by the family.

FAMILY ASSESSMENT

A multidisciplinary team composed of social workers, psychologists and psychiatrists carries out the assessment. By means of interviews and tests conducted at the agency or during home visits, the assessment process provides ample opportunity for the family members to express themselves with different people in different settings. The team has up to six months to facilitate communication amongst the parties concerned in an effort to define the problems and to propose potential solutions. Some time before the end of this period, the assessment team reports its conclusions to the judge in writing.

The court-mandated assessment takes into account the family history. In an attempt to understand the family environment, it raises questions about family composition, housing, budget, employment, schooling, leisure activities, etc. It also explores issues relating to deficient parenting, marital conflict, social isolation, academic failure, unemployment, physical or mental illness, suspected or alleged abuse or neglect.

Either the judge prescribes specific tests – psychological, psychiatric, medical, academic or vocational – or he/she simply enjoins the team to use some or all of the means at its disposal. Since the purpose of the testing is to help the judge reach a decision, the judge is considered competent to request the material he/she deems necessary. Whatever the means employed, the overall purpose is to evaluate the difficulties encountered by the child and the family, to measure their capacity for change, to determine whether further treatment is necessary within a judicial context and, if so, what type of treatment.

The assessment period allows the judge, to remain open and flexible, rather than form a hasty opinion of the family and the child. Although the judge recedes into the background for the six-month period, he/she nevertheless remains ultimately responsible for the child's protection and for taking emergency measures, as the need arises. The judge's presence acts as a safety net, freeing the assessment team to continue its work despite the possible vicissitudes of the family situation.

At the end of the six-month period, the Judge holds a hearing in the presence of the family and the social workers involved in the case. The family can be assisted by an attorney and has the right to free legal services. A court-appointed children's lawyer can also assist the child. When there is a conflict of interest between the child and his/her parents or legal guardians or if charges have been pressed against the parents or caregivers, an "Ad Hoc Administrator" represents the child's interests. At the time of the hearing, the Judge is obliged to enlist the cooperation of the family. When making a decision concerning the child, the Judge is also required to take into consideration the religious and cultural preferences expressed by the family.

After the initial six-month period, the Judge can mandate a child protection services agency to provide ongoing supportive services aimed at allowing the child to remain within the family. This is a form of constraint on parental authority, insofar as the supportive services are obligatory and remain under the Judge's control. The Judge also has the power to place the child outside the family: in the custody of the extended family, with the Child Welfare Department, or with a non-profit organization. In such cases, parents retain their parental authority, within certain limits determined by the Judge. Parents must be informed of the location of their child's placement and of the child's development over time. Whenever possible, contacts between the parents and child are maintained and encouraged because the ultimate goal of any placement is the return of the child to the family.

ADMINISTRATIVE PROTECTION

The Departments, with the aid of the voluntary sector, control administrative protection (i.e., non-judicial or non-coercive protection services). French legislation concerning the family and social welfare requires the Departments to develop social welfare programs and to provide supportive services to children and families facing difficulties that "threaten to seriously compromise their equilibrium." This allows for diverse forms of assistance at the request of parents, caregivers, or professionals as needed to ensure the health, well being, and education of child. According to French law, it is the responsibility of the Department to:

- Provide financial, educational, and psychological assistance to children and their families facing social problems that threaten to "seriously compromise their equilibrium"
- Organize collective actions, such as parenting programs or after-school centers, aimed at preventing marginality and at facilitating the social integration of children and their families
- Provide emergency assistance
- Provide for the needs of children placed in the care of social service agencies at the request of their families
- Take measures in preventing child abuse and neglect.

Departmental Social Services are composed of generic social workers, each responsible for a geographic territory covering approximately 5000 inhabitants Caseloads tend to be heavy, but not necessarily overwhelming. The generic social workers do not work with families on a long-term basis. These are the "general practitioners" of social action.

The Child Welfare Department consists of caseworkers, group workers, psychologists, mother's helpers, and home visitors all of whom provide specialized preventive and protective services, including placement in children's shelters, to children at risk. Further responsibilities of the Child Welfare Department include providing pre or post natal care to young mother encountering social problem and providing care for abandoned children, children with no administrative status, or children placed in view of adoption

Mother and Infant Care Services is a public health service for pregnant women, mothers and children under the age of six. Its purpose is to help families in difficulty and to prevent child abuse and neglect. It is composed of pediatricians, midwives, and baby nurses working under the supervision of a medical director. Home visits are an important component of Mother and Infant Care Services.

These various forms of administrative protection concern situations where the child protection professionals provide appropriate help within the context of a voluntary, contractual relationship with the family, devoid of major tensions. Judicial protection is solicited when there is a clear and present danger for the child and a refusal on the part of the family to enter into a contractual relationship. In such cases, recourse to a higher authority makes it possible to impose obligatory protective measures.

POSITIVE AND NEGATIVE ASPECTS OF THE FRENCH SYSTEM

Common points in the legal foundations of both the administrative and judicial child protection systems make it possible for parents, caregivers, children, and professionals to directly request either form of protection in situations where children are considered to be "at risk" or "in danger." The French child protection system is characterized by the ease with which it is possible to pass from the administrative framework to the judicial framework, and back again. It is a highly flexible system that provides individualized responses adapted to each child's needs.

However, legal texts that employ terms such as "problems tending to compromise the child's equilibrium (or mental health) or refer to children being "raised in conditions that are gravely compromised" lend themselves to broad interpretation. The complexity of the system and the ambiguity of the underlying texts can lead to confusion amongst families and professionals. Parents do not always have a clear idea of what child protection professionals expect of them. Nor do professionals always have a clear idea of what constitutes help in raising children.

The relative ease with which child protection professionals can obtain the intervention of a Children's Judge tends to make them overly dependent on the judiciary system. As one French Children's Judge stated, "If there exists a notion that will never be precisely defined once and for all, it is the notion of 'danger'."

CONCLUSIONS

In conclusion, the French system opens the way to intensive judicial intervention in private family life and also to a never-ending debate on the limits and respective legal capacities of the administrative and judicial authorities. The French system puts civil justice in the position of making up for deficits in parental authority.

REFERENCES

[1]   Amiel C, Garapon A. Justice négociée et justice imposée dans le droit français de l'enfance. Actes 1986;56:18-2. [French]
[2]   Chaillou P. L'Enfant et sa famille face à la justice. Toulouse: Privat, 1992. [French]
[3]   Grevot A. Voyage en protection de l'enfance une comparaison européenne. Vaucresson: CNFE-PJJ, 2001. [French]
[4]   Manciaux M, Gabel M. Enfances en Danger. Paris: Edition Fleurus, 1997. [French]
[5]   Ministère Délégué à la Famille et à l'Enfance. La Politique de la France en faveur de l'enfance. Paris: La documentation française, 2002. [French]

In: International Aspects of Child Abuse and Neglect   ISBN: 978-1-60876-703-8
Editors: H. Dubowitz, J. Merrick pp. 131-138   © 2010 Nova Science Publishers, Inc.

Chapter 13

CHILD PROTECTION IN NORWAY: CHALLENGES AND OPPORTUNITIES

Tine K Jensen and Elisabeth Backe-Hansen

NOVA-Norwegian Social Research, Norwegian Ministry of Education and Research,
Oslo and Norwegian Center for Violence and Traumatic Stress Studies (NKVTS),
Oslo, Norway

The aim of this chapter was to describe the Norwegian system for child protection and the regulating laws. Although combating all kinds of violence and neglect against children is a high priority for the government, there are still a vast number of youth that experience violence, abuse and neglect. One important characteristic of the Norwegian system is that child welfare problems are seen as a whole, thus services or interventions are aimed towards all children, irrespective of the reason for the intervention. A low threshold for contacting the child welfare authorities and for receiving preventive services is one of the objectives of the present Child Welfare Act. Thus preventive services address a continuum of situations, ranging from fairly limited needs to long-term intensive and comprehensive services aimed at avoiding out of home placement. Strenghts and challenges of the system are described.

INTRODUCTION

Norway is a small country with only 4,8 million inhabitants, where 26% are less than 20 years old. Approximately 10 % are immigrants, mostly from other European countries (1).

Health care and dental care is free for children and all children below school age are invited to regular controls as part of our welfare services. The offer of pre-school care is extensive, and Norway is close to reaching the goal of complete coverage for all children from one years of age, with a fairly low maximum monthly cost. The school system is public and free, and schooling is mandatory between the ages of six and sixteen. In addition young persons have the right to three years' secondary schooling until they reach 24 years of age. Pre-school care differs from the school system in that more than half of the places offered are private, albeit in principle subject to the same control as public kindergartens.

Despite the fact that Norway is one of the richest countries in the world, child abuse and neglect remains a relatively large social problem. Combating all kinds of violence and neglect against children is a high priority for the Norwegian government. According to the UN Children's Rights Convention (CRC) the State is to protect children against physical or mental abuse, neglect, or exploitation by their parents or other caregivers (section 19). In accordance with this the Department of Justice issued a White Paper for Children (2) summarizing a series of services and projects aimed at helping and protecting children who have been victims of abuse or neglect, as well as preventing abuse and neglect. These efforts are country-wide, and established at either regional or municipal levels. They also come in addition to interventions through the child protection authorities, which we will describe in more detail below.

In addition the Department of Justice (in 2008) has issued a Plan of Action against violence in close relationships, covering the years 2008-2011(3). The Plan covers 49 different activities and a series of departments are responsible for their implementation. Among these activities are a 24-hour free telephone service for child victims, reviewing the need for an increased legal protection through the Penal Code for children exposed to violence in their families, better treatment services directed at perpetrators as well as victims, and efforts to increase the awareness of violence and abuse among professionals who have daily contact with children and young people. As part of this national plan to protect abused children, the Norwegian government has in addition decided to establish six Children's Houses throughout Norway, one in each health region. The purpose of this service is to establish a setting where children who have been physically or sexually abused, are victims of domestic violence or where there is suspicion of such abuse, can receive coordinated services in one place. The centres offer forensic interviewing, medical examinations, case consultations, psychological assessments, and short term therapy if needed. The idea is that the families and children shall not need to go from place to place to receive help, thus lessening the burden on the child and family. Also, the intention is that coordinated action and cooperation between services is easier to achieve when they are located in the same house. This model is inspired by Iceland where such houses have already existed for several years, with promising results.

The total Plan of Action must be seen in relation to a former initiative from the Department of Children and Families (in 2005), a Strategy against sexual and physical abuse against children (4). This strategy includes prevention, disclosure of abuse, help and treatment, knowledge development and dissemination. Here again the outlook is general, and the child welfare authorities play a specified role within the totality of services.

The Norwegian efforts must be seen in a larger context. During the last years, the Council of Europe has developed a programme called "Building a Europe for and with children" (5). This programme included endorsement of former draft Policy Guidelines on National Integrated Strategies for the Protection of Children against Violence, and promotion of national, integrated strategies on children's rights and violence against children in member States. As a member of the Council of Europe, Norway has both helped promote the development of this programme, and taken on the role of being a test country for the programme together with Romania. The above mentioned plan and strategy must thus be seen in relation to Norway's European commitment on this score.

Abuse and neglect are old phenomena within a child welfare context. What is new in Norway is the increased focus on the phenomena from the State and government, and the increased activities to counteract them on a broad basis, not only within the context of child welfare agencies. However, these activities of course influence the work of the child welfare authorities as well, since they also become more conscious of the damage involved, and develop more competence in disclosing and dealing with these problems. We will now describe the definitional and legal foundations for this work more in detail, in the context of how Norwegian child welfare work is organised.

THE DEFINITION OF CHILD ABUSE AND NEGLECT

Three laws in particular address and define child abuse and neglect in Norway. One is the Penal Law of 1902 with several later revisions, the second is the Child Welfare Act and the third is the Children's Act. In Norway all corporal punishment of children, including spanking, has been prohibited by law since 1982 and Norway was one of the first European countries to effect such legislation. The Children's Act states that a child should not be exposed to violence or in any other way be treated so that it's physical or psychological health is harmed. A suggested amendment to the existing legislation, proposed late in 2008, strengthens the ban on corporal punishment even further. In the proposal the following is added: All use of violence towards children, both physical and psychological is illegal. This applies also to cases where the physical and/or psychological violence is meant to be part of child rearing.

The legal definition of child sexual abuse (CSA) sets the age limit at 18 years, when the child is in care of an adult. 16 years is the age limit for sexual activity. The law also defines sexual abuse with children below14 years as more serious then abuse between the ages of 14 and 16. Sexual abuse is defined according to the kind of activities involved and is legally divided into three groups of behavior. The most serious includes all kinds of penetration of vagina and anus. The next category involves all forms of fondling of genitals, breasts and buttocks. Kissing is also included in this category. The mildest form refers to acts such as exhibitionism where there is no actual physical contact. Sexual exploitation through prostitution and involving children in pornography is also illegal.

All sexual contact between persons with a familial relationship is illegal regardless of age. This does not only pertain to biological relationships, but also to adoptive children and stepchildren or other children in the perpetrator's care. With regard to siblings, only intercourse is defined as illegal.

THE PREVALENCE OF CHILD ABUSE AND NEGLECT

Very few studies on the prevalence of child abuse and neglect have been conducted in Norway. For child sexual abuse, two national surveys have been conducted which reported the prevalence to be 16% (6) and 2.8% (7). These studies used different definitions of CSA that mostly accounts for the difference in prevalence rates.

The prevalence of physical child abuse in Norway is not well documented either. A recent study involving 7033 eighteen to nineteen year olds reported that 20% girls and 14% boy had experienced at least one violent episode during their lifetime. Approximately 2% reported being beaten more than ten times during childhood. Furthermore10 % of the youth reported witnessing at least one violent episode between their parents (8). In another study 15,930 youth aged 15-16 years were asked whether they had been physically or sexually abused during the last year. The results indicate that 4,6% of the girls and 3,3% of the boys had experienced violence from an adult. The rates for sexual abuse were 6,1% for the girls and 1,6% for the boys. In the study the children were not asked who sexually abused them (9).

In 2007 there were approximately 25,000 reports to the child welfare agencies in Norway. Of these 50% resulted in interventions. 2.75% of the child population between the ages 0-17 years thus received some kind of child welfare interventions. Four out of five receive preventive services, and one of five is placed outside their homes. When looking at the statistics for new children receiving interventions in 2007, it appears that not more than 4% of the interventions were initiated because of child abuse and neglect. However, is thought that these figures are probably somewhat misleading since other causes may often be registered such as parental drug abuse or mental illness, or the conditions of the home (1).

CHILD WELFARE WORK IN NORWAY: A GENERALIST MODEL

All child welfare work in Norway is regulated by the Child Welfare Act from 1992, superseding the former Act from 1953. One important characteristic of the Norwegian system is that child welfare problems are seen as a whole, thus the Act sanctions services or interventions towards all children and young people included, irrespective of the reason for the intervention. The same law applies whether a child needs preventive services in the guise of a place in kindergarten, or needs to be placed in foster care.

Child welfare work is reactive in the sense that others notify the authorities that a child may be living in a detrimental care situation, or a youth may be out of control. The idea is that anybody can notify, while the child welfare authorities assess the situation and decides whether to suggest interventions or not. As mentioned above interventions are initiated in about half of the reported cases. Actually a series of persons and services report possible child welfare cases yearly. In 2007 as many as 19 different services or persons reported cases to the child welfare authorities that actually resulted in some kind of intervention, prominent among them the parents themselves. Among the almost 12,000 new cases resulting in interventions in 2007 the parents were the most frequent reporters, in one fifth of the cases. This reflects that children of primary school age or youth are more frequently reported than small children, and that the reports then concern the children's and young people's behaviour and the parents' need for help. Cases reported from the school comes second to those initiated by the parents where children of primary school age are concerned, while cases initiated by other child welfare authorities or children's health services come second and third to those initiated by the parents of younger children. And when a case involved a young person, the most frequent initiators of the case besides the parents were the school and the police (1).

Reporting to the child welfare authorities is mandatory in cases of suspected serious child abuse or neglect, but the authorities will still have to assess the child's situation independently. Nor is reporting to the police mandatory for the other services who are in contact with children, young people and their families.

Child welfare authorities have much informal power, in that this body decides whether to suggest interventions in a particular case or not. But the law regulates quasi-legal as well as legal procedures aimed at ensuring in particular the parents' rights, enabling them access to all documentation in their case, the right to be consulted, and last, but not least the right to free legal advice if they do not agree with the proposal made by the child welfare services in the more serious cases. The latter becomes particularly important, when there is conflict about possible out of home placement, where, in addition, parents have unlimited appeal rights. In addition young people are entitled to free legal advice for themselves if forcible placement of them in residential care is proposed. This system necessitates that child welfare workers pay attention to the legal aspects of their work, particularly when out of home placement becomes actualized, and have to tailor their arguments to fit the formulations in the law (10). In other settings this process is often referred to as juridification, which signifies, amongst other things, a limitation of the scope of professional discretion in single cases.

A central principle in both the former and the present Act is that interventions are supposed to be as non-invasive as possible. Thus, preventive services directed towards the child and his or her family have to be tried properly before out-of-home placement is considered. The child welfare services must be then able to justify that preventive services will not be sufficient to ensure that the child's care situation improves sufficiently in order to have an out-of-home placement sanctioned by the Board of Child Welfare, the first formal decision-making body in these cases. This principle is reflected in the yearly statistics, which, as mentioned above, show that children and young people receiving preventive services regularly outnumber those placed outside their homes by about four to one.

Preventive services are used in a plethora of situations, reflecting huge variations in the life situations of the children, young people and families involved. Indeed, a low threshold for contacting the child welfare authorities and for receiving preventive services is one of the objectives of the present Child Welfare Act. Thus preventive services may be understood as addressing a continuum of situations, ranging from fairly limited needs, for instance for a place in kindergarten, to long-term intensive and comprehensive services aimed at avoiding out of home placement.

The most important preventive service for young children is pre-school care and kindergartens are obliged by law to accept a child in these circumstances. The fee will then often be paid by the child welfare authorities. Other preventive services are, for instance, economic support of various kinds which plays a prominent role, support persons or mentors, having a family to visit at week-ends, a consultant to help out at home, home-based interventions like Multisystemic Therapy (MST) or Parent-Management Training (PMTO). The more serious the child's situation the more likely it is that several services will be used in combination over time. It might, however, be said that the scope of preventive services within child welfare is only limited by the creativity of the child welfare worker (11), and, it might be added, the economic situation of the municipality.

Another important characteristic is the importance attributed to collaboration with the parents. When investigation of a case does not lead to services being offered or an intervention being proposed, this is quite often because the parents do not wish to receive such services (12). We also acknowledge that preventive services within the family of origin rarely succeed unless a working relationship with the parents is possible to develop and maintain. And enforced services are not possible to effect unless a case is very serious.

The UN Convention of the Rights of the Child was incorporated in Norwegian legislation in 2003, and is given preference whenever there is conflict with other legislation. This means that children are to be included in the decision-making process in child welfare cases from the age of seven, and become independent legal actors at the age of fifteen. The obligation to include children was present earlier as well, but is significantly more focussed on after 2003. Since child welfare interventions may take place in situations where there in a conflict of interests between parents and children, this development also signifies a shift away from prioritizing the parents, which is very easily done, towards paying more attention and even acting on children's views.

It is important to bear in mind that cases of child abuse and neglect have to follow the same procedures as all other child welfare cases even though a substantiated suspicion of in particular physical or sexual abuse may lead to a more rapid processing of the case. Reporting these cases to the police which in turn may but often do not lead to court cases according to the Penal Code, is not mandatory. Nor do we in Norway have a mandatory child abuse register. So while it is mandatory for others, like professionals in other helping services or in schools and kindergartens, to report cases of suspected serious abuse or neglect to the child welfare authorities, whether the police is notified or not will then depend on discretionary judgments made by the professionals within the child welfare system.

Norway's social and medical services for children are mainly public with relatively scant contributions from NGOs or other private initiatives. And most child welfare services, with the exception of more specialised out-of-home services, are organised at a municipal level. Indeed the presence of municipal child welfare authorities is regulated by law. And the number of child welfare professionals in a municipality varies greatly, depending on size. One recent survey of aftercare in Norwegian municipalities shows that the number of employees working with child welfare cases in a municipality varies from 0.2 to 100 (13). With few employees, it is very difficult to offer specialist services. Rather those present have to deal with the whole plethora of cases, and develop general skills. This may be one of the reasons why child abuse and neglect is so rarely the reason given for child welfare interventions.

THE STRENGTHS OF THE SYSTEM

One important strength of the system is its accessibility. The existence of child welfare authorities in every municipality, with a wide mandate and a primary focus on preventive services, makes the threshold for contacting the services fairly low. Although there will always be potential conflict, particularly if out of home placement of a child becomes imminent, some surveys show that parents in child welfare cases actually become more pleased with the services they receive over time. After a while the rates are on a par with the level of satisfaction with other services (14). Related to this is the access to services that are of real help to children, young people and their families. As long as the child welfare services have sufficient funding to pay for places in kindergarten, support persons, holidays for children, etc., these services can make a difference.

A second strength is the strong focus on parents' and children's rights, coupled with the accessibility of free legal advice in cases of conflict between authorities and clients. In addition comes several possibilities of appeal, which enables fair hearings of individual cases. And this is a strength although cases may take too long before a final decision is made, or individual decisions may be wrong from the perspective of the child welfare authorities.

A third strength is the focus on competence and knowledge on the part of the State. First, the Ministry of Children and Equality has initiated practice-relevant research activities in collaboration with the Directorate of Children, Young People and Families, where the explicit aim is to increase amount of practice that is knowledge-based or even evidence-based. As part of this strategy an electronically based library has been established, with easy access to existing literature. In addition short descriptions of particularly important issues, like foster home breakdown or talking with traumatized children, have been commissioned specially. Second, the Ministry has appointed an expert group to assess the need for restructuring the education of child welfare workers, in all probability ending with a recommendation to increase the length of the basic education to four or maybe even five years.

MAJOR CHALLENGES

As mentioned at the beginning of this article about 10% of Norway's population are immigrants. Although most of them come from other European countries, a sizeable proportion are for instance Pakistani, Afghan, Sri Lankan, Vietnamese, Turkish, Moroccan or Somali. One major challenge is, thus, how to develop culturally sensitive child welfare interventions and services while at the same time ensuring that children from ethnic minorities are guaranteed the same rights as others. Incidentally the same pertains to children from national minorities. One reason why the incidence and prevalence of physical abuse is thought to be fairly small is that corporal punishment is not very frequent in Norway, and, indeed, surveys showed that most Norwegian parents were against this form of punishment even before it was banned in 1982. Then conflicts arise when the child welfare authorities are confronted with child-rearing practices from other cultural settings, where spanking, for instance, may be acceptable.

Challenges and strengths tend to go hand in hand. While a focus on increased competence is a strength of the system, lack sufficient competence, particularly at the municipality level, is also a challenge at present. This entails all kinds of knowledge, about laws and regulations, methodologies, and research. This challenge is difficult to overcome, not in the least because Norway has so many very small municipalities with few professionals.

A third very serious challenge is lack of good and efficient interprofessional and inter-departmental collaboration. The Norwegian welfare state has primarily been built up since World War II, a process which has entailed the development of lots of different services with differing objectives. At the same time clients are whole persons, and there is a great need to counteract the fragmentization we see alongside greater specialization of services. The challenge in essence concerning a shift in focus from being service-led to being client-led, and of utilizing a life-course perspective in the work with children and young people. This is virtually impossible as long as the different services do not collaborate towards a common goal, related to the client.

REFERENCES

[1]   Statistics Norway www.ssb.no, 2009.

[2]   Department of Justice. The Children's White Paper No. 1 (2008-2009). On violence and abuse against children. Oslo: The Department of Justice.
        Available at: http://www.regjeringen.no/upload/JD/Vedlegg/Barnas_stortingsmelding_web.pdf

[3]   Department of Justice. Plan of action against violence in close relationships (2008-2011). Oslo: Dept Justice, 2008

[4]   Department of Children and Families. Strategy against sexual and physical abuse of children (2005-2009). Oslo: Dept Child Fam, 2005.

[5]   Building a Europe for and with children. 2009-2011 strategy: www.coe.int/children.

[6]   Sætre M, Jebsen E, Holter H. Tvang til seksualitet : en undersøkelse av seksuelle overgrep mot barn. [Forced sex: A study of child sexual abuse]. Oslo: Cappelen, 1986. [Norwegian]

[7]   Tambs K. Undersøkelse av seksuelle overgrep mot barn.[A study of child sexual abuse]. Oslo: Norwegian Health Ins,1994. [Norwegian]

[8]   Mossige S, Stefansen K, eds. Vold og overgrep mot barn og unge. [Violence and Abuse against children and adolescents]. Oslo: NOVA rapport, 2007. [Norwegian]

[9]   Schou L, Dyb G, Graff-Iversen, S. Voldsutsatt ungdom I Norge. [Youth and violence in Norway]. Oslo: Norwegian Health Inst, 2007. [Norwegian]

[10]   Backe-Hansen E. Rettferdiggjøring av omsorgsovertakelse. En beslutningsteoretisk analyse av saksbehandlernes argumentasjon i en serie saker om små barn. [The justice of out of home placement]. Oslo: NOVA, rapport 2/01, 2001. [Norwegian]

[11]   Gjerustad C, Grønningsæter A, Kvinge T, Mossige S, Vindegg J. Bare fantasien setter grenser? Om kommunenes bruk av hjelpetiltak i barnevernet. [Only fantasy sets the limits? The use of interventions within child protection agencies]. Oslo: Fafo-report 545, 2006. [Norwegian]

[12]   Christiansen Ø, Havnen K, Havik T. Mellom vern av barn og støtte til foreldre. Hva Vektlegger barnevernsarbeidere ved beslutninger i undersøkelsessaker? [Between child protection and help to parents]. Bergen: Barnevernets Utviklingssenter Vestlandet, report nr. 1, 1998.[Norwegian]

[13]   Oterholm I. Barneverntjenestens arbeid med ettervern. In: Bakketeig E, Backe-Hansen E, eds. Forskningskunnskap om ettervernet. [Research on after-care]. Oslo: NOVA, rapport 17, 2008. [Norwegian]

[14]   Sandbæk M. Barn og foreldre som sosiale aktører i møte med hjelpetjenester. [Children and parents as social actors in their meeting with services]. Oslo: NOVA, Report 14, 2002. [Norwegian]

In: International Aspects of Child Abuse and Neglect   ISBN: 978-1-60876-703-8
Editors: H. Dubowitz, J. Merrick pp. 139-148   © 2010 Nova Science Publishers, Inc.

Chapter 14

CHILD PROTECTION IN POLAND

Olga Kudanowska [*]
Nobody's Children Foundation, Warsaw, Poland

This chapter presents the Polish reality in the field of child protection, both in legislative terms and in respect of good practices. It discusses both the accomplishments and the weaknesses of the Polish child protection system, such as legislative gaps that make it difficult to combat child abuse and neglect effectively. Such gaps and imperfections require not only legislative amendments, but also a substantial change in attitudes among persons who learn about cases of child abuse or are responsible for prevention. The chapter emphasizes a strong need for systemic changes concerning not only intervention in cases of child abuse, but also what comes before and after such intervention. Only a comprehensive approach to the family and the child within the family may provide a basis for effective efforts.

INTRODUCTION

The issue of children's wellbeing and the protection of children's rights has grown in significance in recent years. Certainly, the main contributors to the promotion of children's right to protection from abuse have been numerous social campaigns initiated both by NGOs and government bodies and institutions, such as: "Childhood without Violence", organized by: State Agency for Prevention of Alcohol-Related Problems (PARPA), Nobody's Children Foundation, National Helpline for Victims of Domestic Violence "Blue Line" (2001); "Childhood under Protection", organized by: Ministry of Labour and Social Policy (2007); "See It, Hear It, Say It", organized by: Nobody's Children Foundation (2007); "I Love – I React", organized by: National Competence Centre Foundation, Ministry of Labour and Social Policy, Nobody's Children Foundation (2009).

Child protection efforts in Poland are decentralised. On the central (government) level issues related to minors are handled by the Ministry of Justice (efforts concerning child

[*] *Correspondence:* Olga Kudanowska, Nobody's Children Foundation, ul. Walecznych 59, 03-926 Warsaw, Poland. E-mail: olga.kudanowska@fdn.pl

victims of crime), the Ministry of Health (health care), Ministry of Labour and Social Policy (work with the family, social welfare services, and preventing domestic violence), Ministry of Education. Efforts for the benefit of children are also initiated by the Ombudsman who intervenes in specific cases and makes inquiries to government institutions concerning the protection of these children's rights. The institution obligated to protect children's rights is the Children's Ombudsman (CO). Pursuant to the act regulating the CO's work, the person in this position may examine specific cases and demand that adequate proceedings be instigated (1). However, the CO's competence is still insufficient to protect children's rights effectively. Therefore, child protection efforts remain spread across many institutions and services, with a substantial proportion of them having been taken over by NGOs.

DEFINITION OF CHILD ABUSE AND NEGLECT

In the Polish law there is no clear definition of child abuse or neglect. The broad concept of child abuse includes offences against children and threats to their wellbeing (e.g., by neglecting a child).

OFFENCES AGAINST CHILDREN

The Polish Penal Code (3) penalizes a number of offences against a minor, including:

- Maltreatment of a minor or another family member by deliberately inflicting physical pain or moral suffering on the person (mental or physical maltreatment; article 207);
- Causing damage to someone's health (articles 156 & 157), e.g., by beating a child;
- Exposing a child to an immediate danger of loss of life / severe damage to health (article 160), e.g., by starving a child, extreme health neglect, or leaving a young child under dangerous circumstances without supervision;
- Abandoning a minor under 15 years (article 210) – deliberate abandonment by a person obligated to care for the child (actual caregiver, parent, foster family, etc.);
- Violation of personal integrity (article 217), involving any instance of hitting another person, jerking, pushing, etc. Although violation of child's integrity formally can be interpreted as a crime, it is still not considered as a form of abuse or neglect in Poland.

The following sexual offences should also be listed:

- Rape (article 197), i.e., subjecting another person to a sexual intercourse or making him/her submit to another sexual act or perform such an act by force, illegal threat or deceit;
- Abusing a relationship of dependence (article 199), which plays a significant role in institutional abuse. This offence involves subjecting another person to sexual intercourse or making him/her submit to another sexual act or perform such an act by

abusing a relationship of dependence or taking advantage of the victim's critical situation;

- Paedophilia (article 200) or having a sexual intercourse with a child under 15;
- Pornography (article 202), including: distributing, producing, recording, possessing, disseminating or public presentation of pornographic material involving a minor (so called hard pornography).

THREAT TO A CHILD'S WELLBEING

The Family and Guardianship Code (4) does not define the concept of a threat to a child's wellbeing. It only provides that if a child's wellbeing is threatened, the family court shall make appropriate decisions concerning the child's parents. Neglecting a child by a person obligated to care for him/her (e.g., by malnutrition, educational neglect, or health-related neglect) constitutes such a threat.

THE EXTENT OF THE PROBLEM

Despite a growing number of facilities that help abused children, Poland still does not have a national system of institutions offering assistance in all cases and forms of abuse, in accordance with common standards. Consequently, there are no national records (registers) helpful in the assessment of the scale and prevalence of child abuse in Poland. The only available data are police and court statistics.

According to the police statistics in 2007 more than 45,000 children under 18 years in Poland, including 31,000 children under 13 years, experienced domestic violence. The police records also show that between 1999 and 2007 the number of child victims of sexual abuse was relatively stable and amounted to 1,500-2,000 cases annually.

Corporal punishment of children seems an established child-rearing method in Poland. Only 35% of parents think that this form of punishment should never be used against children. Fifty percent believe that corporal punishment is sometimes justified and 13% express the opinion that parents may beat their children whenever they see it as an effective child-rearing method (5).

Corporal punishment is a commonly used disciplinary measure in Polish families – only one fifth of adult Poles did not experience this form of punishment in their childhood. Today's parents report using different forms of corporal punishment against their children, including spanking (80%), beating with a belt (25%), and slapping on the face (8%). Five percent of the respondents (parents) admit that they have beaten their child severely, causing an injury; most of them describe such events as rare (6).

Forty four percent of adult Poles believe that the scale of child sexual abuse in Poland has grown during the past 10 years (6). This may result from increased media coverage of the problem – since 2000 the number of press articles on child sexual abuse has grown nearly tenfold (7). However, the number of recorded criminal offences defined by article 200 of the Polish Penal Code has been relatively stable; in 2006 1687 such offences were recorded in criminal files.

Sixteen percent of adult women and 12% of men reported in a retrospective survey that they experienced various forms of sexual abuse by adults (penetration, touching, indecent exposure, presentation of pornographic material) before the age of 15 years (6).

In 2004, 8% of institutionalized children aged 15-18 experienced rape or forced sexual intercourse. Most of the victims (79%) reported that they knew the perpetrator. Forty three percent described the perpetrator as their peer. Ten percent of the respondents had sexual intercourse with an adult when they were under 15 years (7).

THE SYSTEM OF RESPONDING TO CHILD ABUSE AND NEGLECT

Under the Polish law it is obligatory for everyone to inform law enforcement bodies about offences and to notify the family court about threats to children's wellbeing. It is so called "social obligation", so a person who fails to fulfil it will not bear any liability. This obligation arises from article 572 of the Code of Civil Procedure (8) and article 304 of the Code of Criminal Procedure (9). These articles impose also a legal obligation to report child abuse to appropriate bodies. This responsibility lies primarily with organizations and facilities providing care for children, as well as government and local-authority institutions that have learned about child abuse in the course of their work. This obligation has been reinforced by article 12 of the Family Violence Prevention Act (10) which provides that any person who, while performing his/her professional duties, suspects that an offence has been committed with the use of violence against family members (including children), should report the case immediately to the police or the prosecutor.

In the Polish legal system a failure to fulfil this obligation does not translate directly into clearly defined legal consequences. However, if it has been neglected by a public officer, the person may be penalized for the offence of failing to comply with statutory obligations. It also appears that a failure to fulfil the mandatory reporting obligation may result in disciplinary responsibility of the person (e.g., a school or kindergarten staff member or a nurse).

The system of responding to child abuse comprises a number of intervention paths. If a child's wellbeing is threatened (by neglect), a civil intervention should be taken in a family case, with the goal to supervise the persons who exercise the parental authority or take care of the child. If an offence against a child has been committed, both the criminal and civil paths are appropriate. The criminal path aims at holding the perpetrator responsible for the illegal act. As already stated, such an intervention should be initiated by the person who has learned about an instance of child abuse (by submitting a notice of an offence or a request to examine the child's situation). However, if a criminal court develops a suspicion of child abuse while conducting its proceedings, it should also notify a competent family court about the case.

Apart from the strict legal intervention in cases of child abuse, there is also social intervention, regulated by the Social Welfare Act (11). Social workers may, even ex officio, i.e., without a motion submitted by an authorised person, provide social welfare services, not only in the form of financial or non-cash benefits, but also by supporting the family and working with its members. Therefore, information reported to the local Social Services Centre is sufficient for social workers to initiate efforts to help a family in need. Social services are provided on the basis of a family assessment conducted by a social worker. The goal of the assessment is to learn about the family's life circumstances and to diagnose problems that can be addressed by the social welfare services. Importantly, providing any social help depends on the beneficiary's (the family's) willingness to cooperate. Lack of such cooperation constitutes a basis for a refusal to provide social services (12). As mentioned earlier, the following institutions may take part in interventions in cases of child abuse: prosecutor's office / police (criminal path), family court (civil path), and Social Services Centre (social intervention).

Despite these three services' possible involvement, there are no centralised efforts for the benefit of children. There is no one, dedicated institution to guide the child through all the procedures and to monitor the child's situation during the intervention and afterwards. To fill the gap, interdisciplinary groups (often informal ones) have begun to be established in Poland to work out comprehensive solutions for particular families. These groups consist of police officers, social workers, lawyers, psychologists, and representatives of NGOs and local-authority organizations. Their composition may change depending on the requirements and circumstances of specific cases (13). The interdisciplinary approach enables comprehensive assessment of the problem, which is impossible for either the criminal court or the family court acting alone, because it exceeds the competence of each of these bodies.

RESPONSE TO REPORTED CHILD ABUSE AND NEGLECT

When an offence against a child is reported, criminal proceedings should be instigated. The obligations of the police and the prosecutor's office depend on the type of the offence committed. Generally speaking, there are three types of offences in the Polish legal system:

- prosecuted ex officio,
- prosecuted upon complaint (by the offended party),
- prosecuted upon private accusation.

In case of offences prosecuted ex officio, law enforcement bodies have an obligation to instigate and conduct proceedings and if the suspected offence is confirmed, they are required to bring indictment and substantiate it before the court. Most offences listed in the penal code are prosecuted ex officio.

In case of offences prosecuted upon complaint, law enforcement bodies cannot instigate any proceedings unless it is requested by the victim. A child is represented by his or her statutory representative – a parent with the parental authority or a guardian. If the guardian/parent is the perpetrator of the offence and does not file a request to instigate proceedings, the family court may appoint a guardian ad litem to take this particular action. Rape in one example of an offence prosecuted upon complaint. If a child under 15 years of age is the victim of rape, the offender commits two crimes – rape and paedophilia. Then the complaint is not needed.

In case of offences prosecuted upon private accusation, the bill of indictment is brought to the criminal court by the victim (or – on behalf of a child victim – by his/her statutory representative). This category of offences includes violation of bodily integrity or causing disturbance of health for a period shorter than 7 days.

For instance: if the child is a victim of paedophilia, prosecutor has a legal obligation to instigate and conduct criminal proceeding (offence prosecuted ex officio). But if the child is over 15 years of age (so paedophilia doesn't occur) and is a victim of rape, the parent of a child, before prosecutor instigates the proceeding, has to file a petition for conducting his proceedings. Otherwise a prosecutor has no right to conduct it (offence prosecuted upon complaint). In the case where the child is a victim of a violation of personal integrity (e.g. hitting without any serious injuries), a public prosecutor will not conduct the proceedings at all. The role of private prosecutor will be played by the legal representative of a child, e.g. his/her parent. Notice of an offence prosecuted ex officio or upon complaint (after the complaint is filed) makes it obligatory for law enforcement bodies to instigate proceedings. The prosecutor or the police supervised by a prosecutor should take adequate action in order to determine whether an offence has been committed and to identify the perpetrator. This is accomplished in the course of evidentiary proceedings. If the suspected offence is confirmed, the prosecutor's office brings indictment to the criminal court and argues the case in the court. During the court proceedings the whole evidentiary procedure is repeated – in accordance with the rule that the court has to handle each piece of evidence directly.

In cases of sexual offences against children and violence in the family, a new article, 185a, has been introduced to the Code of Criminal Procedure. It ensures that already at the stage of preparatory proceedings the judge interviews a child victim with the participation of a psychology expert. Such an interview does not need to be repeated during the court trial. However, this mode is applied only in situations when the victim is under 15 at the time of interviewing. Such an interview should be recorded and can then played back in the court room (14).

In order to enhance child protection in criminal proceedings, the Nobody's Children Foundation has initiated a programme called "Child Victim Advocate" in 4 Polish towns and cities (Warsaw, Szczecin, Bialystok, and Grudziadz). The goal of the programme is to provide knowledge and support for child victims' parents and caregivers. Moreover, volunteers working in the programme prepare the child to participate in the legal procedure by offering psychological support and accompanying him/her in court (15). Such efforts will be also incorporated in the Ministry of Justice's new initiative – a programme called "Help Network for Victims" (16).

The perpetrator's responsibility for the committed crime is not limited to the conviction and the sentence (e.g., a fine, restriction of liberty – community work, or imprisonment). In some cases the court may apply other measures, such as:

- a ban on holding certain positions, practicing certain professions, or running certain types of businesses;
- a ban on running any activity associated with child rearing, health care, education, and other care services;
- an order to stay away from certain environments and places, an order prohibiting any contact with certain persons (including the victim) or a ban on leaving the current place of residence without the court's permission.

Undertaking civil intervention in a family case may involve filing a request to examine the situation of the family or the child. Such a request should include information about threats to the child's wellbeing. Having received such information, the court should order an assessment to evaluate the family's life circumstances and determine whether there has been any neglect or abuse. Then the court may instigate proceedings – ex officio – concerning the rights of the child's parents or caregivers. The main directive that should be followed by the court is to act in the best interest of the child.

Pursuant to article 109 of the Family and Guardianship Code, when a child's wellbeing is threatened, the court may obligate his/her parents to certain behaviour; specify which actions may be taken by the parents without the court's permission; or subject the exercise of the parental authority to permanent supervision. As a rule, the court should limit parental rights gradually – starting from the most lenient measures to apply more severe ones only if there is no desirable effect. The most extreme measure involves placing the child in a foster family or a residential care institution.

It is also possible in the Polish legal system to deprive a child's parents of the parental authority, especially if they abuse their power or grossly neglect their parental obligations. This measure, however, is applied only in extreme situations, e.g., when a parent has committed an offence against his/her child. It is also possible to prohibit parents being in touch with a child.

Unfortunately, after placing the child in a foster family or a residential care institution, the family is not provided with any special support or social assistance. Because of that the level of its educational / child-rearing abilities or coping skills does not improve. Consequently, the chances for the child's return to the family are poor. Such cases require intense work with the biological family, professional training, and parenting skills workshops to prepare the family for the child's return. Unfortunately, often biological families from which children have been removed, are not provided with comprehensive support.

It should be also mentioned that Poland does not have adequate substitute care resources to provide appropriate family conditions for abused children. In 2007, there were nearly 44 thousand foster families in Poland, providing care for almost 65 thousand abused children. Still, there were more than 700 residential care institutions (17), in which children were placed. Several systemic problems (e.g., lack of support, insufficient training for foster families, difficulties to obtain the status of a professional foster family) result in a small number of candidates. Consequently, future development of foster care in Poland is uncertain (18).

It is worth mentioning another mode of placing a child outside his/her family – the urgent mode. The family court is competent to ensure a child's safety immediately, e.g., by placing him/her in a foster family in the protection mode. Also, the police are authorised to remove a child from his/her family in the urgent mode. Legislative work is underway to introduce amendments that will grant this authority to social workers as well, when there is an immediate threat to a child (19). A child removed from his/her family in the urgent mode is usually placed in an emergency shelter or a foster family acting as an emergency family care service. The child's placement in such an environment should be later legitimised by the family court. Such a situation should always lead to instigating legal proceedings ex officio – it is a signal for the family court that something seriously wrong has been happening in this family.

STRENGTHS OF THE SYSTEM

The main strength of the Polish child protection system is that the law clearly specifies a legal obligation to report child abuse, including the obligation to exchange information among various services (e.g., the criminal and family court). The public awareness of this obligation – including among professionals who work with children – has been increasing.

Moreover, the legal system enables NGOs to play a growing role in combating and preventing child abuse, by ensuring great flexibility of their actions. NGOs, which are resistant to transient political influences, may significantly improve the situation of abused children by acting directly for the benefit of children and their families, and through training and lobbying activities.

WEAKNESSES AND CHALLENGES OF THE SYSTEM

Despite these strengths, the Polish system of responding to child abuse is still seriously lacking and likely to fail. Despite the legal obligation to report child abuse and the growing public awareness of this obligation, it continues to raise doubt, especially among professionals. Employees of institutions such as schools, kindergartens, hospitals, and health care clinics seem to have low motivation to intervene in cases of suspected child abuse. The reasons for failing to undertake intervention in such cases include a fear of making a mistake, being afraid of the perpetrator, lack of clear principles of responding to suspected child abuse, and – if the perpetrator is another professional – reluctance to denounce a colleague. This lack of motivation results in a small number of reported cases and, very frequently, a failure to intervene in cases that clearly require intervention.

Another weakness of the Polish system is the lack of specialised child protection services, which leads to frequent incompetence and diffusion of responsibility for the wellbeing of children and their families. There is still no place to report child neglect or abuse, except to police and the court. In most cases these institutions do not make a quick assessment and they are not able to act effectively.

Practice also shows that there is no comprehensive collaboration among various services for the benefit of a child and his/her family. The emerging interdisciplinary approach encounters legal obstacles, e.g., difficulties associated with regulations concerning the protection of personal data. Legislative changes cannot keep up with practical advances.

CONTROVERSIES

A person who has found out about child abuse almost always has some doubt about whether to intervene. In many cases two conflicting values need to be balanced: cohesion of the child's family and the objective wellbeing of the child. On the one hand, the child's family poses a threat to his/her wellbeing, but on the other hand, there is a concern that the child may be taken away from the biological family and – if no foster family is found – placed in residential care.

As mentioned earlier, another problem involves choosing the right manner of intervention, i.e., deciding whether the suspected case of child abuse should be reported only to social services or to the court, too. Such decisions are often wrong, i.e., either the police or the family court are notified when there is no basis for doing so, or the obligation to inform these institutions is neglected in situations when they should intervene. For instance, a social worker may not report a suspected case of physical violence against a child in spite of obvious evidence, e.g., characteristic bruises on the child's back and legs. Such a social worker may limit his/her intervention to working with the violent parent, whereas in cases of evident violence there should be no barrier to reporting abuse to the police.

Another problematic issue involves the timing of intervention. For example, should a professional who works with an abused child and his/her family, wait for the effects of this social work, or rather undertake intervention immediately? It is very difficult to identify the right moment. Some interventions, however, are clearly belated, for example, when employees of a school report that a child is beaten by his/her parents after having observed evidence of such violence for two years!

PREVENTION OF CHILD ABUSE

Regrettably, efforts to prevent child abuse are insufficient in Poland.. There is not a dedicated government programme defining firm steps to be taken to ensure effective prevention. Much of the preventive work is done by NGOs that offer services for families at risk of child abuse. One example is a programme carried out by the Nobody's Children Foundation, "Good Parent – Good Start." Within the programme, professionals conduct workshops for parents with young children, train other professionals in identifying risk factors, and initiate cooperation among services to ensure more effective prevention (20). As part of the programme, close cooperation between local health care facilities and Social Services Centres was established in one Warsaw district. This cooperation involves exchange of information about families at risk, which enables a fast response and makes it possible to prepare a set of services to meet each family's individual needs. In this way, the risk of child abuse in the future is significantly reduced.

CONCLUSIONS

In sum, the Polish child protection system is still far from perfect and requires enormous work and effort, including legislative changes and the development of good practices. Raising public awareness of the need to respond to child abuse, and teaching people how to identify abuse and make decisions appropriate to the actual risk, are the main challenges that are still faced by government and local-authority institutions and NGOs in Poland. These institutions and organisations also have to face the need for comprehensive, multidisciplinary work aimed at prevention and responding optimally to child abuse and neglect.

ACKNOWLEDGMENTS

Monika Sajkowska is thanked for her important contribution to this chapter.

REFERENCES

[1]   Ustawa z dnia 6 stycznia 2000 r. o Rzeczniku Praw Dziecka, Dz.U. Nr 6, poz. 69 ze zmian. [Act of 6 January 2000 on the Child's Ombudsman. J Laws 2000;6:69, with amendments].

[2]   Olszewska A., Kudanowska O. „Prawa dzieci-ofiar przemocy w rodzinie – analiza", „Polski Raport Social Watch 2008. Czas na prawa", Warszawa: Koalicja KARAT 2008.

[3]   Ustawa z dnia 6 czerwca 1997 r. - Kodeks karny, Dz.U. Nr 88, poz. 553 ze zmian. [Act of 6 June 1997, Penal Code. J Laws 1997;88:553, with amendments].

[4]   Ustawa z dnia 25 lutego 1964 r. – Kodeks rodzinny i opiekunczy, Dz.U. Nr 9 poz. 59 ze zmian. [Act of 25 February 1964, Family and Guardianship Code. J Laws 1964;9:59, with amendments].

[5]   Research of FDN & OBOP, 2005

[6]   Fluderska G, Sajkowska M. Problem krzywdzenia dzieci. Postawy i doswiadczenia doroslych Polaków. Raport z badan, Fundacja Dzieci Niczyje, Warszawa, 2001.

[7]   Sajkowska M. Wiktymizacja wychowanków domów dziecka, Fundacja Dzieci Niczyje, 2005.

[8]   Ustawa z dnia 17 listopada 1964 r. - Kodeks postepowania cywilnego, Dz.U. Nr 43, poz. 296. [Act of 17 November 1964, Code of Civil Procedure. J Laws 1964;43:269, with amendments].

[9]   Ustawa z dnia 6 czerwca 1997 r. - Kodeks postepowania karnego, Dz.U. Nr 141, poz. 1181. [Act of 6 June 1997, code of Criminal Procedure. J Laws 1997;141:1181, with amendments].

[10]   Ustawa z dnia 29 lipca 2005 r. o przeciwdzialaniu przemocy w rodzinie, Dz.U. Nr 180 poz. 1493. [Act of 29 July 2005 about Family Violence Prevention. J Laws 2005;180:1493, with amendments].

[11]   Ustawa z dnia 12 marca 2004 r. o pomocy spolecznej, tekst jednolity: Dz. U. 2008 r. Nr 115, poz. 728. [Social Welfare Act of 12 March 2004, consolidated text. J Laws 2004;115:728, with amendments].

[12]   Decision by the Supreme Administrative Court of the Republic of Poland of 2 October 2008, I OSK 38/2008, http://orzeczenia.nsa.gov.pl.

[13]   Drozdowski L., „System Opieki nad Dzieckiem i Rodzina - od modelu do realizacji". In: „Systemowa pomoc dzieciom - ofiarom przestepstw, krzywdzenia i zaniedbywania. Dziecko krzywdzone. Teoria. Badania. Praktyka" No. 23/2008.

[14]   Wesolowska A. „Regulacje prawne dotyczace ochrony maloletnich w toku postepowania karnego", Warszawa: Fundacja Dzieci Niczyje, 2007.

[15]   Podlewska J., „Opiekun dziecka - ofiary przestepstwa" Warszawa: Fundacja Dzieci Niczyje, 2006.

[16]   http://www.ms.gov.pl.

[17]   Statistics of the Polish Ministry of Labour and Social Policy for 2007, http://www.mpips.gov.pl.

[18]   Dobrzynski L., „Raport o problemach rodzicielstwa zastepczego w Polsce", Warszawa 2006 (unpublished).

[19]   Draft amendment to the Family Violence Prevention Act submitted by the Ministry of Labour and Social Policy, accepted by the Council of Ministers on 3 February 2009 and submitted to Sejm (the lower chamber of the Polish Parliament), http://www.mpips.gov.pl.

[20]   http://www.dobryrodzic.pl.

In: International Aspects of Child Abuse and Neglect
Editors: H. Dubowitz, J. Merrick pp. 149-160

ISBN: 978-1-60876-703-8
© 2010 Nova Science Publishers, Inc.

Chapter 15

CHILD MALTREATMENT IN RUSSIA

Tatiana N Balachova, Barbara L Bonner, and Irina A Alexeeva

Center on Child Abuse and Neglect, Department of Pediatrics,
University of Oklahoma Health Science Center, Oklahoma, United States of America and
New Steps, Saint Petersburg Foundation for Crisis Psychological Help for Children and
Youth, Saint Petersburg, Russia

The aim of this chapter is to discuss the evolution of child protection and the development of services for abused and neglected children and families in Russia. The chapter begins with an introduction that brings an historical prospective to the discussion. Definitions of child abuse and neglect and laws related to child maltreatment and child protection are described. Although the incidence and prevalence of child maltreatment in Russia are unknown, available statistics indicate that children in Russia experience physical and sexual abuse, neglect, and psychological maltreatment similar to children in other regions of the world. Changes in the laws and services that have been made recently to improve prevention and services for children and families are discussed. The authors conclude that the absence of an organized child abuse reporting and investigation, systems, established policies for case management, and a system to monitor parental progress limits the implementation of laws and the ability of professionals to intervene and prevent child maltreatment. Child abuse and neglect is an interdisciplinary problem and an integrated response and coordinated work by professionals from different disciplines is necessary to advance child protection in Russia.

INTRODUCTION

Until the late 1980s, statistics on social problems such as child maltreatment were not publicly known in Russia, and data on negative issues were not allowed to be published in the press or in professional literature. Children in Russia were experiencing physical, sexual abuse, neglect or psychological maltreatment similar to children in other regions of the world, but there was no recognition of child abuse in families or in institutions. If a child was abused by a parent the termination of parental rights was the only legal action available, as restriction of parental rights was not a legal option, even on a temporary basis. Only cases of severe neglect, typically along with parental alcohol addiction, would be investigated and lead to termination of parental rights. Terminating parental rights was a long and complicated procedure and the child could not be removed from the parents until their rights were terminated. The milicia (police) were responsible to care for street children and children who ran away from their families or institutions, and Police Collection and Distribution Departments were established to house children found on the streets. After identification, a child would be referred for permanent placement in an institution, such as a Children's Home, or sent back to their parents, typically without recognition and investigation of possible child abuse or neglect. There were no transitional programs or shelters to provide services for these children.

At the beginning of "Perestroika" in the late 1980s, information about these issues became available for the public and professionals. The term Child Abuse and Neglect (CAN) was introduced in Russia in the early 1990s and the first training on child abuse and neglect for Russian professionals was conducted in St. Petersburg in 1991. In 1990, Russia signed the United Nations Convention on the Rights of the Child (UNCRC). Since the 1990s, public awareness and professional knowledge about CAN have increased and the Russian government has initiated actions designed to reduce juvenile delinquency, address the needs of families with children, and increase birth rates in the country (1,2).

HOW ARE THE DIFFERENT TYPES OF CAN DEFINED?

There are currently a number of laws and acts related to child protection in Russia. However, there are no uniform legal definitions or special statues focusing specifically on CAN. There are no specific definitions for different types of abuse; maltreatment is addressed in separate articles of various laws and codes.

An early example of child protection in Russia was a statute introduced in the Russia Code on Marriage and Family in 1968 (3) that included improper child rearing as one of the legal justifications for termination of parental rights. Since the 1990s, a number of laws, government resolutions, and regulations have been signed to implement the UNCRC. The major documents, the 1995 Family Code of the Russian Federation (4) and the Federal Law on Basic Guarantees of the Rights of the Child in the Russian Federation (5), included improper rearing but did not specify forms of CAN. More recent laws include "On the Prevention of Child Neglect and Juvenile Delinquency" (6). In its recent additions, the law defines a "beznadzornii" (neglected) child – a child who is lacking control on his behavior because of parents or others who, by law or because of job duties, are responsible for childrearing, but do not perform the duties for childrearing, education, and/or support; a child in danger as a child who is at risk for harm to health or life because of neglect or street life or a situation that does not meet the child's needs, or conducts delinquent or antisocial acts; and a family in social danger as a family with children in a precarious social situation or one in which the parents or legal representatives of minors do not perform their duties in rearing their children, such as providing an education, supporting them, negatively affecting their behavior, or being cruel to them (6).

The Family Code states that parental rights may not take precedence in a conflict with the child's rights and "parents may not harm the physical or mental health or moral development of the child. Child rearing should exclude neglect, abuse, vulgar, degrading treatment, insulting or exploitation of children" (4). Grounds for terminating parental rights are defined as follows: "neglecting to perform parenting duties, including paying child support; abandonment of a child at a maternity or other hospital; abuse of parental rights; abuse of the child by conducting physical or mental violence against the child or violating child's sexual integrity; parental alcoholism or substance dependency; or intentionally committing crimes against the life or health of the child or the spouse" (4).

Several aspects that affect the definitions of CAN can be found in the Russian Criminal Code (7). These include Failure to perform parenting (childrearing) duties and Leaving in danger, which address the endangerment of a child as well as a person with limited abilities because of age or disability. Failure to perform parenting is defined as failure or improper performing of child rearing responsibilities by a parent or other person responsible to care for the child, as well as teachers or other persons working in education, childcare, medicine, or any institution that is obliged to supervise minors if the act involves abuse (cruelty) toward the minor. The Code includes torture which is defined as causing physical or mental suffering through systematic beatings or other violent acts against a minor or a person known to be in a helpless state of either material or other dependency on the perpetrator, as well as individuals who are kidnapped or taken hostage. Other articles relevant to the abuse of both adults and children are kidnapping of a person, illegal deprivation of freedom, the use of slave labor, and trafficking.

Sexual abuse of minors is covered in the Criminal Code in special articles focused on sexual crimes against minors, including sexual intercourse and other acts of a sexual nature and debauchery with a person younger than 16 years by a person 18 or older. In addition, several articles include sexual crimes against both adult and child victims with more significant punishment for crimes against minors. These include rape of a person known to be a minor, other acts of a sexual nature with the use of force, coercing a person to perform acts of a sexual nature, and involving minors in prostitution. Rape, according to the Code, is sexual intercourse accomplished by force or the threat of force to a victim (female) or any other person or by using a vulnerable state of the victim. In addition, the Criminal Code includes involving minors in conducting criminal or antisocial behaviors, which are defined as systematic use of drugs, alcohol, or other substances; prostitution; vagrancy or begging; and other actions which violate the rights or legitimate interests of others.

In summary, while professionals working with maltreated children and their families use the definitions recommended by international organizations such as UNICEF, the World Health Organization, and the International Society for the Prevention of Child Abuse and Neglect (ISPCAN.org), CAN is not a formally defined and utilized term in Russian law. The maltreatment of children is addressed in Russian law, but the separation of different aspects across multiple laws and statutes weakens the overall recognition of CAN as a major problem. This lack of clarity and a specific legal definition of CAN significantly affects the recognition of abuse and the protection of children.

WHAT IS KNOWN ABOUT THE EXTENT OF THE PROBLEM?

The incidence and prevalence of child maltreatment in Russia are unknown. No major studies have been conducted to date to formally estimate the occurrence of child maltreatment; its magnitude can only be estimated indirectly. There is no reporting or federal registration system for CAN cases and consequently there are no official numbers. Statistics on different aspects of the problem are provided by different ministries. In 2004, the Ministry of Health and Social Development of the Russian Federation reported that 65,200 children were deprived of parental care because their parents' rights were terminated (8). Since termination of parental rights represents only the most severe cases of CAN, that figure can be seen as the minimum number of children experiencing CAN. It can be estimated that the number of CAN cases that are investigated but do not have parental rights terminated is significantly higher than the number of terminations. Additionally, as in all countries, it is known that the number of cases that are never reported is much higher than the number of known cases.

While there are no official figures for the incidence of child maltreatment in Russia, some data indicate significant problems for children: an estimated 730,000 children live without parental care, over 180,000 children live in institutions and between 20,000 and 100,000 children live on the streets,. The Moscow Helsinki Group indicated that each year approximately two million children under 14 years of age are victims of domestic violence and approximately 50,000 children run away from home to avoid this problem (11). In Moscow, 78.6% of street children reported that they experienced corporal punishment at home, and of these, 44.4% reported injuries and wounds as a result (12). Another survey of street children reported that 92% of children reported running away from home because of physical or other abuse (13).

There are a number of indications that different forms of child maltreatment may be widespread in Russia. Every year approximately 15,000 minors under age 14 die, with 50 per cent of them dying of unnatural causes, and more than 2,000 from murder or severe physical abuse (8). Frequently, these deaths are the result of the failure of parental care and supervision (9). The majority of physical abuse cases are committed by parents, including 1,080 documented murders of children by parents between 2000 and 2005 (10).

The recognition of child sexual abuse is limited in Russia and different government agencies and ministries report data separately. The Ministry of Interior's Government Analytical Information Centre reported almost 6,000 crimes of a sexual nature committed against minors in 2004 (9). The report stated that six adolescents were victims of murders connected with sexual violence; 2,091 children were raped; 2,103 children faced violence of a sexual nature; and 1,086 children faced indecent treatment of a sexual nature. The involvement of children in prostitution, sex tourism, child pornography, and sexual exploitation on the Internet has been an increasing concern. One out of five street children reported being sexually harassed by adults (14) and between 20 and 30% of street children under the age of 18 reported being involved in prostitution or the production of pornography (14).

Child neglect is a major factor in child deprivation and termination of parental rights. There is a strong association between neglect, poverty, and parental substance abuse and Russia is a country with very high rates of alcohol use (15). A survey of street children reported that many children "did not want to go home because their parents were alcoholics and their homes had been turned into underworld hangouts" (14). Many children who experience chronic neglect and parental exploitation leave home and live on the streets. A survey of experts working with children in Moscow indicated that there were between 30,000 and 50,000 street children; 50 to 60 percent of them were under 13 (14). In 2004, 32,600 children voluntarily left their homes because of difficult situations in the home, 61,600 children were missing (8), and the Russian Deputy Prosecutor-General reported that the number of street children in Russia continued to increase (10).

THE SYSTEM(S) TO ADDRESS CAN

Since the concept of CAN is not clearly defined, recognized, and investigated, a comprehensive infrastructure dedicated to CAN, such as state and federal child protection agencies, trained investigators, etc., has not been developed. However, changes have been made in the laws that can expand the protection of children. During the 1990s, the Russian government signed more than 140 laws designed to prevent juvenile delinquency, improve the protection of children, and bring Russian legislation into line with the Convention on the Rights of the Child (CRC) (16). Several important changes in Russian legislation have been made recently, including criminalization of trafficking or involving a child in producing pornography, strengthening punishment of adults for sexual solicitation and sexual contacts with children, and raising the age of sexual consent from 14 to 16 years old. However, the lack of a clear legal definition of child pornography and barriers to law enforcement to hold organized crime groups liable for the selling of child pornography leave children vulnerable to sexual abuse and exploitation (9).

Federal laws assign the provision of prevention measures and assistance for children to a wide range of agencies and commissions. They are obligated to ensure the rights and legitimate interests of minors and implement measures to protect them against all forms of discrimination, physical or psychological abuse, insult, rude treatment, and sexual or other exploitation. There are three agencies that have the authority to act in situations of child maltreatment, including 1) the Commission for Juvenile Affairs and Protection of their Rights: this commission may issue a warning to a parent, order a parent to pay a fine, and/or prepare and submit documents to a court for termination of parental rights; 2) the Offices for Guardianship and Custody (OGC): these offices may remove children from a family if there is a threat for their life or health, or prepare and submit documents to a court for termination of parental rights; and 3) the Offices for Internal Affairs: this office may remove a child from a family if there is a threat to the child's life or health.

If the circumstances are beyond the parent's control, such as a mental disorder, chronic disease, or a combination of difficult circumstances, the parents' rights may be restricted rather than terminated. In 1995, the Family Code first allowed for a child to be removed from parents/custodians by the OGC in extreme cases or when a direct threat to the life and health of the child is found. Such child protection actions were new for Russia and laws and policies are still undergoing revisions. Termination of parental rights is a more common practice than restricting parental rights and there is no system in place to provide and monitor services for families with restricted rights. The restriction of parental rights is a relatively new type of court intervention for Russia. Restriction of parental rights is intended to provide parents some time to correct conditions that caused the child to be removed from home.

The latest revision of the law indicates that the prosecutor should be notified immediately and a "deprived child" hearing should be conducted within seven days of removal (4). In April 2008, a new law On Guardianship and Custody was signed. This law introduced "host families" who can provide temporary emergency placements for children who have been removed. In Russia the term foster families refers to families that take a deprived child, intending to adopt or provide a permanent placement. Host and foster families typically receive financial assistance and substantial services, and there is a procedure to remove a child and take another child if the placement does not work well. Under the 2008 law, the OGC is responsible for placing orphans and deprived children in host and foster families (4). If the parent does not change the behaviour within six months after the court decision, the Office for Custody and Guardianship files a petition for termination of parental rights. The petition may be filed earlier if this is in the best interests of the child.

In accordance with the Family Code, parental rights that have been terminated may be restored if the parent files a petition to the court and demonstrates changes in behavior, lifestyle, and (or) attitudes toward parenting and such action is in the best interests of the child. The Office of Custody and Guardianship is involved in such cases; if the child is older than ten, restoration of parental rights is possible only with the child's consent. Parental rights may not be restored if the child has been adopted by another family.

However, this important law has not been implemented effectively. Termination remains more common than restriction of parental rights, and cases of restoration of parental rights are rare. There are no regulations or practices to provide court-ordered treatment for families when parental rights are restricted or terminated, and there is no child protection system in place to monitor parents' progress in treatment. As a result, in 2006 the family reunification rates were similar to those of 2001: the rights of parents of 1,993 children were terminated compared to only 25 cases of restoring parental rights, and 73 cases of restricting parental rights in St. Petersburg, a ratio of 1 restriction case to 27 terminations. These statistics show a stable but problematic trend in the ratio of the restriction of parental rights compared to terminations: the ratio was 1 restriction to 15 terminations in 2003 and 1:20 in 2005 (17). The implementation of this law has not led to an increase in family reunifications; termination of parental rights has risen in Russia by 40 percent between 1999 and 2004 (8).

HOW DOES THE SYSTEM WORK REGARDING REPORTING OF SUSPECTED CAN?

The absence of a child abuse reporting and investigation system significantly hinders the ability of professionals to intervene and prevent further abuse, even when it is recognised. However, some changes to the basis of a legal framework of child protection have been made. The Family Code established important directives, such as a requirement for professionals and other citizens who become aware of danger to the health or life of a child or violations of a child's rights or lawful interests, to report this to a local Office of Guardianship and Custody OGC (18).

Although the Family Code provides for mandatory reporting, a mechanism for the implementation of this article has not been established. Professionals have not been made aware of the reporting requirements, the implementation of the laws is very limited. Sanctions for failure to report or failure to act do not exist, and a definition for evaluating the "threat to life and health… or a violation of the child's rights…" has not been established. Procedures for removing a child by making a report to an OGC or to the milicia (police) have been established in most regions of Russia, but these are typically used only in the most severe cases. In cases of less severe CAN, actions are determined mainly by the initiative of the professionals who handle the case and the level of the local child protection system. Because policies and a mechanism of professional collaboration have not been established in most regions and professionals are very limited in resources and actions that they can take alone, CAN cases are often just registered in the professional's records and are not reported or investigated further. Assistance or intervention for the family is often limited to a voluntary conversation with the parent who is told to take care of the child or to treat them "properly."

THE NATURE OF THE "TYPICAL" RESPONSE BY THE RESPONSIBLE AGENCY

Yury, a 12-year-old boy, is beaten by his father repeatedly. Typically, the beatings occur when the father is under the influence of alcohol. The family, including the father, mother, Yury and his younger sister, share one room in a hostel, a dorm where factory workers live; they do not have a private bathroom and share a kitchen with other families. The majority of the adults in the hostel abuse alcohol. Sometimes Yury's parents do not let the children into the room, especially when they are drinking, and sometimes make them stay away from the room for several days. Yury often comes to school with bruises from the beatings, and appears sleep deprived. The school contacted the Commission on Juvenile Affairs and the family was issued a warning, but the beating and locking the children out of the home continued. However, other basic needs of the children were being met: the parents fed them, dressed them, monitored their school attendance, and the father started attending the school's parents' meetings. The school continued to report the problems periodically to the local Commission for Juvenile Affairs. In spite of the ongoing abuse, no additional measures were taken. It was believed that there was not sufficient evidence to file for a criminal action under the Criminal Code Article 156, "Failure to perform child rearing duties," due to a lack of documentation. Municipal social welfare service workers attempted to visit the family a few times, but the parents did not want to communicate with them, refused to receive any help except financial assistance and clothing, and the social welfare workers' visits stopped.

The necessary elements of child protection, such as a child abuse reporting line and professionals designated to screen reports, investigate, provide case management and services, and monitor parental progress in treatment, simply do not exist in Russia. As a result, the majority of abused children do not receive necessary interventions or legal actions (9).

STRENGTHS OF THE RUSSIAN APPROACH/SYSTEM

There is a tradition of universal preventive services for children and families rooted in the Soviet period when there was strong governmental control on parental compliance with state regulations. The services included home visitations by pediatricians and nurses for all new parents, mandatory immunizations, and medical and dental check-ups monitored by school personnel. In the 1990s and early 2000s, dramatic social, political, and economic changes and a decrease of government funding for social services disrupted this social safety network for many families. More recently, the government has taken action to improve the situation. New regulations and programs that reintroduced the state's control of children's school attendance and other services for children and families have been developed. The Ministry of Education and its agencies are responsible for the registration of school-age children and school enrolment. The Russian public school system has sufficient personnel resources with thousands of well-educated teachers, nurses, pediatricians, and school psychologists who serve the entire population of children. Medical insurance and education are provided for children and families registered at a permanent residence - at no charge. In Russia, registration is necessary to receive a medical insurance card for free medical services provided by the state and for children to be enrolled in school. Children's centers and many schools provide sports, art, and other activities; some of the services are free. All of these measures play an important role in providing for the basic needs of children, support to families, and oversight of parental care for children.

WEAKNESSES/CHALLENGES IN THE RUSSIAN APPROACH/SYSTEM?

The lack of an established definition, specific laws related to CAN, and a CAN system for reporting, investigating, providing services, and monitoring families results in a significant lack of child protection in Russia. Other problems to be addressed include:

- Limited public awareness about child maltreatment;
- Lack of resources for low income families;
- Lack of education on CAN for professionals in medicine, law, law enforcement, education, mental health, and social services;
- Lack of standardized investigation procedures and interview protocols;
- Lack of agencies to provide specialized treatment and case management;
- Lack of systematic follow-up on children reported for abuse;
- Need for foster families and placements other than state-run institutions; and a
- Lack of interagency collaboration and communication.

A system of identification, collaboration, and service provision has not been developed or is not functioning adequately in most regions of Russia. In the majority of cases, services for maltreated children and their families are limited to fines, issuing warnings to parents, and providing limited financial assistance.

MAJOR CONTROVERSIES

There are few openly recognized controversies in child protection in Russia. While there are laws in place to address CAN, they are divided among ministries and agencies with no single governmental agency responsible for their implementation. Across Russia, there are no CAN reporting services, established child welfare investigation units, and no consequences for not reporting suspected abuse, or not taking action when a child is maltreated. In different regions, the same agencies under the same Ministry or Commission operate very differently and there is a lack of communication between agencies in order to establish common procedures.

The new laws on termination/restoration and restriction of parental rights have not served the purpose of promoting family preservation and reunification. The law on restoration of parental rights after terminating parental rights by the court and the requirement for parents to file a petition to court on their own are confusing and do not accomplish its purpose. To be implemented effectively, these laws need to be supported by procedures of assigning voluntary or court-ordered treatment plans, close monitoring of the parents' progress on correcting the conditions by child protection/child welfare agencies, and evaluating and reporting the parents' progress to the court.

PREVENTION EFFORTS - PRIMARY, SECONDARY, AND TERTIARY

Primary prevention efforts typically focus on educating the public to prevent a problem before it occurs. While there are currently several aspects or events occurring in Russia that would be designated as "primary prevention," there is no organized approach by the government or any Ministry to inform the public about preventing CAN. Listed below are aspects that are considered primary prevention:

- In some schools, children are introduced to the Convention on the Rights of Child (CRC), but this is not a mandatory part of school education;
- Brochures for children and parents on the prevention of violence, primarily on sexual abuse, are widely distributed; and
- There are periodic news reports and documentaries about victims of abuse.

Secondary prevention programs are aimed at intervening with members of the population that are at-risk for experiencing a problem. In Russia, there are clearly children and families at-risk for maltreatment: children living on the streets or in institutions, and families in which substance abuse, poverty, or domestic violence occurs. Agencies and programs have been established in Russia to work with these children and families, but there is not an overall, planned approach—the services are dependent on governmental and international funding and the level of services varies widely across Russia.

Some promising aspects include:

- The numbers of agencies providing social services for children and families reached 2,744 in 2002 (19);

- Increasing numbers of regions, such as St. Petersburg, Moscow, and Kalugu, have children's rights ombudsmen;
- The government is promoting deinstitutionalization and providing special attention to families of children with disabilities (20);
- Low-income families receive financial subsidies, and the children receive free breakfasts and lunches at school, free school supplies, and a school bag at the beginning of the school year;
- The government is increasing financial support for families from a child's birth to 18 months (21); (Note: Concerns have been reported that while this may benefit families with very young children, it may place older children at increased risk for maltreatment or abandonment); and
- A number of charities and international organizations, such as IREX/USAID, UNICEF, and WHO, have established relationships with the government and are providing services to street children and children with special needs. In 2003, the Russian National Foundation for the Prevention of Cruelty to Children (NPPCC), with support from IREX/USAID, initiated programs in child welfare reform in several regions of Russia (http://www.sirotstvo.ru/fond/) (22). NPPCC conducts programs to prevent social abandonment such as assistance to orphans, prevention of abandonment of newborns by HIV positive mothers, and the development of effective models in child protection. Some of the prevention measures reported 50 to 100% success in preventing child abandonment (23).

Tertiary prevention focuses on providing services to those affected by a problem and preventing its reoccurrence. Services for children and families have been expanded in Russia, but large numbers of maltreated children continue to receive no intervention. For example, in 2001, the St. Petersburg Department of Internal Offices reported that 51% (n=28,174) of children taken to police stations were in "social danger" and in need of protection by the state, but only 6% (n=1,803) were provided emergency social assistance (24).

CONCLUSIONS

The absence of an organized child abuse reporting and investigation system, established policies for case management, and a system to monitor parental progress significantly hinders the ability of professionals to intervene and prevent further abuse, even when it is recognised. Despite major advancements in the legal framework of child protection, there are still missing pieces of legislation, such as a special article on CAN, which would integrate the various laws relating to child maltreatment. Most importantly, services for families need to be integrated with the court and child protection procedures. That can be achieved by implementing voluntarily or court-ordered treatment plans for parents whose parental rights are restricted temporarily. In summary, there are laws, physicians, law enforcement officers, psychologists, and social workers in Russia, but there is no integrated legally-based child protection system. Child abuse and neglect is an interdisciplinary problem and coordinated work by professionals from different disciplines is crucial for positive outcomes for children and families.

REFERENCES

[1]   Balachova T, Bonner B, Levy . Street children in Russia: steps to prevention. Int J Soc Welfare 2008 Mar 07, epub ahead of print.

[2]   Ministry of Labor and Social Development of the Russian Federation. [Information on actions to straighten prevention of homelessness and neglect of underage children, Electronic version]. 2002 Oct 07. Message posted to http://www.mintrud.ru/press/

[3]   Volkova E, ed.) [Protection of Children from Abuse]. Saint Petersburg: Piter, 2007.

[4]   [Family Code of the Russian Federation] available at http://www.kodeks.ru/noframe/com-pus-FullLegRF?d&nd=9052456&nh=1

[5]   [Federal Law on Basic Guarantees of the Rights of the Child in the Russian Federation] available at http://www.kodeks.ru

[6]   [Federal Law N 120 "On the prevention of Child Neglect and Juvenile Delinquency"] available at http://www.kodeks.ru/noframe/com-pus-FullLegRF?d&nd=901737405

[7]   [Criminal Code of Russian Federation] (1996, with May 27, 2008) Available at http://www.kodeks.ru/noframe/com-pus-FullLegRF?d&nd=9017477

[8]   Ministry of Health and Social Development of the Russian Federation. [Situation of Children in the Russian Federation, 2006]. Moscow, 2006.

[9]   UNICEF. Situation analysis of children in the Russian Federation 2007. Retrieved 2007 Sept 09, http://www.unicef.org/russia/media_7522.html

[10]   [Deputy Prosecutor-General of Russia Sergei Fridinsky's interview to ITAR-TASS]. Retrieved 2007 Sept 16, http://www.genproc.gov.ru/ru/managament/interview/index.shtml?item_id=58

[11]   US Department of State. Russia: Country Reports on Human Rights Practices- 2006. Bureau of Democracy, Human Rights, and Labor. Retrieved 2007 Aug 20, http://www.state.gov/g/drl/rls/hrrpt/2006/78835.htm

[12]   Sidorenko-Stephenson S. Street children in Moscow: Using and creating social capital. Sociol Rev2001;49:530-47.

[13]   Basu B. The health of street children in Moscow and St. Petersburg. Unpublished honours thesis. Stanford, CA: Stanford Univ, 1998.

[14]   International Labour Office (2002). In-depth analysis of the situation of working street children in Moscow 2001. ILO/IPEC working paper. Moscow: Intl Labour. Retrieved 2006 Jan 03, http://www.streetchildren.org.uk/reports/Moscow_Report_Eng_1.pdf

[15]   WHO. Alcohol policy in the WHO European region: Current status and the way forward. (Fact Sheet EURO 10/05). Copenhagen: WHO, 2005.

[16]   Korop E. [Kremlin Orphans]. Izvestia. Retrieved 2005 Oct 12, http://izvestia.ru/politic/article12705

[17]   St. Petersburg Committee on Labour and Social Protection. [Analytical materials on children in St. Petersburg in 2006]. St. Petersburg: St. Petersburg Committee Labor Social Protection. Retrieved 2008 Jul 07, http://www.homekid.ru/childinspb/kidspbpart11.html

[18]   Mamai V. [Commentary to the Family Code of Russia]. Moscow: PRIOR Publ Expert Bureau, 1998.

[19]   Kupriayanova G. The information of the Department on Youth Policy of Ministry of Education of Russia and Ministry of Labor and Social Development of the Russian Federation about a situation in the Russian Federation with children and youth of group of risk: A history, development of rehabilitation work, the establishments working in this sphere, the current situation, programs and projects. Meeting "Children on the Street", Ministry of Education of the Russian Federation, Council of the Baltic Sea States – Working Group for Co-operation on Children at Risk, Moscow, Abstract retrieved 2005 Dec 24, http://www.childcentre.info/projects/street_children/dbaFile11655.html

[20]   Government of the Russian Federation. [Information for Press. Bill #79-p on Children of Russia Federal target program for 2007–2010, Electronic version]. Government meeting press release. http://www.government.ru/government/governmentactivity/rfgovernmentdecisions/archive/2007/01/31/1125147.htm

[21]   President of Russia. [V. Putin Address to the Federal Assembly]. Retrieved 2007 Sept 09, http://president.kremlin.ru (http://www.kremlin.ru/text/appears/2006/05/105546.shtml)

[22]   US Agency for International Development. Assistance to Russian orphans 2 Program (ARO).Final Report. International Research & Exchanges Board, 2006.

[23]   US Agency for International Development. Community reintegration of street and neglected children. Center for Fiscal Policy. Doctors of the World summary report, 2007.

[24]   St. Petersburg Committee on Labor and Social Protection. [Analytical materials on children in St. Petersburg in 2002]. St. Petersburg: & Regional Center Family St. Petersburg state agency of social help for families and children, 2002.

In: International Aspects of Child Abuse and Neglect
Editors: H. Dubowitz, J. Merrick pp. 161-169

ISBN: 978-1-60876-703-8
© 2010 Nova Science Publishers, Inc.

Chapter 16

CHILD WELFARE IN THE USA: IN THEORY AND PRACTICE

Howard Dubowit and Diane DePanfilis

Division of Child Protection, Department of Pediatrics,
University of Maryland School of Medicine
University of Maryland School of Social Work, Baltimore,
Maryland, United States of America

The United States has approximately 80 million children living in 50 states and the District of Columbia. In general, the responsibility for protecting children from abuse and neglect lies with state and county governments. There is enormous variability. Even within a state, resources, policies and practice may vary considerably. It is thus difficult to describe the overall situation regarding child welfare in the US. The focus of this paper is on the abuse and neglect of children within their families. In conclusion, the child welfare system is reasonably developed in the US, although major problems persist. In the broadest sense, there has been striking progress. Children are no longer, for example, forced to work under unbearable conditions in coal mines, as they did just 70 years ago. There is wide acceptance of children's need (and right) to be protected from abuse and neglect, and society's responsibility to protect them. At the same time, national leadership has been weak, and in most of the country, resources to address child abuse and neglect are far short of what is needed. Much remains to be done.

INTRODUCTION

The United States has approximately 80 million children living in 50 states and the District of Columbia. In general, the responsibility for protecting children from abuse and neglect lies with state and county governments. There is enormous variability. Even within a state, resources, policies and practice may vary considerably. It is thus difficult to describe the overall situation regarding child welfare in the US, many generalizations are necessary. As is often the case, there are also frequent and big gaps between what exists in theory or on paper, and what is practiced. Some states have independent groups monitoring the public agencies and contributing to the services families and children receive. For example, in Maryland, there is a committee that reviews the situation of each child in foster care every six months to help ensure their needs are met and that they are not lingering in an uncertain situation. The need for such "watchdog" groups is very clear; we need many more of them.

The focus of this paper is on the abuse and neglect of children within their families. Related problems such as homelessness, poverty, inadequate access to health care and sexual exploitation deserve separate papers, and are beyond the scope of this brief overview.

HOW THE DIFFERENT TYPES OF CHILD ABUSE AND NEGLECT ARE DEFINED

There are four major types of maltreatment considered in the United States child welfare system: physical, sexual and emotional abuse, and neglect. The focus is on parents or caregivers, including for example school teachers or sporting coaches. In contrast, bullying by a peer or sibling, and assault by a stranger are not labeled "abuse" and are handled differently if at all by the public agencies.

Physical abuse refers to inflicted injuries such as bruises, burns, bites, fractures, and head and abdominal trauma (1). Corporal punishment is permitted, unless it results in such injuries. Sometimes bruising may not cross the threshold for abuse, such as when a parent strikes an adolescent's arm. Sexual abuse refers to all forms of sexual contact between a child and an adult or older child (2). Sexual acts include direct contact ranging from fondling over clothes to full intercourse. Indirect acts such as exposing a child to pornography may be considered abusive, although the public agencies seldom become involved. Engaging a child in the production of pornographic materials would, however. There is no need for a physical injury or sexually transmitted infection. Emotional abuse is included in some state laws, but is seldom acted upon. There may be a requirement to demonstrate how a particular abusive behavior is harming a child. Professionals and lay persons worry that this is likely the most damaging form of maltreatment, but it is difficult to quantify. Acts in this category include terrorizing, humiliating and belittling a child – repeatedly. Clearly, other forms of abuse often also involve emotional abuse.

Neglect is defined as omissions in care by a parent or caregiver that actually or potentially harm a child (3). The focus is on unmet physical needs such as food, clothing and health care ("failure to provide"), and, lapses in supervision ("failure to protect"). Mostly, the public agencies require actual harm, such as when a lack of medical care results in health problems (ie, medical neglect). Most states, however, allow parents not to seek regular medical care for a child, if for religion reasons. Christian scientists, for example, believe in faith healing and prohibit medical care. Eleven states exclude circumstances due to poverty in their neglect laws. An alternative definition of neglect focuses on children's basic needs; when these are inadequately met, children experience neglect - regardless of the cause (4). This broader, child-focused perspective offers a more constructive and less blaming approach. It encourages consideration of a broad range of circumstances, and by encouraging contributory factors in addition to parents' behavior, it fosters a comprehensive approach to addressing the problems.

WHAT IS KNOWN ABOUT THE EXTENT OF CHILD MALTREATMENT?

In 2006 in the US, 3.3 million referrals, involving the alleged maltreatment of approximately 6 million children were made to Child Protective Services (CPS) programs (5). Of those, approximately 905,000 children were confirmed as having been abused or neglected. Child neglect continued to represent the largest category of maltreatment confirmed by CPS with 64 percent of maltreated children experiencing neglect, 16 percent identified as physically abused, nine percent confirmed as sexually abused, seven percent confirmed as psychologically maltreated, and two percent identified as medically neglected. Approximately equal numbers of males and females were identified. The youngest children (birth to 3 years) had the highest rate of victimization (14.2 per 1,000 children). A special analysis of infant child maltreatment (6) identified 91,278 infants under the age of one year in 2006; most were classified as neglected (68%). And, a large percentage of the infants were less than one month old (39%) and of these, most (84%) were less than one week old. The majority of the newborns reported were on the basis of their mother's use of illegal drugs prenatally, the drugs being present in the mother and/or baby at the time of birth.

It is well established, however, that reports of child abuse and neglect are only the tip of the iceberg. A national incidence study that has been repeated in the US three times has established that many more children are known to have been abused or neglected than those that are actually reported (7). Surveys of nationally representative samples of children and youth have also established higher rates of child abuse and neglect than the number of children actually reported to CPS programs. One study suggested that more than one in seven of the child and youth population in the U.S. experienced maltreatment (138 per 1,000) (8).

HOW DOES THE SYSTEM WORK REGARDING REPORTING OF POSSIBLE CHILD ABUSE AND NEGLECT?

A combination of federal and state laws and policies guide the reporting of child abuse and neglect and provide the structure for the formal system responses to children and their families. Originally, passed in 1974 by the US Congress, the Federal Child Abuse Prevention and Treatment Act (CAPTA) (42 U.S.C.A. §5106g) as amended by the Keeping Children and Families Safe Act of 2003, (SP.L. 93-247) provides minimum standards for defining physical child abuse, child neglect, and sexual abuse that States must incorporate in their statutory definitions in order to receive Federal (national) funding for related programs. These funds are quite limited; thus, some states have decided not to follow Federal guidelines. While Federal legislation sets minimum standards, each State is responsible for delineating the response to child abuse and neglect within civil and criminal laws.

- Mandatory child maltreatment reporting statutes (civil laws) provide definitions of child maltreatment to guide those individuals mandated to identify and report suspected child abuse. These reports activate the child protection process. All states require most professionals interacting with children to reported suspected maltreatment; some states include all citizens as mandatory reporters.

- Juvenile or family court jurisdiction statutes provide definitions of the circumstances necessary for the court to have jurisdiction over a child alleged to have been abused or neglected. When the child's safety cannot be ensured in the home, these statutes allow the court to take custody of a child and to order specific intervention and treatment services for the parents, child, and family; recent statutes also allow agencies to forego the provision of services to some families based on the type and severity of maltreatment.
- Criminal statutes define the forms of child maltreatment that are criminally punishable. In most jurisdictions, child maltreatment is criminally punishable when one or more of the following statutory crimes have been committed: homicide, murder, manslaughter, false imprisonment, assault, battery, criminal neglect and abandonment, emotional and physical abuse, pornography, child prostitution, computer crimes, rape, deviant sexual assault, indecent exposure, child endangerment, and reckless endangerment.

Together, these legal frameworks define the standards of care and protection for children and serve as important guidelines for professionals who are required both to report and respond to reports of child abuse and neglect.

WHAT SYSTEM(S) OR INFRASTRUCTURE EXISTS TO ADDRESS CHILD MALTREATMENT?

CPS programs within public child welfare agencies have the primary responsibility for assuring that children are safe from abuse and neglect (9). At the state and local levels, professionals assume various roles and responsibilities ranging from prevention, identification, and reporting of child abuse and neglect to investigation and assessment, intervention, and treatment (10). State laws determine which professionals who come in contact with children have a responsibility to report suspected instances of child maltreatment. CPS agencies, along with law enforcement, are responsible for receiving and investigating official reports of child abuse and neglect. In some communities, teams comprised of health care professionals (physicians and nurses), social workers, and law enforcement are used to conduct comprehensive interdisciplinary investigations, particularly in cases of sexual abuse and serious physical abuse. Many community professionals (including health care providers, mental health professionals, educators, and legal and court system personnel) are involved in responding to child abuse and neglect and providing needed services. In addition, community-based agency staff, substance abuse treatment providers, domestic violence victim advocates, clergy, extended family members, and concerned citizens also play important roles in supporting families and keeping children safe.

THE NATURE OF THE "TYPICAL" RESPONSE BY THE RESPONSIBLE AGENCY(IES)

The typical response usually involves someone making a phone call to the CPS agency expressing concern that a child is suspected to have been abused or neglected. The person taking the call is responsible for making a decision whether the information being reported actually meets the state definition of child abuse and neglect. If the report is screened in, then an investigation proceeds with or without the assistance of law enforcement (depending on the nature and severity of the alleged maltreatment). A process of interviewing all children in the home, all family members, and others who may have information about the alleged maltreatment proceeds to determine whether there is sufficient evidence to classify the report as substantiated or founded. It is also the responsibility of the CPS worker to assess the immediate safety of the child and to assess the risk of future maltreatment. Based on the findings of this investigation, decisions are made whether to provide continuing services to the child(ren) and family. Most (approximately 80%) maltreated children remain at home and families may be provided continuing CPS in-home services to help ensure the safety of children and reduce the risk of future maltreatment. Referrals may also be made to a variety of community programs, such as a drug treatment program or a food pantry.

In cases when children have been determined to be unsafe and if services cannot be implemented to keep the children in the home, decisions may be made to place the children in out-of-home care. In those instances, petitions must first be filed in Juvenile or Family Court. When children are placed out of home, the first approach is generally to seek suitable family members who are willing and able to care for them (ie, kinship care). Following placement, continued efforts are made toward reuniting the child with his or her immediate family. When such efforts fail, parental rights may be terminated and the child adopted.

In recent years, more than half of the states in the US have begun to implement alternate ways to respond to concerns about children who may be at risk of child abuse or neglect. Referred to as alternative response, differential response, or dual track systems, these new practices involve triaging reports of child abuse and neglect so that the response varies depending on the presenting risk to children. Instead of a forensic approach to investigate a report of child maltreatment, alternative responses are characterized by an emphasis on the assessment of the needs of families and children, with less emphasis on the allegation of child maltreatment (11). Preliminary evaluations suggest that this approach is preferred by both CPS staff and families, and that the children do not appear to be at added risk of harm.

THE STRENGTHS OF THE US APPROACH AND SYSTEMS

A major strength of the U.S. child welfare system is that the importance of protecting children is established in law, recognizing the governmental or public right to intervene when parents or caregivers abuse or neglect children. There has been much media attention to this problem over the past 45 years, increasing public awareness of this problem. Many professionals involved with children now recognize possible maltreatment and refer families to CPS. Pediatric conferences, for example, often include training on child maltreatment.

Another strength is the extent to which the responsible public agencies, particularly CPS, law enforcement and the judicial system have been developed to help address the problem. For example, anywhere in the country a concerned citizen can – and in some states must – report a situation of possible maltreatment to CPS. As outlined above, a professional investigation or assessment follows in order to ensure a child's safety. Regarding suspected sexual abuse the evaluation is often interdisciplinary in a child advocacy center. Interdisciplinary work has become the standard in many settings.

Despite some strengths there is also widespread recognition of our child welfare system's shortcomings. Evaluations of services and programs have led to recommendations for reforming the system. Some of these evaluations have resulted from class action law suits against states, alleging gross failures to protect children. Consequently, there may be pressure and interest to improve the system. A promising development, for example, is the experimentation with a less forensic and more therapeutic approach to cases involving neglect and "minor" physical abuse. Alternative Response Systems, described above, focus more on engaging families, comprehensively assessing their needs, and supporting them to better protect their children. Finally, some government policies and programs that address children's needs, directly and indirectly, help prevent child maltreatment. For example, low income families may qualify for government health insurance, food programs, and housing subsidies. Some states have funds for prevention programs via Children's Trust Funds, perhaps from a small fee people pay when marrying, or divorcing. A number of relatively small private organizations, such as Prevent Child Abuse America, also advocate for prevention programs, while many provide direct services, such as home visiting, parenting groups, and substance abuse treatment.

THE WEAKNESSES IN THE US APPROACH AND SYSTEMS

One major challenge is the vastly inadequate availability of resources to address enormous needs. For example, CPS agencies often have inadequate staff that are undertrained and overwhelmed. Too often, simplistic knee-jerk responses occur instead of skilled interdisciplinary assessment. This is particularly worrisome given the major ramifications of these assessments: children may be removed from their families; people may be prosecuted – inappropriately. CPS agencies often suffer from low morale, and have difficulty attracting and retaining competent professionals.

There is also much room for improvement concerning related disciplines and professionals, particularly in the health care, educational, law enforcement and judicial systems. Training in this difficult field is minimal; not surprisingly, for example, many pediatricians are not comfortable assessing a child for possible sexual abuse (12). Many judges have little training in child development, resulting in decisions that are not always good for children.

Another weakness is the extent to which resources have been directed to forensic evaluations, while prevention efforts have been meager, and support and treatment services for children and families are in short supply. For example, it is often difficult to find mental health services for an abused child. The emphasis on investigating families to establish fault detracts from efforts to understand and help them – especially concerning neglect. Therefore, relatively few families actually receive services, even when maltreatment is substantiated.

Finally, an important shortcoming is the focus on the symptom of maltreatment, without enough attention to the underlying systemic problems. For example, there is ample evidence demonstrating the direct and indirect ways that poverty jeopardizes children's health, development and safety, and, how it is linked to abuse and neglect (7,13). Yet, efforts to tackle this problem remain inadequate. Approximately one in six US children lacks health insurance (14). Given the costs of health care, it is no surprise that uninsured children, with increased health problems, receive less health care than those with insurance. When their medical needs are neglected, is it fair to hold the family responsible, or US society?

THE MAJOR CONTROVERSIES IN THE US REGARDING CHILD WELFARE POLICY AND PRACTICE

One controversy results from media attention to gross system failures (and seldom to successes) so that some hold the view that the system is useless and perhaps harmful. For example, CPS may be severely criticized when, despite their involvement with a family, a child dies. In contrast, others acknowledge system shortcomings, but think that it still helps protect many children and supports their families.

A second controversy concerns the scope of the child welfare system's roles and responsibilities. Some, concerned with their limited resources, advocate for a narrow CPS role – to protect children in danger. Adequate care and safety are the goals. Others counter that that perspective is too limited; the agency should also be concerned with children's health and development – especially once they become involved. Arguably, for the twenty percent of children with substantiated maltreatment reports removed from their families, the state has a moral obligation to provide exemplary, not just adequate, care.

A related controversy concerns the placement of children with relatives (kinship care), rather than foster families. Some argue that it is in children's interests to remain within the family. Others question the ability to rely on a family that has raised the parent who is now deemed abusive or unable to adequately care for his or her child. There is also skepticism that kinship care may be a convenient way for CPS to shirk its responsibility, instead "dumping" the child with a relative – usually a grandmother. Many of these grandmothers have marginal finances, health problems, and may feel obligated - albeit poorly prepared and supported - to care for their grandchildren. And, frequently the child welfare system does not provide adequate services to support their care of children in their care.

PREVENTION EFFORTS (PRIMARY, SECONDARY, TERTIARY)

There is relatively little in the US by way of primary prevention – to a broad population not necessarily at risk for maltreatment. There are occasional public education campaigns, for example, on topics such as the hazards to children of second hand smoke or the importance of car safety restraints. Most of the limited prevention efforts are secondary, targeting those considered at risk for maltreatment, before the problem has occurred. Government policies and programs that provide low income families with health insurance, child care and housing subsidies, food programs, and tax benefits may – directly or indirectly – help prevent child maltreatment. The most widely used and best evaluated strategy involves nurses or paraprofessionals visiting families with new babies (15-19). Some of these programs begin prenatally and continue until the child is two or three years old. They aim to support the parents emotionally, enhance their parenting skills, and link them to community services they may need, such as substance abuse treatment. The most promising findings in terms of promoting parental functioning and preventing child maltreatment have been with nurses; programs using paraprofessionals have not been found to be effective. Many communities have other programs to support parents and families, such as parenting groups, food pantries, homeless shelters and mental health clinics, which help prevent maltreatment. As stated earlier, there remains a considerable gap between what the above policies and programs provide and what is needed.

Finally, tertiary prevention targets those where child maltreatment has occurred (ie, treatment), aiming to prevent its recurrence and its potentially harmful impact. Here the efforts of CPS together with the related disciplines and agencies comprise the overall response. Medical care is generally available, but as already noted, mental health services for adults and especially for children are often difficult to find.

CONCLUSIONS

In conclusion, the child welfare system is reasonably developed in the US, although major problems persist. In the broadest sense, there has been striking progress. Children are no longer, for example, forced to work under unbearable conditions in coal mines, as they did just 70 years ago. There is wide acceptance of children's need (and right) to be protected from abuse and neglect, and society's responsibility to protect them. At the same time, national leadership has been weak, and in most of the country, resources to address child abuse and neglect are far short of what is needed. Much remains to be done.

REFERENCES

[1]   Dubowitz H. How do I determine whether a child has been physically abused? In: Dubowitz H, DePanfilis D, Handbook for child protection practice. Thousand Oaks, CA: Sage, 2000:143-5.

[2]   Adams JA. How do I determine if a child has been sexually abused? In: Dubowitz H, DePanfilis D, Handbook for child protection practice. Thousand Oaks, CA: Sage, 2000:175-9.

[3]   Dubowitz H, Black M. Child neglect. In: Reece RM, Christian C, Child abuse: Medical diagnosis and management, 3rd ed. Washington, DC: Am Acad Pediatrics, 2009.

[4]   Dubowitz H, Black M, Starr R, Zuravin S. A conceptual definition of child neglect. Criminal Justice Behavior 1993;20:8-26.

[5]   U.S. Department of Health and Human Services, Administration on Children, Youth and Families. Child maltreatment, 2006. Washington, DC: US Gov Printing Office, 2008.

[6]   United States Center for Disease Control and Prevention. Nonfatal maltreatment of infants: United States, October 2005 - September 2006. MMWR 2008;57(13):336-9.

[7]   Sedlack AJ, Broadhurst DD. Third national incidence study of child abuse and neglect: Final report. Washington, DC: US Dept Health Hum Serv, 1996.

[8] Finkelhor D, Ormrod R, Turner H, Hamby SL. The victimization of children and youth: A comprehensive, national survey. Child Maltreat 2005;10:5-25.

[9] DePanfilis D, Salus M. Child protective services: A guide for caseworkers. Washington, DC: US Dept Health Hum Serv, 2003.
Acessed 2008 Apr 13 from http://www.childwelfare.gov/pubs/usermanuals/cps/

[10] Goldman J, Salus M. A coordinated response to child abuse and neglect: The foundation for practice. Washington, DC: US Dept Health Hum Serv, 2003. Accessed 2008 Apr 13 from http://www.childwelfare.gov/pubs/usermanuals/cps/

[11] US Department of Health and Human Services, Administration for Children and Families/Children's Bureau and Office of the Assistant Secretary for Planning and Evaluation. National Study of Child Protective Services Systems and Reform Efforts: Findings on local CPS practices. Washington, DC: US Gov Printing Office, 2003. Accessed 2008 Apr 13 from http://aspe.hhs.gov/HSP/cps-status03/

[12] Lane W, Dubowitz, H. Primary care pediatricians' experience, comfort and competence in the evaluation and management of child maltreatment: Do we need child abuse experts? Child Abuse Neglect, in press.

[13] Parker S, Greer S, Zuckerman B. Double jeopardy: The impact of poverty on early child development. Pediatr Clin North Am 1988;35:1227-40.

[14] Cover the insured. www.covertheuninsured.org. Accessed 2008 Sep 19.

[15] Olds DL, Sadler L, Kitzman H. Programs for parents of infants and toddlers: recent evidence of randomized trials. J Child Psychol Psychiatr 2007;48:355-91.

[16] Olds DL, Robinson J, Petit L, Luckey DW, Holmberg J, Ng RK, et al. Effects of home visits by paraprofessionals and by nurses: Age-four follow up of a randomized trial. Pediatrics 2004;114:1560-8.

[17] Duggan A, McFarlane E, Fuddy L, Burrell L, Higman SM, Windham A, Sia C. Randomized trial of a statewide home visiting program: impact in preventing child abuse and neglect. Child Abuse Neglect 2004;28:597-622.

[18] Caldera D, Burrell L, Rodriguez K, Crowne SS, Rohde C, Duggan A. Impact of a statewide home visiting program on parenting and on child health and development. Child Abuse Neglect 2007;31:829-52.

[19] Gomby DS. The promise and limitations of home visiting: Implementing effective programs. Child Abuse Neglect 2007;31:793-9.

In: International Aspects of Child Abuse and Neglect   ISBN: 978
Editors: H. Dubowitz, J. Merrick pp. 171-189   © 2010 Nova Scienc

172 /

Chapter 17

AN OVERVIEW OF THE CHILD WELFARE SYSTEMS IN CANADA

Pamela Gough, Aron Shlonsky, and Peter Dudding

Centre of Excellence for Child Welfare, Factor-Inwentash Faculty of Social Work, University of Toronto, Toronto, Canada

Canada is physically the second-largest country in the world, but a relatively small population of approximately 33 million people, of which 7 million are children and youth under the age of 18 years. Under Canada's federal structures, the ten provinces and three territories are responsible for providing health, education, and social services, including child protection. The child welfare systems across the country are reasonably well developed and share common features including mandatory reporting, a respect for the primary role of the family in raising children, a paramount objective of protecting children from harm, and a focus on the best interests of the child being taken into consideration when decisions need to be made regarding child safety. While there are many differences in policies and practice from one part of the country to another, Canadian child protection systems, as they are currently structured, are funded to respond to reports of child maltreatment, or risk of maltreatment, but are generally not well funded to take action in areas of social service that would prevent maltreatment from happening in the first place. Aboriginal children and youth, although a relatively minor part of the overall child population, are vastly overrepresented in the child welfare system, with current estimates of the chances of a First Nations child being in child welfare care being approximately one in ten, compared with one in 200 for non-First Nations children in Canada. Despite Canada's affluence as a nation, many families with children continue to live in poverty.

INTRODUCTION

Canada is physically the second-largest country in the world, surpassed only by Russia, and is a high-income northern country characterized by abundant natural resources, vast distances of unpopulated space, and relatively small numbers of people. Stretching over 5,200 km (3200 miles) from the Atlantic Ocean to the east to the Pacific Ocean to the west, and another 5,000 km (3100 miles) from the southern border to the Arctic Ocean in the north, Canada's area is 9.9 million square km (3.8 million square miles). The Canadian climate varies from temperate in the south to subarctic and arctic in the far north. Canada's population of approximately 33 million people is clustered to the south (90% of the population lives within 160 km of the U.S. border), and is increasingly urban. However, there are people living throughout the breadth and width of the nation up to the high Arctic and, for those in northern, rural, and remote areas, delivery of social services can be difficult and is often less than adequate. This is especially true for the proportionately small Aboriginal population, some of whom live in areas so remote that there are no roads, and all supplies must be delivered by air. Economically and technologically, Canada has developed in parallel with its neighbour to the south and major trading partner, the United States of America. Canada became a self-governing democracy in 1867, but has retained its ties to the British crown and is a parliamentary monarchy with an independent judiciary. Politically, Canada is divided into ten provinces and three northern territories (1). It is a bilingual country, with French and English the two official languages, and has a multicultural population with a liberal immigration policy. Canada has approximately 7 million children and youth under the age of 18 (2). The provinces and territories fund universal public education up to the end of secondary school, and literacy rates are high (97-99% of the population aged 15 and over) (3).

Child welfare in Canada, with the exception of some services to Aboriginal peoples, is a provincial responsibility rather than a federal one. Each of the provinces and territories has separately enacted laws to protect the well-being of children at risk of maltreatment. There is no legislation at the federal level to provide overall national standards for the prevention and treatment of child abuse and neglect. In the absence of a federal body or commission with a duty to define the best interests of children and oversee their health and well-being on a national level, the responsibility for protecting children from abuse and neglect is placed at the provincial and territorial level, where structures and practices vary to a considerable extent. The situation is made even more complex by the fact that the mainstream provincial systems in several provinces have parallel child and family service systems for Aboriginal peoples.

Legislative standards for key aspects of child welfare practice are also variable across Canada. One example is the legal definition of whether a person at risk of maltreatment is a child. Although the United Nations Convention on the Rights of the Child (UNCRC) defines a child as under 18 years of age, the age at which a child ceases to be a child for the purpose of receiving protective services in Canada is different across provinces and territories. The age of majority for the purposes of child protection is 16 in Nova Scotia, Saskatchewan (although in Saskatchewan, children up to 18 can be adopted) and Newfoundland and Labrador. In Ontario, the Northwest Territories, and Nunavut, the age of majority is also 16, although children up to 18 can receive child protection social services if they have already been taken into the care of the state. British Columbia defines a child as someone under the age of 19, but has different practices for the provision of child welfare services for youth between the ages of 16 and 19 than for those under 16. The other provinces and territories define a child as under the age of 18 (4).

The definition of the term "child welfare" is variable across Canada as well. If "child welfare" is taken to mean responding to child maltreatment, the child welfare systems in Canada respond to maltreatment, but do not prevent its initial occurrence, or the risk of initial occurrence. In some jurisdictions, the term used for the concept of child welfare is more properly "provision of child protection services" (CPS). The systems are built around the protection and safety of children, but only after they have been reported for maltreatment or risk of harm. Other jurisdictions, such as Quebec, take a more expansive view of child welfare – one that includes preventing child maltreatment and also includes aspects of youth justice, mental health, and health in its definition. As a step in this direction, several provinces have recently implemented alternative response models to provide a broader range of services. This more expansive approach to services, though, is less developed, and can be seen as the exception rather than the rule. While there are many differences in policies and practice from one part of the country to another, Canadian child protection systems, as they are currently and historically structured, are funded to respond to reports of child maltreatment, or risk of maltreatment, but are generally not well funded to set up structures to prevent maltreatment from happening in the first place.

Any discussion of the child welfare system within Canada must include the unique and difficult history and current social location of Aboriginal peoples (First Nations, Métis and Inuit), who account for 4% of Canada's population (5) but are vastly overrepresented throughout the Canadian child welfare system. Jurisdiction over First Nations health and social services is complicated, and is rooted in 19th century Canadian colonial history and statutes. At that time, Canada was forming as a nation and evolving from a colony to a European-style constitutional monarchy, and federal treaties began to be made with the sovereign Aboriginal peoples.

Federal laws of this era exerted governance over the original Aboriginal peoples in Canada. The federal Constitution Act of 1867 designated First Nations peoples and the lands reserved for them (called "reserves") to be the responsibility of the federal government. The Indian Act, another 19th century federal statute, is the primary piece of legislation that addresses First Nations peoples, and federal policy regarding the provision of child welfare services status First Nations people across Canada arises from this very early statute.

Colonial societies, especially the missionaries, condemned Aboriginal practices of child rearing. In the early 20th century, the churches, with the support of the federal government, established a residential school system with the purpose of assimilating First Nations people into European-Canadian society. The experiences of the children and youth in these schools was characterized by emotional, physical and sexual abuse, social and medical deprivation, and cultural dislocation. The psychological trauma continues to the present day, although the residential schools were largely closed down in the 1950s and 1960s. In 2008, the federal government issued an official apology and established a compensation program and a Truth and Reconciliation commission for the former inmates of the residential schools. Many of the children who attended the Indian residential schools suffered profound, long-term, negative psychological consequences and a substantial erosion of their cultural identity. The harm to Aboriginal communities was compounded by the loss of large numbers of children to adoption in the 1960s (an era called the "Sixties Scoop"). Today, many Aboriginal people living on the reserves experience high rates of poverty, isolation, substance abuse, and a chronic lack of health and social service supports.

Aboriginal control over delivery of culturally appropriate services to their communities has been evolving over the last thirty years as a result of a move towards increased Aboriginal self-government, and this field represents one of the most quickly changing areas of child welfare policy and jurisdiction in Canada (6).

How Are the Different Types of Child Abuse and Neglect Defined?

The term "child abuse and neglect" in Canada generally pertains to physical abuse, sexual abuse, emotional abuse and neglect, with exposure to domestic violence increasingly being recognized as a form of emotional abuse. There is no single definition of child abuse and neglect that applies across Canada, since, within the federal framework, federal criminal statutes and provincial/territorial civil laws define various aspects of abuse and neglect. Although most laws and services pertaining to child welfare fall under provincial and territorial jurisdiction, the federal Criminal Code establishes that it is a crime to sexually abuse or physically assault a child.

In situations in which parents use physical force against children, the Criminal Code specifically excuses the use of physical punishment in the context of discipline as long as it "does not exceed what is reasonable under the circumstances" (7). Legal challenges led the Supreme Court to specify new limits on the definition of the use of reasonable force in 2004. According to the judgment, parents may only use minor corrective force of a transitory and trifling nature, while the following kinds of parental behaviour are considered unreasonable use of force against children and would therefore be considered assault:

- physical punishment of children younger than two and older than 12;
- the use of objects or sharp blows to the head;
- the use of force on a child incapable of learning from it because of disability or some other contextual factor;
- force used as a result of the parent's frustration, loss of temper, or abusive personality;
- degrading, inhuman, or harmful conduct.

In addition, the Supreme Court also ruled that teachers may apply force to remove a child from a classroom or secure compliance with instructions, but not as corporal punishment. This ruling on the physical punishment of children is contentious and is one of the elements of debate and controversy among those working in, and with, child welfare services in Canada.

Under the Criminal Code, it is also an offence for a parent or guardian to fail to provide a child with "necessaries of life" or to abandon a child under the age of 10 (8). Criminal investigations for matters that fall under the Criminal Code are handled by the police, and cases are tried in criminal court.

In practice, since many situations involving child abuse and neglect are often nuanced, hidden, take place over long periods of time, and may involve child witnesses testifying against parents, it can be difficult to prove guilt to the highest legal standard (beyond "reasonable doubt"), as required by a criminal proceeding, without subjecting children to further harm and trauma. This is clearly problematic for those involved in protecting the best interests of children. Child welfare agencies and police often have a protocol or joint policy to guide investigations in criminal cases, and it is generally more common for child abuse or neglect to be investigated in civil proceedings, under provincial and territorial laws, rather than in criminal court using the "blunt instrument" of the federal Criminal Code (9).

Despite the fact that there are many differences in the provincial/territorial laws pertaining to child welfare across the country, all of these laws generally share some common features. These include:

- the best interests of the child must be considered when a child is found to be in need of protection;
- the state respects family autonomy and the parent's primary responsibility for child rearing;
- it is recognized that continuity of care and stability is important for children;
- the views of children are seen as important to take into consideration when decisions are being made that affect their futures;
- cultural heritage should be respected, especially for Aboriginal children; and
- protecting children from harm is the paramount objective of child welfare.

Although there are variations within each province and territory, some generalizations in terminology are possible. The following can be used as "working definitions" of child abuse and neglect in Canada (10):

Child abuse refers to the violence, mistreatment or neglect that a child or adolescent may experience while in the care of someone they either trust or depend on, such as a parent, sibling, other relative, caregiver or guardian. Abuse may take place anywhere and may occur, for example, within the child's home or that of someone known to the child. There are many different forms of abuse and a child may be subjected to more than one form:

- Physical abuse involves the deliberate use of force against a child such that the child sustains or is at risk of sustaining physical injury. Physical abuse includes beating, hitting, shaking, pushing, choking, biting, burning, kicking or assaulting a child with a weapon. It also includes holding a child under water, or any other dangerous or harmful use of force or restraint. Female genital mutilation is another form of physical abuse.
- Sexual abuse and exploitation involves using a child for sexual purposes. Examples of child sexual abuse include fondling, inviting a child to touch or be touched sexually, intercourse, rape, incest, sodomy, exhibitionism, or involving a child in prostitution or pornography. Child sexual assault and sexual exploitation are criminal offences in Canada.
- Neglect is often chronic, and it usually involves repeated incidents. It involves failing to provide the basic necessities for the physical, psychological or emotional

development and well being of a child. For example, neglect includes failing to provide a child with food, clothing, shelter, cleanliness, medical care or protection from harm. Emotional neglect includes failing to provide a child with love, safety, and a sense of worth.

- Abandonment refers to an unjustified failure to provide adequately for the financial support for the child and an unjustified failure to maintain, or attempt to maintain, contact or a parental relationship with the child for a certain period of time. .

- Emotional abuse involves harming a child's sense of self. It includes acts (or omissions) that result in, or place a child at risk of, serious behavioural, cognitive, emotional or mental health problems. For example, emotional abuse may include verbal threats, social isolation, intimidation, exploitation, or routinely making unreasonable demands. It also includes terrorizing a child, or exposing a child to family violence. Exposure of a child to domestic violence is increasingly being seen as a category of child abuse.

WHAT IS KNOWN ABOUT THE EXTENT OF THE PROBLEM?

All provincial and territorial child welfare laws require any person who suspects that a child is being maltreated to make a report to the appropriate child welfare authority (mandatory reporting). Yet many situations of child abuse remain undisclosed, either because a child does not, or cannot, tell anyone what has happened to them, or because no one reports the abuse to the authorities (10).

Although many cases of abuse are still not reported to either police or child welfare agencies, data from these authorities are still the most important source of information about child abuse. The most comprehensive and reliable data on the extent of child abuse in Canada come from the Canadian Incidence Study of Reported Child Abuse and Neglect (CIS) (11), which estimates the extent of reported child abuse in Canada. The CIS initiative, which collects nationally representative data from child welfare agencies in five year cycles starting from 1993, is an important milestone in providing a national picture of child abuse. The 2003 Canadian Incidence Study of Reported Child Abuse and Neglect showed that an estimated 235,315 child investigations were conducted in 2003, of which nearly half were substantiated, for an incidence rate of 18.67 cases of substantiated maltreatment per 1000 children. The key findings of the CIS-2003 include:

- Child deaths: The number of children seriously harmed or killed by their parents in Canada has remained constant over the past 30 years. Less than 3% of known victims, accounting for under 3000 cases in 2003, are seriously physically harmed and an average of 35 children a year are killed (12).
- Physical abuse: In 2003, about one quarter (24%) of substantiated investigations involved physical abuse as the primary reason for the investigation. Physical abuse was confirmed in 25,257 investigations, a rate of 5.31 cases of confirmed physical abuse for every 1,000 children in Canada.
- Sexual abuse: In 2003, 3% of substantiated investigations involved sexual abuse as the primary reason for the investigation. Sexual abuse was confirmed in 2,935

investigations, a rate of 0.63 cases of confirmed physical abuse for every 1,000 children in Canada.

- Neglect: Neglect was the most common form of substantiated child abuse in 2003. Thirty percent of substantiated investigations involved neglect as the primary reason for the investigation. Neglect was confirmed in 30,366 investigations, a rate of 6.38 cases for every 1,000 children in Canada.

- Emotional maltreatment: In 2003, 15% of substantiated investigations involved emotional maltreatment as the primary reason for the investigation. Emotional maltreatment was confirmed in 15,369 investigations, a rate of 3.23 cases of confirmed physical abuse for every 1,000 children in Canada.

- Exposure to domestic violence: In 2003, 28% of substantiated investigations involved exposure to domestic violence as the primary reason for the investigation. Exposure to domestic violence was confirmed in 29,370 investigations, a rate of 6.17 cases of confirmed exposure to domestic violence for every 1,000 children in Canada.

Aboriginal children are vastly overrepresented in the Canadian child welfare system. Recent reports from provincial and territorial ministries of child and family services estimate that 30-40% of children living in out-of-home care in Canada are Aboriginal, yet Aboriginal children number fewer than five percent of children in Canada (13). In Western provinces, overrepresentation is shockingly high. In Manitoba, for example, Aboriginal children made up more than 80% of children living in out of home care in 2000 (14). Neglect is, by far, the most prevalent category of substantiated maltreatment for Aboriginal children and youth. The CIS-2003 found that 60% of the Aboriginal children in the child welfare system had maltreatment substantiated due to neglect, compared to 30% of non-Aboriginal children (15).

Similar to the US and other nations, children in the Canadian child welfare system are disadvantaged and do not tend to fare as well as their peers in the general population. The emerging profile of the children and youth in Canada's child welfare system shows a high rate of mental disorders and multiple disabilities. An Ontario study of a random sample of 429 children who were permanent wards of the Crown (16) found that more than a third (37%) of children had mental disorders. In a Manitoba study done in 2004, 33% of children in child welfare care had a disability and, of this group, 75% had an intellectual disability and 56% were diagnosed with, or suspected to have, a mental health disability. Multiple disabilities were common, and Fetal Alcohol Spectrum Disorder (FASD) was diagnosed in 11% of all children in care, most of whom were Aboriginal (17).

In 2003, the Law Commission of Canada funded a research report to measure the total economic costs of child abuse to Canadian society in the year 1998. The yearly cost of child abuse, measured by estimating costs in six major categories: judicial, social services, education, health, employment and personal, was a staggering $15,705,910,047 (18).

WHAT SYSTEM(S) OR INFRASTRUCTURE EXISTS TO ADDRESS CHILD ABUSE AND NEGLECT?

Child and family service agencies have the primary responsibility for investigating maltreatment reports and taking appropriate steps to protect the wellbeing of children. Each province and territory is covered by a network of these local agencies (or government offices serving the same purpose), and their workers respond to reports of child maltreatment or risk of maltreatment. Law enforcement agencies and emergency service providers may also be involved, depending on the circumstances. Provincial and territorial statutes stipulate the overall framework that defines when a child is considered to be at risk of maltreatment, and they also define the areas of practice in which child and family service agencies operate. The definition of the factors that constitute abuse and neglect, and the situations that need to be considered by agencies in relation to the best interests of the child, vary to some extent from one province and territory to another.

The provincial/territorial administrative structures for child and family service agencies have evolved in different ways across Canada. In Newfoundland and Labrador for example, child protection services operate within a broad provincial framework of health delivery. Regional health authorities, working within departments of the provincial government, deliver health and social services throughout the province. Each authority has a director who oversees the delivery of a range of child, youth and family services, including child protection, within the region. Children who need to be removed from their families for protective intervention are placed in the legal guardianship of the directors of the regional authorities, who delegate their responsibilities to the social workers in their agencies.

In Ontario, by way of contrast, child protection services are delivered by non-profit, community-based agencies called Children's Aid Societies, which work under locally appointed boards of directors. Children's Aid Societies receive provincial funding, and work under provincial legislation, policy and standards, but are independent agencies working in association with one another and a provincial secretariat. The large urban centre of Toronto has four child and family service agencies that provide child protection: an Aboriginal agency, a Jewish agency, a Catholic agency and a general agency.

In Quebec, child welfare services are provided by provincially funded "youth centres" which range across 18 administrative regions across the province. Quebec differs from the other provinces and territories in that children and youth with serious behavioural problems, such as those with involvement in drug abuse, or who have been running away from the parental home, can come under the purview of directors of youth protection if the security or development of the child might be in question (19). Quebec's child welfare laws define the range of situations that can harm a child from the point of view of the child's security and development.

Many of the provinces have special provisions for Aboriginal child welfare. Aboriginal cultures take a uniquely holistic view of children as being not only members of their families, but also of their communities. The preservation of cultural and community identity are important factors for the best interests of First Nations children, who have special legal status and rights under federal charters and legislation. For Aboriginal children living off reserves, provincial laws require, as a minimum, that the child's cultural heritage be taken into account for planning of service provision. Social workers working with Aboriginal children and families notify the child's tribal band of court proceedings, and the band is often involved in planning for the child. First Nations have mounted significant advocacy for rights of self-government over child welfare programs for their children, families, and communities. Tribal bands living on reserves began developing their own child and family service agencies in the 1970s. The Canadian Charter of Rights and Freedoms recognizes and affirms the rights of Aboriginal peoples and since its passage in 1982, the federal and provincial/territorial governments have given increased recognition to the needs and status of Aboriginal children. In this context, First Nations child and family service agencies are increasingly being established in the present day. These take the form of several models, the most common being a "tripartite delegated agreement" in which the provincial and federal government enter into an agreement with a First Nations or Tribal Council that delegates authority for the provision of child welfare services to the band. The terms of these agreements require that the First Nations observe provincial legislation, policy and standards in the creation of their practice, and the federal government provides full or partial funding.

Of all the provinces, Manitoba provides the broadest range of child welfare services to Aboriginal people. As a result of the recent Aboriginal Justice Inquiry-Child Welfare Initiative (20), there are now four child welfare authorities for Manitoba: two First Nations (northern and southern), one Métis, and one mainstream. People receiving child welfare services select the authority they prefer at the time of entry into the system.

Throughout Canada, Aboriginal self-government is emerging as a major third option for providing child and family services by, and for, Aboriginal peoples. Although a First Nations self-government model has yet to be fully implemented anywhere in Canada, provincial and federal governments are moving in this direction, particularly in British Columbia.

CHILD ADVOCATES

All of the provinces, with the exception of Prince Edward Island, have established offices of child advocacy, separate from the child welfare agencies and at arm's length from the provincial governments. The mandate of the offices of the Children's Advocates is to act as independent advocates for children involved in the protection process or in the legal care of a protection agency. In some provinces, the responsibility of the office of the children's advocate is combined with other roles. In New Brunswick, for example, the office of the Child and Youth Advocate is combined with the office of the provincial Ombudsman.

The role of the child and youth advocates is not to provide legal representation for children in court, but to act as independent voices on their behalf in the context of the child protection system, point out the problem areas, and advocate for change in the child welfare system. For example, in February 2009, the Saskatchewan Children's Advocate published a controversial report on the foster care system in that province, claiming that many children in the care of the province were suffering harm due to foster homes that were overcrowded and were being run in non-compliance with provincial policies and standards. In the most extreme example, a foster home that should have had just four children was instead looking after fifteen (21). Other child and youth advocates conduct periodic reviews of services for children and youth within the province and gather statistical profiles or longitudinal studies to determine such indicators of outcomes as school success rates, overall health and well-being, and criminal justice figures.

The establishment of the offices of the children's advocate reflects a political concern that the bureaucratic nature of the child welfare services within the provincial government's administrative structures may result in situations where the needs of the children and youth at risk of maltreatment are not being fully met (9).

All of the advocates are now independent officers reporting directly to elected members of the provincial legislature, with the exception of Alberta, where this matter is currently under review. The powers of the advocates do not include representation for Aboriginal children and youth living on reserves.

How Does The System Work Regarding Reporting of Possible Child Abuse and Neglect?

Throughout Canada, legislation requires that everyone has a responsibility to report suspected child abuse or neglect perpetrated by a parent, caregiver, or guardian to the relevant child welfare agency or to the police, and those who report in good faith have immunity from prosecution. In some provinces and territories, the responsibility of professionals who work with children is specifically identified (4).

This duty to report suspected child maltreatment supersedes the ethical and legal obligation to maintain confidentiality, however every province but Newfoundland and Labrador provides an exemption for solicitor-client privilege (4). In all jurisdictions except Newfoundland and Labrador, if a person discloses child abuse to his or her lawyer, the lawyer is not obligated to report it.

The "Typical" Response by the Responsible Agencies?

Child and family service agencies have two basic functions: child protection (or family services) and arranging temporary (or permanent) care for children who are not safe at home. In some agencies, workers have both child protection and child care responsibilities. Other agencies are more specialized and have intake departments with child protection workers to deal with initial investigations and crisis situations; if ongoing service is needed, cases are transferred to family service workers after the initial intake investigation is completed.

Reports of suspected child abuse and neglect are made by members of the community to child welfare service agencies. The legislation of each province and territory determines the time frame in which the agency must undertake an investigation. Often, the response time is dependent on the nature of the call, as assessed by the intake worker, with the most severe situations being taken care of the most quickly. In Ontario, for example, the response time ranges from 12 hours to 7 days (4). If the situation being reported is a clearly defined criminal act such as child physical abuse and/or sexual abuse, police are notified and a joint criminal investigation will take place with a team composed both of child welfare workers and police.

Many of the provinces use a standardized model of risk assessment, such as the Ontario Family Risk Assessment, or a structured safety assessment, such as the New Brunswick Immediate Safety Assessment. Rates of substantiation vary from a low of 20% for child sexual abuse to a high of 76% for exposure to domestic violence, with physical abuse, neglect and emotional maltreatment being substantiated at rates of 37%, 40%, and 44% respectively (22).

The presence of large numbers of unsubstantiated reports have led several jurisdictions, the first being Alberta, to adopt a differential response system (23) whereby the level of urgency is assessed first, and the type of investigation that takes places depends on the assessment of urgency or risk to the child. If it appears that the situation is not urgent, and the child is not at immediate risk of harm, a decision is made as to whether the child's needs may be met through providing the family with enhanced community services. In these situations, a caseworker will bring together a multidisciplinary team that may include representatives of a child and family service agency, a delegated First Nation agency (if applicable), early intervention services, and other services such as the school or local health authority. The purpose of the team is to help the family address challenges (e.g., mental health problems, substance abuse issues, and poor parenting skills) so that the child can live in a healthy family environment (24). Not all provinces and territories have developed differential response systems to the degree that Alberta has, but all require that child welfare systems investigate reports of child maltreatment, substantiate child abuse and neglect situations, carry out protective intervention, and work with children and families to alleviate risk.

If a maltreatment investigation determines that the child is at imminent risk of harm, provisions exist in each province and territory to immediately take the child into protective custody (some jurisdictions require a warrant for this). Child apprehensions are followed by a court application for temporary or permanent wardship (4). Typically, temporary wardship can last up to 24 consecutive months before a decision to return home or apply for permanent wardship is made. This time period can be shorter in the case of young children.

Whether or not a child is apprehended, if there is substantiated or indicated maltreatment, the child and family service agency will provide services to the child or youth with the aim of preventing further harm and reducing risk. Parents may voluntarily consent to work with the child welfare agency, or, if the family is unwilling to volunteer and if the situation warrants it, the agency may make use of the family court system to require children and parents to receive services under "supervision orders." In some provinces, such as British Columbia, the services that are provided will be tailored to the age of the child, so that if the child is over 16 and under 19, a plan is developed in collaboration with the youth to allow him or her to live independently with some supervision from the agency and with financial support, albeit often very limited, from other community services (4). The age limit for protective intervention varies across provinces and territories from age 16 to age 19 years, although most jurisdictions have extension provisions to age 21 years.

In some jurisdictions, arrangements for temporary care by agreement or special needs agreement can be made to provide care for children who are not in need of protection.

Child welfare agencies are also responsible for arranging adoptions, although in many areas there are private adoption agencies or licensees that are involved in arranging adoptions as well. Adoption statistics are difficult to determine, due in large part to the provincial and territorial mandates surrounding child welfare and the various reporting mechanisms of the provinces and territories. As of 2004, however, it was estimated that there were 78,502 children in care in Canada, of which 30,717 were legally available for adoption, and an average of 2,336 children are adopted every year (25).

WHAT HAPPENS TO CHILDREN WHO ENTER FOSTER CARE?

Child welfare agencies have responsibility for children who are taken into care on either a temporary or permanent basis. Typically, children are cared for in family-like settings in non-related foster homes or in the home of relatives or kinship caregivers. In some cases, children are placed in treatment foster care, group care, or residential care, but these placement types are generally reserved for children who have fairly substantial emotional, behavioural or health challenges. Child welfare workers have a liaison role with foster parents, relatives, and group home staff; and they also develop permanency plans to enable the child, as much as possible, to live in a family environment with a lifetime continuity of relationships. Children are placed into care environments that match their needs as closely as possible, in terms of the level of care needed by the child, the continuation of cultural or faith traditions, the level of involvement of the birth family and the preferences of the child.

There are substantial problems with the transition to adulthood for young people exiting the foster care system. The issues of arbitrary age cut-offs, lack of preparation for adult life, lack of support, and lack of funding are well documented (26), but the problems have not been effectively addressed to date.

THE STRENGTHS IN CANADA'S APPROACH/SYSTEM

Canada is an affluent country with a long standing commitment to providing a social safety net for its citizens. Under Canada's public health care model, all children are covered by the universal medical care system. In practice, however, there are inequities and the system is not comprehensive. Children in remote areas, such as the far northern reserves, do not have the same access to medical facilities as those in the south, and very little government funding has been invested in children's mental health care.

Despite provincial/territorial differences, the child welfare system has great strength in that every jurisdiction in Canada has enshrined into legislation the necessity of protecting children and youth who are at risk of maltreatment, and provides immunity from prosecution to those who report child maltreatment. Each child welfare statute had a definition of "child in need of protection" or "an endangered child." This is a key legal concept, since only children within this definition are subject to involuntary state intervention under the law. While there is some variation in how the concept of the "child in need of protection" is defined, all provinces and territories have legislation that speaks to a common set of situations of physical and sexual abuse, parental neglect and abandonment. Throughout Canada, a child may be brought into agency care without the permission of the parents. In all jurisdictions, there is also provision for protection in cases of emotional maltreatment, or if the child is an adolescent and has parents who are having serious difficulties in caring for him or her (9).

There is a growing recognition that evidence-based practice is essential to improving effectiveness in Canadian child welfare. Since 2000, federal funding has supported research and knowledge transfer initiatives such as the Canadian Incidence Study and the Centre of Excellence for Child Welfare, so that national statistics about the rates and types of child maltreatment are available to practitioners and policymakers, and dissemination of other research is conducted. Links between research, policy, and practice are being developed, but much more remains to be done.

The child welfare system is addressing issues of children and families being "in need" by providing tertiary prevention programs such as family support services, family counselling, and respite services to prevent or mitigate child maltreatment. The field of child welfare has been able to attract very committed and passionate people in a variety of professional, paraprofessional and voluntary roles who are motivated by the principle of the best interests of young people and a genuine concern for promoting positive child and youth development. Without this substantial human resources capacity, the child welfare system would not be able to function as well as it does.

The child welfare systems, although separate from the justice systems, have made many efforts to collaborate with one another, especially in situations in which reported maltreatment could lead to a criminal investigation. The development of joint police, child welfare, and health teams, as well as protocols for joint response to child abuse investigations, have also been very positive developments that have taken place over the past 30 years.

There are a variety of service models across Canada (e.g. fully government-administered systems such as Newfoundland and Labrador; government funded, community-based systems such as those in Ontario with the Children's Aid Societies; and Aboriginal models, such as those in Manitoba and on many reserves) that provide an excellent opportunity to learn from different approaches. There has also been a strong community-based focus across all the different delivery systems involving citizens and volunteers. More recently, the emergence of Aboriginal child welfare organizations provides an opportunity to address the unique needs of these populations, and also forms a basis of new learning in areas such as community involvement, family group conferencing, and extended family care (kinship and customary care).

The Child Advocates in all the provinces (except PEI, which has not appointed one) have been vocal and independent critics of the child welfare systems and have served to bring many issues regarding the well-being of children in the system to the attention of the public. The furor aroused by some very tragic deaths over the last decade, notably in British Columbia and Manitoba, has sparked a review and overhaul of some of the systems. These reforms have involved major public consultations and there is a great interest in the ability of the systems to meet the needs of children and families.

WEAKNESSES/CHALLENGES IN CANADA'S APPROACH/SYSTEM?

Canada's physical and human geography presents major challenges that are reflected in its social systems. We are a very large country with a diverse population that is sparsely scattered across rural and far northern areas. Many of the indigenous communities live in extreme poverty and isolation. At the same time, large numbers of Canadians, many of them immigrants, are congregated in a few urban centres.

At the service system level, there is considerable variation across the provinces, territories, and agencies. This diversity has precluded national initiatives on data collection, policy development and cross-Canadian programs. Overall, the service systems are under-funded and face significant capacity challenges in key areas such as human resource development and services to children, youth and families. The lack of funding for prevention of child abuse and neglect is a chronic and growing problem, and scant attention is being paid to the health and social implications of child maltreatment. The child welfare system often operates in relative isolation from other key areas that are important to the lives of young people (e.g., health, education, mental health, recreation, and justice) and this limits the ability of the system to address the complex needs of vulnerable young people.

Child welfare, as it is currently practiced in Canada, is largely crisis-driven. The data arising from the Canadian Incidence Study of Reported Child Abuse and Neglect indicate that the systems are preoccupied at the front end (investigative services) with a high number of re-opened and multiply opened cases. There is inadequate attention being paid to preventative interventions for families that are at risk of child maltreatment. The service response to children and youth with disabilities, youth with complex behavioural and mental health problems, and youth transitioning out of care, is often not sufficient to meet their needs. The system has been designed with security concerns at the forefront, but the developmental needs of children and youth are not well integrated, nor are they understood by many in the legal and social systems who serve to intervene on behalf of the best interests of children. Other countries, such as England, have a common assessment framework for children in care (such as the Looking After Children initiative) which allows health, school readiness and scholastic success to be tracked simultaneously for individual children in a manner that parallels that actions of a responsible, caring parent. In Canada, although several provinces have begun to work with the Looking After Children model, there is generally very little coordination between the education, justice, health, and child welfare systems, and rules of confidentiality preclude the inter-jurisdictional sharing of important information regarding child development (e.g., the attainment of developmental milestones) that is needed for a coordinated overview of how well the child is doing. Close attention to the developmental needs of children in care is essential if they are to reach standards for the quality of life enjoyed by their more fortunate peers (27).

MAJOR CONTROVERSIES IN CANADA'S APPROACH/SYSTEM?

One of the major debates touching on the child welfare system is why, despite Canada's affluence as a nation, 17-18% of children and families in Canada are living in poverty, and why the poverty rate has not decreased in the early 21st century despite strong economic growth and high rates of employment (28). Although Canada (and the provinces/territories) ratified the United Nations Convention on the Rights of the Child (UNCRC) in 1991, the Senate Standing Committee on Human Rights found in its 2006 report "Children: the Silenced Citizens" (29) that Canada has done a poor job of implementing and monitoring the provisions of the UNCRC. Further, Canada's national action plan for children, "A Canada Fit for Children," (30) released in 2004, lacks specific goals and an implementation monitoring process. In 2007, UNICEF released its Report Card 7, a report on the monitoring of the performance of the world's most wealthy countries, those in the Organization for Economic Co-operation and Development (OECD). In this report, which looked at six dimensions of the well-being of children and adolescents, Canada ranked a surprisingly low 12th place out of 21 OECD countries in overall child well-being (31). Although Canada has a generous and universal public education and health care system, there are great disparities in outcomes for children born in Canada, (32) and there is a lack of political will to deal with issues related to children's well-being at the federal level. There is no federal body or commission, such as a National Children's Commissioner, with a duty to define the best interests of children and mandate to oversee their health and wellbeing.

The under-funding of child welfare systems is a continuing problem in Canada, particularly the lack of funding for prevention programs. The diminishing human resources capacity of the system at all levels is a continuing problem. The lack of research to support the development of effective services is a rapidly growing issue, particularly as accountability expectations grow with respect to meaningful outcomes and increased competition for scarce public resources. The unique resource requirements and capacity building issues for the development of Aboriginal child welfare services includes all of the above identified issues, but must also be considered in light of the profound societal mistreatment and the resulting highly disadvantaged circumstances of Aboriginal children and families both on and off reserves.

The situation with regard to the overrepresentation of Aboriginal children is a source of great controversy. Aboriginal child and family service agencies are working with populations that are growing at the fastest pace of any ethnic group in Canada. Between 1998 and 2006, the Aboriginal population grew by 45%, nearly six times faster than the 8% rate of increase for the non-Aboriginal population (5). Data collected for a recent national policy review show that the chances of a First Nations child being in child welfare care are approximately one in ten, compared with one in 200 non-First Nations children in Canada (33). Approximately 8,000 children are in the care of First Nations agencies, which contribute to an estimated total of 27,000 children First Nations children in provincial agency care (34). This is three times the number of children that were in residential schools at the height of their operation (35) and marks a substantial overrepresentation of children in care with respect to their overall numbers in the population.

There are major concerns regarding the lack of equity in the level of funding provided by the federal government to First Nations child and family services, compared to levels of provincial funding provided to mainstream agencies. In 2008, First Nations representatives made a complaint about the inequitable funding of their child and family service agencies to the Canadian Human Rights Commission, which, at the time of writing, is set to go before a Tribunal Hearing. The federal government has recently established a Child Welfare Early Prevention Fund for First Nations agencies, and is implementing the program on an incremental basis. Although there are plans to expand the program, it is currently being implemented in only three provinces.

Despite the fact that the international community ratified the United Nations Declaration on the Rights of Indigenous Peoples in 2007, setting out human rights standards for indigenous peoples, Canada was not a signatory to the Declaration, citing concerns about the possibility of reopening previously settled land claims.

Moving to other aspects of concerns related to human rights in Canada, the extent to which physical discipline of children constitutes abuse is another ongoing controversy. As mentioned earlier, section 43 of the Criminal Code, which has remained part of criminal law since 1892, defends the assault of certain identified classes of people, and originally included children, apprentices, prisoners, and sailors. Over time, these special exemptions have been repealed with the exception of children, who can still be assaulted providing the force is considered reasonable in the circumstances and is used for the purposes of correction (4). Examination of substantiated cases of physical abuse, as documented in the Canadian Incidence Study of Reported Child Abuse and Neglect, 2003, has shown that one quarter of substantiated cases did not exceed any of the Supreme Court's limits, suggesting that a large proportion of incidents of physical maltreatment are not being captured by the Court's limits on corrective force (36). This section of the Criminal Code continues to come under scrutiny by those concerned with the best interests of children in Canada.

PREVENTION EFFORTS (PRIMARY, SECONDARY, TERTIARY)

Prevention is often categorized into three streams: primary (preventing something before it happens); secondary (preventing something from happening again); and tertiary (treating the problem in the hopes that worse complications will not ensue). Despite having a more preventive approach to healthcare, Canada's child welfare system is structured in a manner that is consistent with what Alfred Kadushin (37) termed a residual model. That is, services are generally provided to families once maltreatment has occurred or is at high risk of occurring. Services are mostly seen as intrusive and costly, and they are provided only when they are perceived as imminently necessary. Similar to the US, this philosophy has translated into a lack of primary prevention efforts in child welfare, with services instead focusing on the secondary prevention of child maltreatment through either providing preservation or maintenance services to birth families or, when these are untenable, placing children into foster care.

The movement, across Canada, toward differential response models may be a step in the right direction, but the focus is still on secondary prevention. The differential response model in Ontario, for instance, uses elements of structured decision-making (including a validated risk assessment instrument) to determine whether families reported for maltreatment should receive community services or standard investigative services. In theory, this model allows more flexibility for agencies to use a less coercive approach. The inclusion of a validated tool likely means that better decisions are made at the front end of service provision, translating to lower recurrence rates. However, entry to the system is still based upon a child maltreatment report, implying that opportunities for primary prevention efforts have long since passed. Tertiary prevention is highly variable and generally comes in the form of foster care and treatment foster care. Targeted services (e.g., behavioral and mental health services) for maltreated youth are provided through individual agencies and high quality, effective services (e.g., Trauma-focused Cognitive Behavioural Therapy) can often be found, but this is not always the case. In rural areas or highly impacted urban areas, access to services can be extremely limited.

Nonetheless, progress in primary prevention has been forthcoming in a number of areas. Quebec offers universal child care at $7 per day. Such a program decreases stress in overburdened families and also provides structured interactions and stimulation for children, some of whom might come from fairly deprived homes. Unfortunately, the federal government withdrew plans for funding to support a national child care system in 2006/2007, and replaced this program with a modest monthly income supplement to parents. A recent UNICEF report found Canada at the bottom of the OECD countries with respect to availability, quality and standards of early childhood services (38).

Multi-level prevention and treatment programs are slowly being implemented in Canada. For instance, some provinces have implemented, and are testing, 'Triple P,' (39) a program based on social learning theory, that operates at three levels: the macro/population level using public announcements and televised parenting shows; the mezzo level, uisng universal parenting education programs; and at the micro level, using more intensive parenting programs for high risk families. In addition, the 'Nurse-Family Partnership' (40) and Webster-Stratton's 'Incredible Years (41, 42) programs have been launched in various sites across the country.

However, greater emphasis needs to be placed on primary prevention and, especially with respect to the Aboriginal population in Canada, the structural issues (e.g., historical oppression, substance abuse, poverty, funding disparities, lack of adequate housing and services) that bring families to the attention of child welfare in the first place. The overrepresentation of Aboriginal children in foster care has led some to propose a complete restructuring of child welfare as part of a reconciliation process (43) that utilizes more traditional forms of caring and encourages high levels of community cohesion. Such movements, if properly funded, have the potential to reshape child welfare as we know it, relying to a greater extent on promoting community cohesion than treating individual pathology.

REFERENCES

[1] US Government. The 2009 World Factbook: Canada. Washington, DC: US Government Printing Office, 2009. Retrieved March 9, 2009 at: https://www.cia.gov/library/publications/the-world-factbook/print/ca.html

[2] UNICEF. Statistics at a glance: Canada. Retrieved March 10, 2009 at:
http://www.unicef.org/infobycountry/canada_statistics.html

[3] One World: Nations Online Project. Canada. Retrieved March 10, 2009
at: http://www.nationsonline.org/oneworld/canada.htm

[4] Regehr C, Kanani K. Essential law for social work practice in Canada. Don Mills, ON: Oxford Univ Press, 2006.

[5] Statistics Canada. Aboriginal peoples in Canada in 2006: Inuit, Métis, and First Nations, 2006 Census highlights. Retrieved March 10, 2009 at:
http://www12.statcan.ca/english/census06/analysis/aboriginal/highlights.cfm

[6] Sinclair M, Bala N, Lilles H, Blackstock C. Aboriginal child welfare. In: Bala N, Zapf MK, Williams RJ, Vogl R, Hornick J, eds. Canadian child welfare law: Children, families and the state. Toronto, ON: Thompson Educ Publ, 2004:199-244.

[7] Criminal Code, R.S.C. 1985. c. C-46, s.43. The constitutional validity of this position was upheld by the Supreme Court of Canada in Canadian Foundation for Children, Youth and the Law v. Canada (2004) S.C. J. 6.

[8] Criminal Code, R.S.C. 1985, c. C-46, ss 215, 218.

[9] Bala N. Child welfare law in Canada: An introduction. In: Bala N, Zapf MK, Williams RJ, Vogl R, Hornick J, eds. Canadian child welfare law: Children, families and the state. Toronto, ON: Thompson Educ Publ, 2004:1-25.

[10]   Department of Justice, Canada. "Child abuse: A Fact Sheet from the Department of Justice Canada." Retrieved March 8, 2009 at: http://www.justice.gc.ca/eng/pi/fv-vf/facts-info/child-enf.html

[11]   Trocmé N, Fallon B, MacLaurin B, Daciuk J, Felstiner C, Black T, et al. Canadian incidence study of reported child abuse and neglect – 2003: Major findings. Ottawa, ON: Min Public Works Gov Serv Can, 2005.

[12]   Trocmé N, Lajoie J, Fallon B, Felstiner C. Injuries and deaths of children at the hands of their parents. CECW Information Sheet #57E. Toronto, ON: University of Toronto Faculty of Social Work. Retrieved March 9, 2009 from www.cecw-cepb.ca/DocsEng/Injuries57E.pdf

[13]   Gough P, Trocmé N, Brown I, Knoke D, Blackstock C. Pathways to overrepresentation of Aboriginal children in care. CECW Information Sheet #23E. Toronto, ON, Canada: University of Toronto. Retreived [date] from www.cecw-cepb.ca/DocsEng/AboriginalChildren23Epdf.

[14]   Aboriginal Justice Inquiry--Child Welfare Initiative (AJI-CWI). (2001). Promise of Hope: Commitment to Change: Child and Family Services in Manitoba Canada. Winnipeg, Manitoba: Executive Committee of the AJI-CWI. Available at: http://www.aji-cwi.mb.ca/eng/Phase3/promiseofhope.html

[15]   Trocmé N, Knoke D, Shangreaux C, Fallon B, MacLaurin B. The experience of First Nations children coming into contact with the child welfare system in Canada: The Canadian Incidence Study on Reported Abuse and Neglect. In: First Nations Child and Family Caring Society, Wen:De: we are coming to the light of day. Ottawa, ON: Author, 2005:60-86.

[16]   Burge P. Prevalence of mental disorders and associated service variables among Ontario children who are permanent wards. Can J Psychiatry 2007;52:305-14.

[17]   Fuchs D, Burnside L, Marchenski S, Mudry A. Children with disabilities receiving services from child welfare agencies in Manitoba. Centre of Excellence for Child Welfare, Canada. Toronto, ON: Faculty of Social Work, University of Toronto. Retrieved [2009 Jan 02] from http://www.cecw-cepb.ca/files/file/en/DisabilitiesManitobaFinal.pdf

[18]   Bowlus A, McKenna K, Day T, Wright D. The economic costs and consequences of child abuse in Canada: Report to the Law Commission of Canada. London, ON, Canada: University West Ontario, 2003

[19]   Lajoie J. Québec's child welfare system. CECW Information Sheet #35E. Montréal, QC: McGill University, School of Social Work. Available at: http://www.cecw-cepb.ca/DocsEng/QueChildWelfareSystem35E.pdf

[20]   Aboriginal Justice Inquiry--Child Welfare Initiative (AJI-CWI). (2001). Promise of Hope: Commitment to Change: Child and Family Services in Manitoba Canada. Winnipeg, Manitoba: Executive Committee of the AJI-CWI.

[21]   Bernstein M. A breach of trust: An investigation into foster home overcrowding in the Saskatoon Service Centre. Saskatchewan Children's Advocate's Office. Retrieved March 5, 2009 from http://www.saskcao.ca/documents/FHOC_Report_022509%20(2).pdf

[22]   Trocmé N, Knoke D, Fallon B, MacLaurin, B. Substantiating child maltreatment: CIS-2003. CECW information sheet 40E. Toronto, ON: University of Toronto Faculty of Social Work. Retrieved March 9, 2009 from www.cecw-cepb.ca/DocsEng/SubChildMaltreatment40.pdf

[23]   Waldfogel J. The future of child protection. Cambridge, MA: Harvard Univ Press, 1998.

[24]   Gough P. Alberta's child welfare system. CECW Information Sheet #46E. Toronto, ON, Canada: University of Toronto Faculty of Social Work. Retrieved March 9, 2009 from www.cecw-cepb.ca/DocsEng/Altachildwelfaresystem46E.pdf

[25]   Pederson S. Adoption Council of Canada. Personal communication, 2009.

[26]   Reid C, Dudding P. Building a future together: Issues and outcomes for transition-aged youth. Ottawa, ON: Centre of Excellence for Child Welfare, 2006. Available at http://www.cecw-cepb.ca/files/file/en/BuildingAFutureTogether.pdf

[27]   Kufeldt K, Este D, McKenzie B, Wharf B. Critical issues in child welfare. In: Kufeldt K, McKenzie B, eds. Child welfare: Connecting research, policy and practice. Waterloo, ON: Wilfred Laurier Press, 2003.

[28]   Campaign 2000. 2006 Report Card on Child and Family Poverty in Canada. Retrieved March 5, 2009 from: http://www.campaign2000.ca/rc/rc06/06_C2000NationalReportCard.pdf

[29] Government of Canada. Children: The silenced citizens: Effective Implementation of Canada's International obligations with respect to the rights of children. Final Report of the Standing Senate Committee on Human Rights, 2007. Available at: http://www.parl.gc.ca/39/1/parlbus/commbus/senate/Com-e/huma-e/rep-e/rep10apr07 e.htm#_Toc164844428

[30] Government of Canada. A Canada fit for children: Canada's plan of action in response to the May, 2002 United Nations Special Session on children. Ottawa, ON: Her Majesty the Queen in Right of Canada, 2004. Available at: http://www.hrsdc.gc.ca/eng/cs/sp/sdc/socpol/publications/2002-002483/canadafite.pdf .

[31] UNICEF. Child poverty in perspective: an overview of child poverty in rich countries, Report Card Innocenti 7. Florence, Italy: UNICEF Innocenti Research Centre, 2007.

[32] Turpel-Lafond ME. Representative for Children and Youth, British Columbia. (personal communication, February 27, 2009). Speech made at UNICEF Canada's "The Best Interests of the Child: Meaning and Application in Canada" conference.

[33] First Nations Child and Family Caring Society of Canada. National policy review phase two report. Retrieved March 5, 2009 from: http://www.fncfs.com/projects/nationalPolicy.html

[34] Assembly of First Nations. First Nations child and family services: Questions and answers. Retrieved March 10, 2009 from: http://www.afn.ca/article.asp?id=3372

[35] National Collaborating Centre for Aboriginal Health. Aboriginal and non-Aboriginal children in child protection services. Retrieved March 4, 2009 from: http://www.nccah-ccnsa.ca/downloads/nccah-factsheet1-childhealth.pdf

[36] Durrant J, Trocmé N, Fallon B, Milne C, Black T, Petrowski N. Physical punishment of children: Assessing the validity of the legal definition of "reasonable force." CECW Information Sheet #71E. Toronto, ON, Canada: Centre of Excellence for Child Welfare. Retrieved March 9, 2009 fromcecw-cepb.ca/DocsEng/PhysPun71E.pdf www.cecw-cepb.ca/DocsEng/PhysPun71E.pdf

[37] Kadushin A, ed. Child welfare services: A sourcebook. New York: Macmillan, 1970.

[38] UNICEF. The child care transition. Innocenti Report Card 8, UNICEF Research Centre, Florence, Italy, 2008.

[39] Sanders MR. The Triple P-Positive parenting program: Towards an empirically validated multilevel parenting and family support strategy for the prevention of behavior and emotional problems in children. Clin Child Fam Psychol Rev 1999;2(2):71-90.

[40] Olds DL. Prenatal and infancy home visiting by nurses: from randomized trials to community replication. Prev Sci 2002;3(3):153-72.

[41] Linares OL, Montalto D, Li M, Vikash S, Oza VS. A promising parenting intervention in foster care. J Consult Clin Psychol 2006;74(1):32-41.

[42] Taylor TK, Schmidt F, Pepler D, Hodgins H. A comparison of eclectic treatment with Webster-Stratton's Parents and Children Series in a Children's Mental Health Center: A randomized controlled trial. Behav Ther 1998;29:221-40.

[43] First Nations Child and Family Caring Society. Wen:De: We are coming to the light of day. Ottawa, ON: Author, 2005. Available at: http://www.fncfs.com/docs/WendeReport.pdf

In: International Aspects of Child Abuse and Neglect   ISBN: 978-1-60876-703-8
Editors: H. Dubowitz, J. Merrick pp. 191-198   © 2010 Nova Science Publishers, Inc.

Chapter 18

CHILD MALTREATMENT IN ARGENTINA

*Irene Intebi**

Private practice, Buenos Aires, Argentina

This chapter describes the child protection system and policies in Argentina. It briefly comments on the types of maltreatment professional have to deal with, including missing children of the late 1970s and the effects on children of the 2001 financial crisis. It depicts the systems that exist to address child abuse and how they work regarding the reporting of possible maltreatment. It also portrays the strengths and the challenges in this approach.

INTRODUCTION

Argentina is a South American country, a federation of twenty-four provinces and an autonomous city. It is second in size on the continent to Brazil and the eighth largest country in the world. Argentina occupies a continental surface area of 2,766,890 km² (1,068,302 sq mi) between the Andes mountain range in the west and the southern Atlantic Ocean in the east and south.

The National Institute of Statistics and Census of Argentina (INDEC) 2001 census showed the population to be 36,260,130. It ranks third in South America in total population and 30th globally. The 2007 estimate is for a population of 40,927,301. Argentina's population density is 14 inhabitants per square kilometer. However, the population is not evenly distributed: areas of Buenos Aires have a population density of over 14,000 inhabitant/km², while Santa Cruz province has less than 1 inhabitant/km². Argentina is the only nation in South America with a net positive migration rate, of about +0.4 persons. According to the 2001 INDEC population census, there are about 12.2 million children and young people under 18, representing 32% of the population.

School attendance is compulsory between 5 and 17 years of age. The Argentine school system consists of a primary or lower school level lasting six or seven years, and a secondary

---

* *Correspondence:* Irene Intebi, MD, Junín 969–9°A, Buenos Aires, C1113AA Argentina. E-mail: ireneintebi@ciudad.com

or high school level lasting between five to six years. Education in public schools (primary, secondary and tertiary) is free. Public education, thought to have been of the best quality during the mid 20th century, is now often perceived as bad and in continuous decline because of lack of funding. Today, the country has a literacy rate of 97%.

Argentina's population is very highly urbanized. About 3.5 million people live in the autonomous city of Buenos Aires, and 12.4 million in Greater Buenos Aires (2007), making it one of the largest urban centers in the world. Illegal immigration has been a relatively important factor in recent years. Most illegal immigrants come from Bolivia and Paraguay, bordering Argentina to the north. Smaller numbers arrive from Peru, Ecuador, and Romania. The Argentine government estimates that 750,000 inhabitants lack official documents.

THE ECONOMY (1990- 2008)

In the last 4 years, Argentina appears to be recovering from the 2001 crisis. It has the highest Human Development Index level and Gross Domestic Product (GDP) per capita in purchasing power in Latin America. The Human Development Index is a summary composite index that measures a country's average achievements in three basic aspects of human development: health, knowledge, and a decent standard of living. Health is measured by life expectancy at birth; knowledge is measured by a combination of the adult literacy rate and the combined primary, secondary, and tertiary gross enrolment ratio; and standard of living by GDP per capita (PPP US$). For further details, visit hdr.undp.org/en/statistics/faq/question,68,en.html. The country is currently classified as an Upper-Middle Income Country or as a secondary emerging market by the World Bank. Argentina's GDP makes it the 31st largest economy in the world.

But, the present 8% annual GDP growth has not had a proportionate impact on equitable income distribution: after four years of such a growth, 10% of the poorest sector of the population has a 73 peso per capita monthly income ($US 21) while the richest 10% has an over 2,200 peso per capita monthly income (about $US 715).

The 1990s represented a period of strong structural imbalance in every aspect of the country economy, especially due to the privatization of companies and resources that had until that time been managed by the government, and, the massive importation of manufactured goods. Following 1989 hyperinflation, a drastic set of reforms were started: national companies and businesses were privatized; an artificial exchange rate was established (US$1=1 Argentinean peso); taxes and protective regulations of local manufacturing were eliminated; and workers' rights were limited. These measures were supposed to bring stability and improve people's welfare led to increased poverty (30% of the population); unemployment (double digit percentages); unprecedented social inequality; recession; and negative growth (1). This imbalance represented a major change in employment opportunities, in working conditions and in the decrease of the working class's income ,triggering deep economic and social transformations. The elimination of welfare policies also aggravated social inequality.

Rural towns become ghost towns when train services ceased and slums (villas miserias) sprouted in the outskirts of the largest cities, inhabited by impoverished lower-class urban dwellers, migrants from smaller towns in the interior, and immigrants from neighboring countries that came during the '90s apparent economic boom.

Thus, economic policies generated a serious deterioration of general population living conditions in a country that was not used nor prepared to face the impoverishment of such a large proportion of its population. This deterioration resulted also in a marked increase in children living in poverty, up to 58.6% of the population under 18. Argentina became one of fifteen countries with the most unfair income distribution in the world.

IMPACT OF 2001 FINANCIAL CRISIS ON CHILDREN

The increase of poverty led to family survival strategies which often involved children in the activities to obtain resources, such as:

- Informal "jobs" on the streets: selling different kinds of cheap merchandise, cleaning windscreens, begging, and looking after their younger siblings while their parents begged.
- At-home "jobs": looking after siblings while adults worked, household responsibilities.
- Work with parents in marginal activities: "cirujeo" (looking for recyclable marketable items –mostly cardboard; metal and plastic items not necessarily usable goods- in the garbage in urban areas)

Universal policies, such as health and education, suffered budget cuts during the crisis; that have become permanent, compromising the administration of crucial programs.

There are very few governmental studies and research related to the current social situation of childhood and regarding the paths the national, provincial and local policies should follow to improve this situation. Most social programs only cover basic and immediate needs in a quasi-paternalist fashion –providing specific resources to children and families following their own requests, without any previously developed plan with strategies and goals, and without investing in long-term outcomes for improving children's and adolescents' lives.

Programs and strategies are usually started without studying actual needs and resources, something very frequent in other areas as well.

TYPES OF CHILD ABUSE AND NEGLECT (CAN)

The types of child abuse and neglect addressed by legislation and policies are mostly intrafamilial abuse (physical, sexual and emotional abuse, and neglect) and extrafamilial sexual abuse.

NGOs and human rights activists report that 19,579 children and young people under 18 years are confined in institutions and police facilities in terrible and humiliating living conditions; some dying of preventable conditions, while many are victimized, beaten and sexually abused. Remarkably, 87.1% of the confinements are due to socioeconomic and "protective" reasons , not to offenses or crimes (2). Based on old legislation, whenever a child living in an institution - as a protective measure - runs away, professionals have to report it to the police and to the criminal system. When the child is found she/he is confined to more restrictive institutions with limited freedom. Some professionals try to avoid such procedures by reporting "abandonment of treatment" to ensure family court intervention instead.

Despite legislation to prevent child labor, many children are in the workforce; 5 to 9% of 5 -13 year olds, 8 to 15% of 10 – 13 year olds, and 20% of 14 to 17 year olds (3).

Unfortunately Argentina has "coined" a recently identified problem: missing children. In March 1976, the military forces led a coup d'état against the democratically elected government and established the Proceso de Reorganización Nacional, a dictatorship that lasted until December 1983. During that period, about 30,000 people who opposed the regime were kidnapped and killed by the military and police.

Sadly, the kidnapping of babies and children was part of this organized terror carried out by the authorities. Seven thousand children and adolescents were victimized by the kidnapping of one or both parents; 450 to 500 babies were born to missing mothers in concentration camps. After the babies were born, the mothers were killed and the babies were "given" to other families. Decisions of where the babies would go or to whom were totally arbitrary, depending of the military leaders of the concentration camps. The closest to legal adoptions happened, when the military abandoned babies and children at hospitals and/or with neighbors. Unfortunately, this was not frequent. More typically, they regarded the children and babies as their booty. They either kept them or gave them as "presents" to military families, to ensure they would "straighten" them up by raising them "correctly."

The non-governmental organization Abuelas de Plaza de Mayo, formed in 1977, aimed to locate the kidnapped children, return them to their legitimate families (although their parents had been killed), and prosecute those responsible, as well as to prevent similar human rights violations in the future. By July 2008, 92 grandchildren were found and contacted by their biological families. The great majority re-established contacts with their families and many – not all- were returned to them.

EXTENT OF THE PROBLEM

There are three main obstacles to measuring the extent of child abuse and neglect in Argentina.

- The vast Argentinean territory and the political organization as a federation of twenty-four provinces and an autonomous city make it difficult to keep reliable and comparable records. This is a difficulty found by many large countries and it is not insurmountable, but the Argentinean information system seems very chaotic to address this issue.
- There are no studies addressing the magnitude of the problem. Governmental or university funded research in the field is practically non-existent. Research depends on individuals or small teams and funding opportunities. This is true not only for child abuse and neglect, but for many other issues related to health and social conditions. This results in many researchers emigrating to pursue their interests.

- There have been very few efforts to define different types of child abuse, to adapting international ones, and to selecting measurable indicators and methods.

In urban areas, the population is moderately aware of the problem, usually based on media attention to the most severe cases. Still, many people support the use of corporal punishment. In Argentina, professionals and community in general know very little about the mid- and long-term effects of moderate or serious child abuse. Few consider child abuse to be a community problem; rather, it is seen as one involving individual families and requiring individual professional responses.

An epidemiologic investigation in a small town in Chubut province (Argentinean Patagonia) showed that 13% of students aged 4-14 years were suspected of suffering some type of child abuse and neglect (4) .

CHARACTERISTICS OF THE SYSTEM TO ADDRESS CAN

The child protection system is undergoing a transition with many blind spots and neglected areas. Mandatory reporting to the civil court system was started in Buenos Aires in 1996 and has expanded to all the provinces. Until 2005, most serious cases were reported to civil courts that could enforce protective measures based on professionals' reports or the risk assessment by the judicial system team. If the civil courts considered that a crime had been committed (severe physical abuse and/or neglect; abandonment; intrafamilial sexual abuse), they reported it to the criminal courts. In the meantime, the child would be protected by civil court measures.

Currently, after new legislation incorporating the United Nations Convention on the Rights of the Child (CRC) standards, was passed - Law 26.061 (Protección Integral de los Derechos de Niños, Niñas y Adolescentes or Integral Protection of Children and Adolescents Rights), there is confusion on implementation. While, it represents a major step forward to ensure children's wellbeing, its implementation has been delayed. NGOs report that the judicial system in some provinces is reluctant to implement the new legislation, including cases where its implementation has been vetoed or suspended.

Regarding child abuse and neglect interventions, there are contradictions or a lack of clarity on who should intervene. In theory, reports should be made to a governmental agency, independent of the judicial system. This agency should assess risks and decide how to intervene (e.g., whether judicial intervention or therapy are needed.)

Although the underlying idea appears promising, the system is facing many problems to intervene efficiently, including:

- Lack of trained and experienced staff in governmental agencies
- Organizational problems (creation of local agencies; lack of staff; poorly trained staff; limited hours of operation)
- Lack of collaboration between agencies in different neighborhoods, municipalities and provinces
- Lack of cooperation between other governmental programs and institutions and the judicial system

- Lack of networks and resources to refer cases for in-depth assessment or for treatment
- Lack of intervention resources

THE "TYPICAL" RESPONSE BY THE RESPONSIBLE AGENCIES

Theoretically, when a case is detected by schools or physicians or, rarely, when a family consults the governmental agency spontaneously, staff from the agency (lawyers, social workers and psychologists) assess the problem and the risk level. They may decide:

a. that the risk is low and refer the case to another service;
b. that the risk is low to medium and refer the case to a child abuse intervention program – if one is available (governmental or NGO; usually in urban areas);
c. that the risk is high and refer the case to civil or criminal judicial system (with or without a referral for treatment)

The governmental agency has no authority to remove a child from home, even if the risk is high. Only the civil courts can do so. In cases of domestic and family violence, however, the courts can remove the offender(s) from the home enabling the victim(s) to stay in their own environment. There are no resources for treating offenders.

A child abuse intervention program performs an in-depth assessment of causes and family dynamics and offers different types of treatment and follow-up.

In light of the transition the system is currently undergoing, there are no intervention protocols in place. This procedure varies according to the program or the individual professional's approach. There is no supervision and very limited professional liability in this respect.

STRENGTHS OF THE SYSTEM (5)

The strengths in the system relate to its potential, based on the national legislation and the incorporation of the CRC into the Argentinean Constitution. The fact that the legislation enables the removal of offender(s) and not the victim(s) is another strength of the system.

WEAKNESSES/CHALLENGES IN THE APPROACH/SYSTEM

The system faces many challenges, including:

- lack of public health policies to address child abuse and neglect;
- lack of awareness among policy-makers of the importance of having a policy to address this problem;
- low or non-existent budgets to address the problem;
- lack of governmental and/or NGO resources;

- lack of collaboration between government authorities & professionals;
- vast geographic area;
- different procedures, approaches and resources depending on location (Buenos Aires, other main cities, rural areas);
- lack of reliable information on the magnitude of the problem;
- lack of training opportunities for frontline workers;
- lack of specific treatment programs for victims, families and offenders;
- lack of awareness in the community, and among professionals and policy makers, of the mid- and long-term consequences of child abuse and neglect;
- blind spots and neglected areas in detection and intervention procedures together with overlapping services in other areas (e.g., there are many municipal and national agencies in the same areas dedicated only to admissions and referral, but very few programs that assess cases and offer treatment)
- lack of national detection and intervention guidelines and protocols
- lack of research

Major Controversies in the Approach or System

There are two major controversies among professionals who intervene in child abuse cases:

- Need to include the judicial system (civil or criminal courts) vs. a family/community-based approach exclusively due to bad experiences and, sometimes, inadequate legal interventions professionals do not trust that effective outcomes will result from legal intervention. This could be improved by mandatory training of all the professionals involved in the child abuse field and of the decision-making professionals in the judicial system.
- Importance of biological bonds vs. a child's wellbeing and protection. Many times in recent years, children have been forced to either live together with or visit their offender(s) just because he/she is a parent or relative. There is no awareness that biological bonds do not ensure that a caregiver adequately protects a child.

Prevention Efforts (Primary, Secondary, Tertiary)

Prevention efforts are few and generally do not address the roots contributors of the problem. They depend mostly on NGOs and individuals. For example, ISPCAN (International Society for the Prevention of Child Abuse and Neglect) has been training professionals in different disciplines and supporting NGOs' child protection projects in Chubut province (Argentinean Patagonia) through the ITPI (International Training Project) since 2000.

REFERENCES

[1]   Bermúdez, I. Argentina: un despegue con marcha atrás. Lo que la década del 90 se llevó. Clarín 2001 Feb 04.
[2]   Secretaría Nacional de Derechos Humanos and UNICEF Report. 2005.
[3]   Trabajo infantil en la Argentina: avances en su medición, Encuesta de Actividades de Niños, Niñas y Adolescentes (EANNA). Last quarter, 2004.
[4]   Malerba T, Canale R, Stiglich K, Barberi C, González de Bisel M. Investigación Epidemiológica del Maltrato Infantil (Sarmiento- Provincia de Chubut). Familias del Nuevo Siglo. Argentina, 2006.
[5]   Intebi, I. Concept paper on the situation of child protection in Argentina presented at ISPCAN Global Summit on Protecting Children from Violence, Abuse and Neglect. Chicago, April 2008.

In: International Aspects of Child Abuse and Neglect   ISBN: 978-1-60876-703-8
Editors: H. Dubowitz, J. Merrick pp. 199-211   © 2010 Nova Science Publishers, Inc.

Chapter 19

CHILD PROTECTION IN BRAZIL: CHALLENGES AND OPPORTUNITIES

Victoria G Lidchi, Daisy Veiga, and Evelyn Eisenstein

The Noos Institute (Instituto Noos)
The Centre of Integrated Studies of Infancy Adolescence and Health or CEIIAS
(Centro de Estudos Integrados Infancia Adolescencia e Saude) Rio de Janeiro, Brazil

Since 1990, Brazil, as a signatory to the United Nation's Convention on the Rights of the Child, has had a statute protecting the rights of children to health, education and safety from harm. This chapter describes how the different forms of child abuse and neglect have been defined in the years following the implemention of the statute and what is known about the problem in Brazil. The Brazilian child protection infrastructure will be outlined, including a desription of the mandatory reporting process and a typical response of the system to child protection concerns. The strengths, weaknesses and controversies surrounding approaches to protecting children are discussed concluding that whilst Brazil has a good legal framework, there are many challenges lying ahead in terms of its implementation.

INTRODUCTION

Brazil covers 39% of South America, covering 8.5 million square kilometers. Of its 186 million inhabitants, 72 million (40%) are children and adolescents aged 0-19 years. Its size and diversity present some unique challenges for the protection of children against violence and abuse. Brazil is both ethnically and socially diverse, with the largest black population outside of Africa, and a large miscegenated population of Caucasians from Europe, Latin American Indians and those from Asian background. In the 20th century Brazil saw waves of immigration including Japanese, German and Italian arrivals. The diversity includes European heritage and influences in the relatively affluent South of the country and the traditions of the Afro-Brazilian culture of the lower income North Eastern States. Brazil also has one of South America's highest Gini coefficients (1) which is a measure of income inequality. Inequality of income distribution and associated poverty, social marginalization and exclusion – referred to as structural violence (2) – has been linked to high levels of interpersonal violence (3).

The profound socio-economic disparities that characterize Brazil are reflected in the contrasts that exist in the skills, knowledge, institutional infrastructure and resources that are available to address violence in all its forms including child abuse and neglect (CAN). However, the Brazilian Child and Adolescent Statute ECA Law enacted since 1990 has committed the government to guaranteeing all children and adolescents the same rights to protection and a healthy development, as an absolute priority and a duty of the family, society and the state. The challenges and innovative initiatives which have arisen as a result of this commitment will be discussed in response to the following questions.

HOW ARE THE DIFFERENT TYPES OF CAN DEFINED?

A number of Brazilian institutions use definitions and models disseminated by international organizations and recent studies have used both the ecological model (4) of violence and the typologies of violence and child abuse and neglect defined by the WHO (5,6). The Brazilian Pediatric Association in collaboration with the Ministry of Justice and leading research institutions produced a professional guide in 2001 containing a definition of maltreatment as "when someone who is in a superior position of "force" (age, social or economic status, intelligence or authority) commits physical, psychological or sexual harm against the wishes of the victim or with the victim's consent, the consent being obtained by inducement or deceitful seduction" (7)). The different categories of abuse recognized in the guide were:

- Physical abuse: defined as "the physical force exerted by relatives or people who are in close proximity to the child with the intention of hurting or destroying the child with or without leaving physical signs" (7) . There is recognition of the "shaken baby syndrome" ("síndrome do bebê sacudido") as "a form of physical abuse that consists of cerebral lesions that occur when the child is usually younger than six months and is shaken by an adult". This is distinguished from the "battered child syndrome" (a síndrome da criança espancada"), which refers to "young children who have suffered injuries such as bone fractures, burns at different times and stages of their development and the explanations given by the parents are inconsistent with the injuries" (8). Finally "Munchausen Syndrome by proxy (Síndrome de Munchausen por procuração) is defined as" a situation in which the child receives medical care for symptoms or signals which have been invented by those responsible for their care. The consequences of this medical care can be conceived of as physical violence (unnecessary medical tests, unnecessary use of medication or the forced ingestion of liquids) and psychological violence (repeated unnecessary medical appointments and hospitalization)."
- Sexual Abuse is "any and all sexual game, relationship (homosexual or heterosexual) in which the aggressor is at a more advanced stage of psychosexual development than the child or adolescent and where the intention is to stimulate or use them sexually to obtain pleasure. These sexual practices are imposed on the child and adolescent through the use of physical violence, threats or influencing them. The acts

vary and include non-contact (voyeurism and exhibitionism) as well as contact (penetration) forms. It includes situations of sexual exploitation such as prostitution and pornography" (7) .

- Psychological maltreatment: includes "all forms of rejection, depreciation, discrimination, disrespect, negative regard and exaggerated punishment or use of the child or adolescent for the needs of the adult responsible for their care. All these aspects of psychological maltreatment can compromise the biopsychosocial development of the child. The subtlety of this type of maltreatment and the absence of immediate evidence of maltreatment makes this type of "violence" one of the most difficult to identify despite its presence within the other types of violence".

- Neglect: is "an act of omission by adults responsible for the care of the child or adolescent, that is a failure to provide for the basic necessities that will safeguard their development" (9) . Abandonment is discussed as an "an extreme form of neglect" where neglect can signify omission of basic care such as privation of medication, necessary medical attention, failure to protect against inclement climatic conditions and not providing the conditions or stimulation necessary, as well as failure to attend school. The Society also refers to the difficulties in identifying the level of intentionality that lies behind cases of neglect, given the social conditions that predominate in much of Brazil. Thus the victim's need for protection needs to be considered independently of the level of intentionality (10).

There is a question about whether there should be another category referring to the intentional killing of children - infanticide. In Brazil, this is not confined to infants, with the case of children involved in organized armed violence (COAV) becoming increasingly common in the "favelas" (urban slums). The scale of the problem of death threats against children has led to the creation by the federal government of a legal project ("PPCAAM") devoted to the protection of such youngsters at risk.

WHAT IS KNOWN ABOUT THE EXTENT OF THE PROBLEM?

There are no nationally held statistics on the extent of CAN in Brazil, however an increasing number of local studies are being undertaken – albeit adopting different methodological approaches, some being of incidence and others of prevalence. A recent large-scale retrospective study of 1685 adolescents in the State of Rio de Janeiro indicated a prevalence of 14.6% of physical violence committed by either the father or the mother. 11.8% of participants witnessed or experienced sexual abuse and 48% psychological abuse, as rated on the Pitzer Drummand Scale (11)).

This study like others emphasizes the link between interpersonal and social conditions in Brazil ("structural violence"), which leave children and adolescents vulnerable to abuse through acts of omission and neglect. Indicators of the effects of violence on youth are the high incidence of death by firearms amongst boys and young adolescent males as well as problems of exploitation, child prostitutions and teenage pregnancy (12). In 2004, 42% of a total of 36,000 deaths by firearms in Brazil occurred in children and adolescents aged between 10 and 19 years and 90% of these deaths were aggressive homicides. The mortality rate for adolescents 10-19 years from external causes, including homicides and "stray bullets" is 46.8/1000 and five times higher in boys (77.2/1000) than girls (15.8/1000) (13) . In the metropolitan area of Rio de Janeiro in the year 2002, the homicide rate for the 15 - 24 age group was 139 per 100,000. (14) , with the rate per 100,000 being 208 for non-white as compared with 65 for white people and 228 for males contrasted with 11 for females. The rate for the same age group is 1.2 per 100,000 considering OECD countries overall - the Organisation for Economic Co-operation and Development (OECD) being an international organisation of thirty countries, that accept the principles of representative democracy and a free market economy. Homicides were often the result of gang conflicts over drug trafficking or of police actions or brutality (12) .

WHAT SYSTEM(S) OR INFRASTRUCTURE EXISTS TO ADDRESS CAN?

Article 227 of Brazil's Constitution (15) explicitly endorses a child's right to education, health care and protection. In addition, Brazil takes pride in being one of the first South American countries to have revised its "Statute" (16) to reflect the principles of the UN Convention on the Rights of the Child (17). The Statute on Children and Adolescents (ECA) of 1990 (18) represented a conceptual shift from the "Codigo de Menores" of 1979 (minors' "Code"), as the Code focused on the social control of poor and needy children and adolescents, "that find themselves in irregular circumstances" . The Statute defines children and adolescents, aged 0-18 years, as "people of a particular developmental status" and "subjects with rights", including the right to "assistance", to be "watched over" and "protected" from harm. The "Lei Ôrganica de Assistência Social" of 1993 ("Social Assistance Law") later reinforced the rights of families, children and adolescents to social assistance.

The Statute represents a comprehensive and progressive statement of child and adolescent rights. However, child protection (CP) also depends upon legal processes involving the civil and penal codes, that unlike the Statute, date back to the 1920's and whose outdated concepts and systems contrast with the progressive emphasis of the Statute (19) . It is the civil and penal codes that determine the conditions under which parental rights are removed and the penalties to be applied to the perpetrator of physical, sexual, emotional abuse or torture. However, the top-level structures, organizations and procedures of the CP system are established according to the Statute's principles. This mandates bodies ("conselhos") at national, state and municipal level to defend children's rights. The federal Human Rights Special Secretary (Secretaria Especial de Direitos Humanos) and National Council for the Rights of Children and Adolescents (CONANDA) have policy advisory and lobbying roles. State councils formulate policies and guidelines within which municipal level councils are to structure their activities.

Decision making about developing, monitoring and implementing policies is therefore devolved to the municipalities who under the statute are responsible for managing and coordinating service provision. Municipal initiatives are required to work in partnership with state and federal programmes most notably, the "Programa Sentinela", a federal initiative focused on multidisciplinary teams that address evaluation and intervention in cases of domestic violence including child and adolescent sexual abuse and exploitation.

How Does the System Work Regarding Reporting of Possible CAN?

The Statute's most significant procedural and organisational contributions were requiring mandatory reporting to the Secretaries of Health of the Municipality and the State and establishing the conselhos tutelares who are responsible for receiving these reports, for legal and social actions of protection. Most municipalities have standard forms available to complete in suspected cases of CAN complete in cases of suspected CAN by professionals and members of the public alike .

In the view of the WHO, an integrated multi-sector framework with a lead agency co-ordinating the efforts is a major step in developing prevention strategies (20). The system currently does not set out the responsibilities of the different sectors involved with children and adolescents in order that they can provide a coherent response. Many professionals do not consider themselves working in a system with clear guidelines and lines of accountability to support them (21).   This suggests that reforms are needed to clarify (i) the roles and responsibilities of different sectors and agencies and (ii) national guidelines that promote inter-agency collaboration and overcome existing fragmentation (22,23). Thus the burden of co-ordinating child protection responses falls to the "conselhos tutelares" – "permanent, autonomous, non-juridical organs," acting as area child protection committees responsible for the protection of children and adolescents. Need is defined broadly covering those who have been maltreated to those who have infringed the law. The conselhos tutelares are responsible for receiving mandatory reports of child abuse and neglect and have the task of assessing the circumstances (including interviewing families and children), requesting appropriate services, initiating any necessary legal proceeding and coordinating the interventions of the different professionals and agencies who become involved.

the Nature of the "Typical" Response by the Responsible Agencies

A form with an accompanying report should be sent to the conselho tutelar ideally with the professional concerned phoning to discuss the case prior to the receipt of the written notification. Notification does not preclude professionals referring families for supportive or therapeutic services at the same time. The flow chart in figure 1 describes the process of receiving and responding to a reported case of child abuse and neglect.

Reporting and Intervention Process:

Suspected and Reported Cases of Abuse and Neglect:

Órgãos de Defesa - Órgãos de Segurança - Serviços de Educação - Serviços de Saúde - Serviços de Assistência

Filling in of mandatory reporting form (information system)

"Conselho Tutelar" (area child protection team) – (Central body of child abuse and neglect reported cases)

Activation of Diagnostic and Investigation Services (Social Services, Health System, Police and Justice System)

Abuse or Neglect Established

Legal Process Initiated (prosecution and protection)

Supportive and Protective Interventions Initiated - Therapeutic and Social Assistance

Figure 1. The Response to CAN Cases In Brazil

However, a survey of participants who participated in training organized as part of the ISPCAN (International Society for the Prevention of Child Abuse and Neglect) ITPI (International Training Initiative) in Rio de Janeiro, during 2005-2006 (24) indicated that the system is "underused" (professionals underreporting) because of interpersonal and structural (social, cultural and economic) factors (25). Factors that influenced non-usage included:

- Awareness. The decentralization of child protection has advantages, but also disadvantages in undermining consistency and levels of awareness of processes and procedures involved in protecting children as well as difficulties in accessing guidelines. Mandatory reporting forms have been produced at both state and municipal levels, are frequently revised, contributing to confusion over the process.
- Lack of confidence in aspects of the child protection framework. Many of the participants preferred not to report cases or to bypass the conselhos tutelares by directly reporting cases to other agencies both formal and informal (such as the legal system and community leaders). Unwillingness to use the conselhos tutelares reflected a perception of their lack of skills in managing complex child protection cases, and that they were overwhelmed and ineffective.
- Potential negative consequences for reported person. Some participants avoid mandatory reporting because of the risks involved, and the lack of agency support in managing the safety or welfare of the child or adolescent post notification.

Mandatory procedures are seen to jeopardise the well being of children and adolescents in places where the poder paralelo (non-official parallel power), is exercised by a gang chief involved in illegal activities such as drug trafficking or extortion. An "agente de saude" (community health worker) described how in the case of a sexually abused adolescent, the mandatory reporting process with the consequent involvement of state authorities was unwelcome to local leaders; it would lead to forced expulsion and loss of livelihood for the whole family. The preferred option was to talk to the girl, her family and to find an alternative placement within the community, without initiating state protection procedures.

- Potential negative consequences for reporting person. Some professionals avoid mandatory reporting because of the risks for the reporter. For example, it is frequent that teachers in the public school system in Rio report threats (sometimes at gunpoint) from parents wanting to avoid interference by police and state authorities.

STRENGTHS IN BRAZIL'S APPROACH/SYSTEM

Working within a poorly co-ordinated and under-resourced system requires commitment and creativity to protect children and adolescents against violence and abuse. Interventions devised in this context have received international recognition (12,26,27) as valuable and innovative, for their understanding of the relationship between interpersonal and structural risk factors, and their focus on fostering local resilience against community and interpersonal violence by building on "social capital" - the attitude, spirit and willingness of people to engage in collective, civic activities, leading to the building of social networks (2). Examples of such initiatives include the creation by Dr. Barreto at the Federal University of Ceara of "Community Therapy" (27), applying systemic family therapy concepts to address the dynamics of social exclusion and the impact this has on communities and families. The therapeutic process allows people to voice their experience of deprivation and exclusion and how this can lead to frustration, manifested as "rule breaking" – that is crime and community violence – and the impact of this behaviour on other interpersonal systems such as families. Community therapy aims to strengthen communities by forming "solidarity networks", "mobilizing" positive individual, family and community experience by revisiting and revaluing the community's heritage - African, Indian and European as well as the individual experiences of group members. The emphasis is not on individual pathology but on community health, stimulating the community to use its strengths to build a new future.

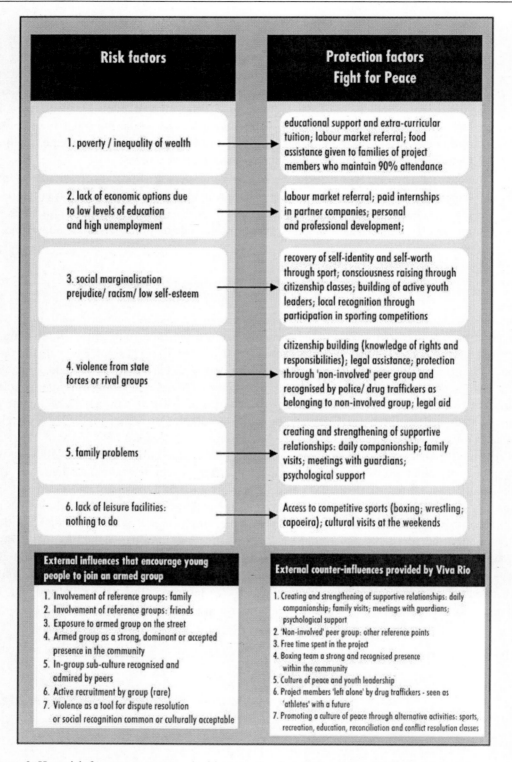

Figure 2. How risk factors are countered with protective factors (reproduced with permission from Dowdney 2005).

Similarly, from its establishment in 2000, Luta Pela Paz (Fight for Peace) project has confronted the problem of "children involved in organised armed violence" or COAV, by using community strategies to prevent youth participation in crime, violence and drug trafficking. The project is based in Nova Hollanda, one of the fifteen favelas of the Complexo da Maré in Rio De Janeiro, where there has been a decade of territorial drug wars between two of the city's largest drug trafficking factions and where openly armed children and adolescents patrol the streets and alleyways to defend the community from invasions and police raids. Luta pela Paz originally started as a boxing project that aimed to provide adolescents aged 12-25 years an alternative to crime and the drug factions. By using sport to discipline and structure their lives, it provides an outlet for aggression and a source of self-worth. Luta pela Paz provided a way to gain insight into the lives of children and adolescents living in the marginalised communities in Rio de Janeiro. This stimulated research, funded by Save the Children Fund Sweden and the Ford Foundation, published as a book "Children of the drug trade: A case study of children in organised armed violence" (12) – a pioneer study into the lives of COAV. It was based on interviews and the analysis of public health statistics (firearms mortality rates within the city), youth crime statistics and police statistics. This analysis highlighted that the firearms mortality rates in the municipality of Rio de Janeiro were above combat related deaths in many modern conflict zones, and demonstrated similarities between the roles of children employed by Rio's drug factions and "child soldiers" participating in armed conflicts. The study grew into an international research project into COAV (children and youth in organised armed violence (28,26) which was part of the UN Secretary General's research project on violence. The research has also provided the foundation for a replicable methodology to promote resilience against involvement in violence, counteracting risk factors with tools promoting resilience (see figure 2).

WEAKNESSES/CHALLENGES IN BRAZIL'S APPROACH/SYSTEM

In the 1990s there was enthusiasm that the Statute and the Social Assistance Law would structure a functioning integrated child protection framework (22). However, the translation of the statute into practice has been slow and "heterogeneous" (23). Obstacles include a lack of resources and trained staff as well as the failure of the required coordinated action of federal, state and municipal governmental agencies together with non- governmental agencies (22) The lack of resources and capacity generates inadequate service responses. The structural violence results in many children and adolescents being out of reach of the statutory services (29). Brazilian professionals realise that they must both address individual manifestations of interfamilial violence or abuse and confront the deeper influences on behaviour of "structural" violence (30). However, the creative initiatives that confront the impact of poverty and social exclusion are insufficient to address the various forms of child and adolescent exploitation they generate - child labour, sexual exploitation and children involved in organized armed violence to mention a few (31). Issues of poverty, ethnic differences, sexism, social inequality and corruption which contribute to the exploitation of children and the infringement of their rights need to be confronted by coherent child and adolescent public policies (32) not only local project initiatives.

Faced with complicated child protection issues, the lack of resources and co-ordination often results in fragmented, crisis-based interventions for cases of CAN (21). The focus is often immediate medical care, removal of the perpetrator if necessary, and the preparation of legal reports for prosecution. Once the crisis is over, the lack of services means that only a small proportion of families have access to therapeutic help.. Even then it will be focused on the victim and not on the system of which they are part - and this is if the mandatory reporting process has been initiated.

MAJOR CONTROVERSIES IN BRAZIL'S APPROACH/SYSTEM

There are currently two issues on the government agenda: (i) reforming the foster and adoption system (33) and (ii) children giving evidence in court using the Depoimento sem Dano (Testifying without Harm) (34). For a number of years the NGO Terre des Hommes has been leading fostering (familias acolhedoras) initiatives to support and formalize the process of fostering children and adolescents. Terre des Hommes has focused on the psychological preparation of families to facilitate incorporation of the child or adolescent, which includes clarification of the legal difference between temporary custody, fostering and adoption. Foster families have been given a small financial incentive to look after children and adolescents – which in 2005 was about 280 reais (the minimum wage earned by unskilled workers) or 100 US dollars per month. However, the process of fostering and adoption remained informal, with neighbours being given "guarda temporaria" or temporary custody of a child at risk without appropriate assessment, support or financial assistance. This system was replaced in 2007 when law 3.029 made it a legal requirement for foster families to be registered, assessed, supported (psychologically and financially) and for foster children and adolescents to be continuously monitored. Clearly it will take time for what is on paper to be translated into practice as (1) there is still a scarcity of families coming forward to foster, and (2) those families who fostered before the 2007 law was instated may not receive the benefits.

Another issue that has become the subject of debate is the "Depoimento sem Dano" which has been implemented in Porto Alegre (35) to minimize the stress to youngsters of repeat interviewing and questioning by different professionals. Children and adolescents are interviewed by social workers and psychologists, and the interviews are taped for the judge and other professionals to view. One of the controversies surrounding the use of the technique regards the function of the psychologist and whether the psychologist merely "assists" by asking questions to obtain the information necessary for the process, or, whether the verbal and non-verbal information gathered in the interview can be "interpreted" and the interpretation considered "evidence" by the court.

PREVENTION EFFORTS (PRIMARY, SECONDARY, TERTIARY)

Local governmental and non-governmental institutions have worked together and with International NGO's such as UNICEF and Save the Children on primary prevention education campaign on issues such as violence, sexual exploitation and most recently the anti-corporal punishment campaign "não bate, eduque". Whilst there is an awareness of the need to develop primary and secondary prevention initiatives, especially pre- and post-natal in high risk populations, the response to CAN, as mentioned previously, often remains on a crisis basis at a tertiary level (36). The Statute states that responses to CAN need to be coordinated at a municipal level in a joint effort between governmental, non-governmental and private institutions. There are many organizations working with different types of violence against different populations – women, children, young people and the elderly – surveys of professionals indicate that these are perceived as fragmented and not matching the demands (37). Professionals are often unaware of the available services as, until recently, there have been few attempts to compile registers either at a Federal, State or Municipal level detailing what is available where. An exception is an initiative by the Instituto Noos that has compiled records on institutions in the state of Rio, categorizing them in terms of the WHO types of violence or neglect and age group in which they specialized. The Noos identified 46 different types of institutions, the majority of which were municipal governmental. Most of the institutions covered urban areas, with rural areas being poorly served, with only 21% of the institutions operating outside the municipality in which they are based. The professionals most commonly involved in service provision are psychologists (72%), social workers (71%) and nurses (34%). The infrastructure of the institutions was described in the study as "poor" - 9% lacked a fixed telephone contact. Most cases take referrals for longer term individual psychotherapy (80%), medical care (76%), legal advice (71%), income generation schemes (52%), educational guidance (48%) and professional training (43%) (38).

CONCLUSIONS

Brazil is committed of its efforts to establishing a strong legal framework relating to child protection and which is consistent with the UNCRC and a system that guarantees children and adolescent rights..It is also committed to creative violence prevention initiatives which address the complex child protection issues that arise from the impact of structural violence on interpersonal violence and CAN. Many challenges lie ahead for the government and the society as a whole regarding implementation.

REFERENCES

[1]   World Bank. Brazil inequality and economic development: Poverty assessment report 2008. Avaliable at www.worldbank.org

[2]   Farmer P. Pathologies of power: health, human rights and the new war on the poor. Los Angeles, CA: Univ Calif Press, 2005.

[3]   Minayo MCS. Violence and health. Rio de Janeiro: Editor Fiocruz, 2006 [Portuguese].

[4]   Belsky J. Aetiology of child maltreatment. Am Psychol 1983;35(40):320-35.

[5]   World Health Organization. World report on violence and health. Geneva: WHO, 2002.

[6]   Assis SG, Avanci, JQ, Silva CMFP, Malaquias JV, Olveira RC. Violence and social representation in adolescents in Brazil. Pan Am J Public Health 2004;16(1):43-51. [Portuguese]

[7]   Deslandes SF. Preventing violence. A challenge for health professionals. FIOCRUZ/ENSP/CLAVES: Rio de Janeiro, 1994. [Portuguese]

[8]   Azevedo VNA, Guerra MA. Victimized children: the small power sindrome. Iglu: São Paulo, 1989. [Portuguese]

[9]   Brazilian Multiprofessional Association for the Protection of Children and Adolescents, (ABRAPIA). Child and adolescent maltreatment. Protection and prevention. A guide for health professionals. Autores & Agentes & Associados: Petrópolis, Brazil. 1997. [Portuguese]

[10]   The Brazilian Pediatric Association (SBP) Latin American Centre for the Study of Violence and Health Jorge Carelli (CLAVES) The National School of Public Health (ENSP) FIOCRUZ the Secretary of State for Human Rights. Guide on how to act in cases of child maltreatment; 2ª Edition. Ministry of Justice: Rio de Janeiro, 2001. [Portuguese]

[11]   Assis SG, Avanci, JQ, Silva CMFP, Malaquias JV, Olveira RC. Violence and social representation in adolescence in Brazil. Pan Am J Public Health 2004;16(1):43-51. [Portuguese]

[12]   Dowdney L. Children of the drug trade: a case study of organized armed violence. Rio de Janeiro: Letras-Save the Children, 2003. [Portuguese]

[13]   Ministry of Health, Brazil. Statistics on death by fire arms. Organised armed violence. Accessed Jan 2008.

[14]   URL: http://www.saude.gov.br, 2005. [Portuguese]

[15]   Walselfisz J. A map of violence IV, youth in Brazil, Brasilia UNESCO, 2004. [Portuguese]

[16]   The Ministry of Justice, Brazil. The Federal Constitution. Brasília, 1988. [Portuguese]

[17]   Rizzini I. The Child and the law in Brazil: revisiting history from 1822-2000. Rio de Janeiro: UNICEF-CESPI/USU, 2002. [Portuguese]

[18]   United Nations. Convention on the rights of the child. Geneva: United Nations, 1990.

[19]   Ministry of Justice, Brazil. The child and adolescent statute: social responsiblity. Brasilia, 1990. [Portuguese]

[20]   Silva Pereira T. The new civil code and intrafamilial violence. In: Piza G, Barbosa GF, eds. The silent violence of incest. Sao Paulo: Imprensa oficial, 2004:20-40. [Portuguese]

[21]   World Health Organization. World report on violence and health. WHO: Geneva, 2002.

[22]   Goncalves HB, Brandao EP. Juridical psychology in Brazil. Rio de Janeiro: Nau Editor, 2004. [Portuguese]

[23]   Frota da Cunha MG. A citizenship of youth and adolescence in irregular child protection situations. In: Carvalho A, Salle F, Guimaraes M, Ude W, eds. Public policies: Belo Horizonte: Editor UFMG, 2003, 13-30. [Portuguese]

[24]   Costa Dinz BL. The changes in the agent of social policy in Brazil and the challenge of inaction: the case of child and adolescence welfare assistance. In: Carvalho A, Salle F, Guimaraes M, Ude, W, eds. Public policies. Belo Horizonte: Editor UFMG, 2003:30-45. [Portuguese]

[25]   Eisenstein E, Lidchi V. Abuses and protection of children, vols I-II, Rio de Janeiro: CEIIAS-ISPCAN, 2006. [Portuguese]

[26]   Leal Pinto ML. NGO's confronting violence. Accessed Jan 2008. URL:

[27]   http//www.geocities/projetopirecema/MariaLuciaLeal.html/2005. [Portuguese]

[28]   Dowdney L. Neither war nor peace: international comparisons of children and youth in organised armed violence. Rio de Janeiro: Save the Children and Iansa, 2005.

[29]   Barretto A. Community therapy, 2007. Accessed Jan 2008 URL: www.abratecom.org.br and ww.4varas.com.brd [Portuguese]

[30]   Pinheiro, SP. World report on violence against children. Secretary General's study on violence against children. Geneva: United Nations, 2006.

[31]   Cunha E, Cunha S. Social public policy. In: Carvalho A, Salle F, Guimaraes M, Ude W, eds. Public policies. Belo Horizonte: Editora UFMG, 2003:50-68. [Portuguese]

[32]   Goncalves HS. Childhood and violence in Brazil. Rio de Janeiro: Nau Editor, 2003. [Portuguese]

[33]   Assis, SG. Children and adolescents victims of violence: past, present and future perspectives. Cadernos de Saúde Pública 1994;10:126-34. [Portuguese]

[34]   Carvalho A, Salles F, Guimaraes M, Ude W, eds. Public policy. Belo Horizonte: Editor UFMG, 2003. [Portuguese]

[35]   Ministry of Justice, Brazil. Law 3.029. Institutes the programme of provisional fostering of children and adolescents. Brasilia, 2007. [Portuguese]

[36]   Ministry of Health, Brazil. The notification of child abuse against children and adolescents: a guide for health professionals. Brasilia, 2003. [Portuguese]

[37]   Justice Tribunal of Rio Grande do Sul (2004). Testifying without harm (Depoimento sem dano). Accessed Jan 2008 URL: http://www.direito2.com.br. [Portuguese]

[38]   Murta SG. Prevention programs for emotional and behavioural problems in children and adolescents – lessons of three decades of research. Psychologica: reflexions and criticisms, 2006;20(1):1-8. [Portuguese]

[39]   Lidchi VG. Reflections on training in child abuse and neglect prevention: experiences in Brazil. Child Abuse Review 2008;16:353-66.

[40]   Instituto Noos. Maping the services networks. 2008. Accessed Jan 2008 URL: http://www.noos.org.br/pesquisa_mapeamentoderedesdeatendimento.html [Portuguese]

In: International Aspects of Child Abuse and Neglect
Editors: H. Dubowitz, J. Merrick pp. 213-219

ISBN: 978-1-60876-703-8
© 2010 Nova Science Publishers, Inc.

Chapter 20

CHILD ABUSE AND NEGLECT IN MOZAMBIQUE

*Berta Chilundo**

Rede Contra o Abuso de Menores, Mozambique

Mozambique is a country located on the south east cost of Africa. The population is 20 million, of which 49% are children. Moçambique was a Portuguese colony, having achieved its independence in 1975. Post independence, Moçambique had a civil war that lasted about 16 years. During this period of instability, Mozambicans experienced gross violations of human rights, particularly the rights of the child. In 1994 a peace agreement was signed, and Mozambicans entered a period of political stability, macro-economy and reconstruction at every level at all levels, mainly in the child protection area. This chapter will briefly explain the key aspects of the protection system in Mozambique.

INTRODUCTION

Mozambique is a country located on the south east cost of Africa. The population is 20 million, of which 49% are children. Moçambique was a Portuguese colony, having achieved its independence in 1975. Post independence, Moçambique had a civil war that lasted about 16 years. During this period of instability, Mozambicans experienced gross violations of human rights, particularly the rights of the child. In 1994 a peace agreement was signed, and Mozambicans entered a period of political stability, macro-economy and reconstruction at every level at all levels, mainly in the child protection area. Recent data confirm that Moçambique has experienced an intensive economic and social growth of about 8.5% between the years of 1997 and 2005.

Even with this impressive progress, today many children's rights are still violated. 49 percent of all children living in absolute poverty being deprived of basic services such as health, education, water, sanitation, information, shelter and nutrition. With regards to the matter of the protection system, significant steps have been taken by the Mozambican

---

* *Correspondence:* Berta Chilundo, Oficial de Programas, Rede Contra o Abuso de Menores. E-mail: mwana.redecame@tvcabo.co.mz

Government to improve the legal and political procedures to protect children against violence, abuse and exploitation and to ensure that the most vulnerable children have access to the basic social services.

In general we can say that the child protection system in Moçambique is currently in a consolidation phase, meaning we are in a process of establishing legal reforms. In 2008, three child protection laws were approved. It is still necessary to clearly define and follow the legal instruments because the theory is not applied in the field as a result of various factors such as the lack of resources (economic, technician, etc.). There are also certain cultural practices that violate children's rights, such as premature marriages or neglect.

This chapter will briefly explain the key aspects of the protection system in Mozambique.

HOW THE DIFFERENT TYPES OF CHILD ABUSE AND NEGLECT (CAN) ARE DEFINED?

Abuse can be defined has the exploitation by someone in power towards someone else who is defenseless or less protected in relation to the prior. The Mozambican judicial system recognizes that children have the right to be protected against physical or psychological abuse, maltreatment, negligence on behave of the parents, tutors, family members, legal representatives or anyone else.

Physical abuse is when a child is hurt due to physical injuries resulting from beatings, burns, poisoning, strangulation, suffocation etc. General, parents and other family members physically abuse their children under the pretence that they are actually educating the child. Physical abuse is only considered to be such, when the child breaks a bone, or suffers from serious burns, or even when a child dies.

Sexual abuse can be defined as the act of forcing a child to participate in sexual activities with an adult or with an older child, in order to obtain sexual satisfaction from such practices. Sexual abuse can be through direct contact with the child, or through indirect contact, for example, by exposing a child to pornographic material. Although there is a clear understanding of sexual abuse in Mozambique, there are still some undefined aspects in the definition. For example; paedophilia, sexual abuse against male children (which is currently viewed as indecent assault, and the sentence for such a crime is from one day up to one year in jail) or child pornography.

Emotional abuse is defined as any action towards a child with harmful intentions that can limit the emotional and psychological growth of the child. For example, not showing love and affection, insulting the child, ignoring or showing lack of attention, lowering his/her self-esteem. This form of abuse is not clearly defined in the Mozambican judicial system, but psychologists agree that this type of abuse can cause irreversible damages to the psycho-social and emotional development of a child. Therefore it is difficult to quantify the dimension of this problem. In Mozambican society, this form of abuse occurs mostly with the families that live in the rural areas/communities and the children are often called names, i.e. you are dumb just like your father, or Dumbo "big ears" (talking down to the child). Society ignores this form of abuse and it use traditional and cultural practices as a scapegoat for their harmful actions towards their children.

Negligence occurs when the child's' needs are not physically and/or psychologically meet, which in turn puts the child's health or development at risk. For example, not providing; affection, food, housing, health care, clothing or preventing interaction with other children. In the Mozambican legislature, negligence in the form of not feeding the child can result in the parents, tutor or guardian facing up to six months in jail. This sentence cannot be converted into a fine.

WHAT IS KNOWN ABOUT THE EXTENT OF THE PROBLEM?

Although there isn't a reliable database that could illustrate the true dimension of the problem of violence and abuse against children in Mozambique, the situation is highly vulnerable because our society is faced with various forms of violence. According to the police reports (the Department of Women and Children), in 2008, 446 children were victims of sexual abuse and rape, there were 58 cases of maltreatment and 164 cases of abandoned children. These figures does not reflect the truth, because the communities are not sufficiently sensitized to report cases of violence against children. They would rather resolve the problem at a family level, in which case the perpetrator of a rape incident would be forced to pay a fee.

A study conducted by OIM on human trafficking in southern Africa, states that there are about 1000 people (women and children) trafficked daily from Mozambique to South Africa. The victims are sold at their destination for R650 to become wives to South African citizens. Others are sold to Kwazulu-Natal and Gauteng brothels for R1000. They live in conditions that are close to slavery.

The Mozambican government and the Mozambican civil society are paying extreme attention to trafficking, regardless whether the end result is for sexual exploitation or human labour. They are developing preventative strategies to combat human trafficking. There is a lot more pressure to address these problems now because of the 2010 FIFA World Cup. This current situation/scenario tends to worsen.

The available information raises concerns on the number of incidences of domestic violence and sexual abuse, including sexual abuse in schools.

- During childhood and during the adolescent year, 30 percent of women and 37 percent of men have witnessed direct violence between their parents. 15 percent of the women and 20 percent of men have been victims of physical abuse inflicted by their own family during their youth, (National Inquiry on Reproductive Health and Sexual Behaviour amongst Teenagers, 2001).
- 34 percent of the women who participated in a study conducted by MMAS in 2004 reported to have been victims of physical violence. This form of violence is frequently perpetrated by the husband, a family member or a known person. 10 percent of the women who participated in this study reported to have been victims of some form of sexual abuse. The women who live in the rural areas suffer high levels of violence than the women who live in urban areas.
- Case studies show that there is a high level of sexual abuse occurring in school. A recent study conducted by Save the Children, CARE International, MEC and Rede

CAME/FDC estimated that 8 percent of the children attending schools have been victims of sexual abuse.

- In a Youth profile session held in 2004 by the Ministry of Youth and Sports, with the support of UNICEF indicated that 20 percent of the girls that participated in the study claimed that abuse is a serious problem in schools. They said they had been forced to choose between having sex, paying money or being expelled from school.

THE SYSTEM(S) OR INFRASTRUCTURE TO ADDRESS CAN

In Mozambique, there is a ministry responsible for addressing issues related to children. It is called the Ministry of Women and Social Action. In order to improve the mechanisms to better protect the children, the Government has approved policies and strategies to intervene in this sector. They were able to establish; a strategy on the social action regarding children, a national plan of action for children (PNAC 2006-2010), and another national plan for orphans and vulnerable children (PACOVS) that highlight various activities to protect children from violence, negligence and sexual exploitation.

At Police stations nationwide, a department was created that only deals with cases related to women and children. This department is called Department of Women and Children (Gabinete de atendimento a Mulher e Criança). They are responsible for providing assistance to children victims of all types of abuse. In this department the officer are responsible for opening and referring the cases to other institutions such as the hospital and medical centres, where the victims undergo the necessary exams for "legal medicine", and in certain cases, in the city of Maputo, they get psychological assistance at CERPIJ, (Centro de Reabilitação Psicológica Infanto-Juvenil) which is a psychological rehabilitation centre for children. Recently, pilot offices for women and children have been created with a temporary shelter and psychological and legal assistance for the victim

In the provincial courts, they are creating special sessions for children because there aren't juvenile courts like in Maputo city. Systems have been created for communities to monitor and to prevent abuse and violence against children. In addition, the Mozambican Government has been receiving support from UNICEF and other partners in testing different models of protection and service offering for vulnerable children. This includes access to birth certificates so that children are not exposed to child labour, arbitrary detention, expropriation of the inheritance, trafficking, premature weddings and other forms of abuse and exploitation.

Recently the Government has been negotiating, alongside civil society, to create a multi-sectorial system to assist children victims of abuse, particularly in creating a uniform reference numbering system to prevent cases form being counted more than once.

On the other hand, it is necessary to identify the victim's social circles, from the communities, to the police, to the hospitals. There is also a need to make all forms of abuse and violence toward children a public crime. We should encourage denouncers to follow through with the entire process and not give up, and decide to resolve the matter within the family.

How Does the System Work Regarding Reporting of Possible CAN? Laws?

The Mozambican constitution was recently approved and it states, in article 47, that the children have the right to be protected and they also entitled to well-being.

Criminal Level- The Mozambican penal code is dated since 1880. It was inherited from the Portuguese system. There are some laws that are related to child abuse in this system, for example, if a twelve year old is violated, the perpetrator is guilty regardless whether the act was consensual or not. A rape case requires that the victim be a female over the age of twelve, no more than 18 year, and the victim must also be a virgin. Pimpery refers to parents, tutors or guardians that put the child in prostitution. Other crimes that fall under this category are; violation, indecent assault and maltreatment. The penal code also charges those who through violence, force or through manipulation remove a child from the care of his/her parents or guardians.

In terms of paternal responsibilities, this legal device protects the children form being abandoned by their own parents. In terms of the negligence law n. 2052 de 22 de Marco de 1952, parents, tutor or guardians can be put in jail for a year.

For parents who do not give food to their children, Law n. 8/2008 (organização tutelar de menores) stipulates that they (the parents) can be jailed for a period up to six months, and this penalty can not be converted into a fine. Recently three new laws were passed that state that any health care practitioner should immediately report to the authorities any signs of maltreatment on a child.

This same law states that the parent, tutor or guardian that puts a child on the streets with no apparent valid reason, will face a jail sentence of up to six months.

The parent, tutor or guardian responsible for the child could still face a jail sentence of up to a year if the child is exposed to continuous abuse or any form of exploitation.

Child trafficking is another form of violence that should be addressed. Recently, The Law Against Human Trafficking was passed. The penalty is 8 to 20 year in prison. This law is stricter on the traffickers, if he/she is a parent, tutor or guardian of the child.

Civil Level – In 2008 a law was passed that obligates all personnel working in health care, social services, education and communication should report all incidences of child abuse to the authorities.

The "Typical" Response by the Responsible Agencies

In the case of rape of a 12 year old girl and of child trafficking, which are both considered to be public crimes; anyone who has any knowledge about the crime may report it.

Cases should be reported to the department of women and children where a specialist will investigate the case. If the nature of the case is sexual abuse, the specialist should refer the case to a health care centre for the victim to be examined in legal medicine. Before that exam, the victim should consult a gynecologist for examination, i.e. to determine the child's HIV status. The victim also receives psychological assistance.

After the report from legal medicine, the criminal investigation police (PIC) would refer the case to the Public Ministry who is responsible persecuting along side the courts.

The specialists in the department of women and children work with various civil society organisations that offer legal assistance to abuse victims. They have recently signed an agreement with the Instituto de Patrocínio e Assistência Jurídica (IPAJ), an institute that sponsors legal assistance. In is in complying with this agreement that the specialists have referred cases to these organizations.

The specialists refer the cases to the Ministry of Social Action when the victims need temporary shelter, for example orphanages, although there are not many orphanages in Mozambique.

STRENGTHS IN MOZAMBIQUE'S APPROACH/SYSTEM

The child protection system in Mozambique, finds itself in a very difficult situation, which means that there is a lot of work to be done, in order to fortify and consolidate the current situation. The following are what we consider to be our strong points:

- The current legal reform has resulted in the approval of 3 child protection laws that are going to contribute to the fortification of the child protection system;
- The network of organisations that work in child rights protection, that provide social, psychological and legal assistance, all contribute to the resolution of child related cases.
- The dialogue that exists between government and civil society has resulted in various partnerships that enabled the establishment of the multi-sectorial approach in the child protection system. There has also been an increased participation from the community leaders and other stakeholders in the prevention, and assisting in child abuse cases.
- Civil society organizations have administered courses to capacitate the specialists from the department of Women and Children on child protection and children's rights.
- The Minister of Health has recently initiated a campaign to place a psychologist and social worker at all health care centers, to provide assistance to child victims of abuse.
- Policies have been put in place to prioritize prophylaxis because of HIV/AIDS.
- Government has created separate sections for children in provincial courts, and they have also created the department of Women and Children who have been abused.

WEAKNESSES/CHALLENGES IN MOZAMBIQUE'S APPROACH/SYSTEM

Given the current situation of the child protection system in Mozambique, there are numerous weaknesses, such as:

- Children assistance services are very limited, for example not all police stations have a department of Women and Children, especially in the districts. There are only two health care centres with psychologists.

- The lack of an integrated reference form to avoid opening a case twice. The poor condition under which the officers from the different departments work under, for example low salaries, poor/no equipment such as photograph cameras, transport, computers, etc. Low number of orphanages.
- There are only three departments of legal medicine, in Maputo, Beira and in Nampula. Many perpetrators are set free because of a lack of evidence that could be collected in legal medicine.
- The general publics lack of knowledge on laws, and the time-consuming process of reporting and the lack of interest on behalf of the family members.
- The referral system lacks financial support; therefore, victims can not be transported to the institution that will best provide the adequate assistance.
- The lack of knowledge on the procedures of reporting and referring child related cases for assistance on behalf of society's employees in general.

PREVENTION EFFORTS (PRIMARY, SECONDARY, TERTIARY)

Various civil society organisations and government, particularly the department of Women and Children, are involved in campaigns to sensitize the communities to prevent and fight child abuse at schools and in the communities. In is important to recognize Rede Came, UNICEF and Save the Children for their work in producing IEC material in the different types of abuse.

Other organisations, such as Forcom, have disseminated information on children's rights and the different forms of abuse, through their children's community radio programmes. These organisations have persuaded police officers, community leaders and religious figures with the objective of involving them in the prevention, reporting and assisting of child related cases.

In: International Aspects of Child Abuse and Neglect   ISBN: 978-1-60876-703-8
Editors: H. Dubowitz, J. Merrick pp. 221-229   © 2010 Nova Science Publishers, Inc.

Chapter 21

CHILD PROTECTION IN SOUTH AFRICA

Joan van Niekerk

Childline South Africa, Durban, South Africa

As a result of a democratic government in South Africa (SA), several international conventions and protocols have been signed and ratified that relate to the rights and protection of children. This has led to a comprehensive reform of national legislation relating to children and families to bring domestic legislation into line with these conventions and protocols and also in line with the National Constitution of South Africa, which includes a section on the protection of the rights of children in South Africa. As a new democracy with deep historical inequalities in service delivery the result has been a compromised safety and development for the majority of its citizens, including children. Dealing with the impact of this history has been further compromised by poverty, the HIV/AIDS pandemic, high levels of crime, and more recently the outbreaks of xenophobic violence. However, the reform of policy and legislation relating to the protection and the realization of children's rights brings hope, as does the more recent spirit of consultation and partnership between government and civil society. This process and development has been reviwed in this paper.

INTRODUCTION

With the advent of a democratic government in South Africa (SA), several international conventions and protocols have been signed and ratified that relate to the rights and protection of children. This has led to a comprehensive reform of national legislation relating to children and families to bring domestic legislation into line with these conventions and protocols and also in line with the National Constitution of South Africa, which includes a section (S28) on the protection of the rights of children in South Africa.

THE LEGISLATIVE REFORM PROCESS

In 1997/8 the South African Law Reform Commission was tasked with proposing new legislation to ensure that domestic legislation affecting the lives and protection of children is in line with international treaties (such as the United Nations Convention on the Rights of the Child, the African Union Charter on the Rights and Welfare of the African Child), and the South African Constitution. Three draft Bills were developed by the Law Reform Commission after a process of in-depth research, comparative analysis of other legislation around the world, and consultation with a broad spectrum of role players working in the field of children's rights. The following draft bills were handed to their respective Ministries:

- The Children's Bill (Department of Social Development - DSD)
- The Criminal Law (Sexual Offences and Related Matters) Amendment Bill (Department of Justice and Constitutional Development – DJCD)
- The Child Justice Bill (DJCD)

Despite the extensive research and consultation, conducted through the SA Law Reform Commission, which included government functionaries, all three Bills were extensively re-drafted by the government departments concerned.

THE CHILDREN'S ACT PROCESS

The redrafted Children's Bill prompted the formation of a coalition of concerned child rights and child protection organizations called the Children's Bill Working Group – presently called the Children's Act Working Group. The reworked Bill was seen to be so inadequate that the Children's Bill Working Group lobbied extensively for the Bill not to be passed in its (then) existing form. Numerous provisions relating to child protection had been removed or "watered down" to the point that they would be ineffectual. For example, a national policy framework to facilitate the implementation of the legislation as well as an Umbudsman for children were removed

In 2004 the Bill was split into two parts – one part (the Section 75 Bill) containing the provisions that had national importance and the second part (the Section 76 Bill) containing provisions relating to provincial and local government responsibilities. After extensive advocacy from civil society organizations, and also on the initiative of government, numerous improvements to the Bills were made and the Section 75 Bill was passed in 2005 (The Children's Act no 38 of 2005) and the Section 76 Bill was passed in 2007 (The Children's Amendment Act no 30 of 2007). However as of May 2008 only about 40 sections of the Children's Act have been implemented. Regulations have still to be finalized. The provisions that relate to Child Protection are not yet implemented.

THE CRIMINAL LAW (SEXUAL OFFENCES AND RELATED MATTERS) AMENDMENT ACT NO 32 OF 2007 (SOA)

The SOA went through a similar process as the Children's Acts – a long period of consultation, research and international comparison culminated in the Criminal Law (Sexual Offences and Related Matters) Amendment Bill (SOB). After the Bill was handed from the SA Law Reform Commission to the Government Department of Justice and Constitutional Development, it was rewritten. Public hearings were held in Cape Town, at one working day's notice, thus effectively limiting the participation in the hearings of civil society who deal with sexual assault. This also limited Parliament's ability to understand the need for additional reforms and protections for child victims and perpetrators of sexual crimes.

For several years no progress appeared to be made on finalizing the Bill, despite ongoing calls from civil society organizations dealing with the sexual abuse of adults and children. The rape trial of Jacob Zuma, the ex-Deputy President of South Africa presented an opportunity for intense lobbying of national government to address the Sexual Offences Bill and in May 2006, the Bill reappeared, once again having been extensively rewritten.

Civil Society organizations called for further public hearings on the Bill. These did not materialize. The result is Sexual Offences legislation that has done little to extend protections for either adult or child victims of sexual assault, couched in terminology that even trained legal professionals have found challenging to interpret and plan implementation.

However, there is light on the horizon for child victims of sexual abuse. The judgment of a senior member of the South African Judiciary, Judge Bertelsman , has declared some provisions of the SOA that amend the Criminal Procedure Act unconstitutional.(1) His judgment provides that all child victims of sexual assault will have access to special protections for witnesses in court to facilitate the hearing of their evidence, and provides for consultation with civil society organizations who work in the field of assistance to sexual assault victims when further policy decisions are made by the national government. Whether his recommendations will be upheld by the Constitutional Court remains to be seen.

THE CHILD JUSTICE BILL

This critical piece of legislation, dealing with children in conflict with the law, remains a Bill, after almost 11 years of drafting, consultation and debate. The latest version of the Bill reflects substantial rewriting using terminology and a format that make the provisions difficult to follow. At the public hearings held in February 2008, the Chairperson of the DJCD Parliamentary Portfolio requested that the legal drafters redraft the Bill in language that they (the Committee) and civil society could understand.

"Why such delays?" one might ask, after more than a decade of child rights law reform processes. Why when children's rights are spoken to so eloquently by politicians in South Africa is legislation that would protect them not prioritized? What are Parliament's priorities? These questions are difficult to respond to – it is clear that political "speak" is not followed by prompt action by government.

Furthermore, within this reform process, as different statutes are the responsibility of different government departments, the standardization of provisions such as those that relate to mandated reporting and the use of standard definitions of child abuse and child pornography has not occurred, despite numerous opportunities for consultation across government departments in the development of the legislation.

THE EXTENT OF THE PROBLEM OF CHILD ABUSE IN SOUTH AFRICA

There is no overarching child abuse surveillance system in South Africa to answer this question. One is being planned in a partnership between CIDA (the Canadian International Development Agency) and the Department of Social Development in South Africa.   The research that does exist does not share a common definition of abuse, and reflects the findings of studies conducted in isolation from each other, using varying research methodologies and thus precluding comparisons of results. However, the following examples reflect that the levels of crime against and abuse of children are very high.

CIETafrica, noted that 50% of all the children in their study (283,000 school children between the ages of 12 and 18 years, across urban and rural areas, including all racial, language and cultural groups in South Africa) had experienced some form of sexual abuse. Of great concern were the attitudes of these children towards sexually abusive behaviour

- 30% of the respondents believed that one had to have sex with their boy/girlfriend to show that they loved them
- 60% said that unwanted touching doesn't count as sexual violence
- 60% said that forcing sex with someone you know is not sexual violence
- 30% said that girls do not have the right to refuse sex with their boyfriends
- 10% said that sex with a virgin can cure HIV/AIDS. (2)

The Centre for Justice and Crime Prevention found that children and youth are disportionately at risk of falling victim to crime, have very few safe places, given the high levels of crime at home and in schools and that the overall victimization rate of children was 41.4% as compared to 22.9% of adults.(3)

THE SYSTEMS AND INFRASTRUCTURE TO ADDRESS CHILD ABUSE AND NEGLECT

The National Child Protection Strategy was developed in consultation with government departments, who have some role in the prevention and management of child abuse, as well as National Civil Society Organisations involved in child protection. This Strategy has not yet been formally adopted despite the fact that its development began in 1996. It is presently being costed.

However, a National Child Protection Committee does exist and has met irregularly in an effort to coordinate child protection issues and activities. This inter-sectoral structure, inclusive of civil society child protection organizations, is on paper, replicated at provincial level. The regularity of meetings varies from province to province and this contributes, along with other factors, to high levels of inconsistency in child protection services to children, both in relation to the numbers of children and families served and the quality of the service.

The bulk of child protection services that are not related to criminal justice system intervention are provided by civil society/non-government organizations. Many of these struggle to consistently provide quality services due to funding challenges related to government policy on NGO funding. Instead of outright purchase of child protection services there is a policy of "financial awards" and "subsidies', providing only a portion of the funding required for these services. Systems and structures are therefore in place, but this does not result in adequate child protection services to children.

MANDATED REPORTING

Legislative reform is in the process of changing mandated reporting obligations. However, several pieces of legislation have mandatory reporting requirements related to specific acts of child abuse. For example:

- legislation relating to the proscription of child pornography requires universal reporting to the police of any form of involvement or negligent exposure of children to child pornography. This could include a child accessing a pornographic magazine left lying around. (4)
- legislation criminalizing child prostitution and all who are involved or benefit from child prostitution requires universal reporting to the police.(5)
- the Children's Amendment Act requires only specific professions and occupations to report child abuse. The wording of the reporting requirement in this Act has caused concern among child protection workers as it may lead to unqualified persons investigating alleged child abuse before reporting. This may be done in order to meet the requirement of "on reasonable grounds concludes that a child has been abused in a manner causing physical injury, sexually abused or deliberately neglected" (6)

All of the above provisions do provide immunity from civil action, where abuse is not confirmed and the reporting has been in "good faith". There is criminal liability if a false report is knowingly made.

THE "TYPICAL" RESPONSE BY THE RESPONSIBLE AGENCIES

Although provincial protocols for the management of child abuse and neglect exist in every province these are not consistently followed. Many child protection workers are unaware of their existence. Most are a decade old and require updating and then inter-sector training to ensure their application. Contributing to the inconsistency of approaches are the following:

- the "decentralization" (in effect the disbanding) of the South African Police Services Child Protection Units resulting in inconsistent and poorly managed responses to children at the point of first reporting to the Criminal Justice System. This has resulted in children being turned away from police stations when reports have been made, poor quality investigations and fewer cases entering the system and fewer referrals to other sectors in the child protection system

- the overloading of the child protection system, particularly state and civil society social services as a result of the HIV/AIDS pandemic which has left several million children without an immediate parental caretaker. As many children in South Africa are raised without the presence of their biological father, the loss of the maternal figure invariably requires the intervention of those organizations and institutions tasked with child welfare, thus diverting resources from the management of cases of child abuse and neglect. Many social workers in child protection therefore carry caseloads of up to 300 children and/or families.

In theory, all cases of child abuse and neglect should be investigated, where appropriate criminal charges are laid and services offered to the child and family as needed.

THE STRENGTHS OF EXISTING SYSTEMS AND APPROACHES

At present child protection systems and approaches in South Africa are undergoing processes of policy, legislation and implementation change. A spirit of consultation and cooperation on change processes and implementation has developed over the past three years.. This is bringing government departments and civil society organizations involved in child protection closer together to address challenges and deliver services.

The need for inter-sector child protection service delivery is widely recognized by the majority of involved professionals. New progressive and comprehensive legislation has been passed. The legislation has been costed which will inform the budgeting for implementation. Implementation planning is well underway.

There are many in the field of child protection who have firm commitments to the rights of children, including the right to protection, as well as much knowledge, skill and competence.

THE CHALLENGES IN THE SOUTH AFRICAN SYSTEMS AND APPROACHES

The challenges are numerous and include:

- Historic inequalities that have not as yet been addressed: the vast majority of children in South Africa live in poverty (68%) and 27% of children have stunted growth, mainly due to malnutrition. Poverty increases the vulnerability of children to child abuse and neglect.(7)
- The HIV/AIDS pandemic: levels of HIV/AIDS infection are high: HIV/AIDS prevalence among pregnant women in South Africa was 29% in 2006 and for children reached 2.1% in 2006 and resulted in the deaths of 44663 children. 21% of all children in South Africa have lost either one or both parents. Orphanhood, caring

for sick parents, and the responsibility of care of siblings compromises the right to childhood and increases vulnerability to abuse and neglect. Futhermore, high levels of orphanhood and the need to place large number of children in some form of care has overloaded the resources within the Child Protection System. Social workers, children's court and the social security system are overloaded with the responsibility of orphan care, thus compromising the care and protection of children who have experienced abuse and neglect unrelated to the HIV/AIDS pandemic.

- High caseloads and scarce skills have contributed to further challenges in the child protection system. Social work competencies have become rare as many professionals have either left the country to work in countries that offer more reasonable workloads with more attractive remuneration or have left the profession. Government is in the process of implementing a retention strategy to attract into and retain more people in social work and the allied professions.

- Government planning and decision making that does not take into account the needs of an integrated inter-sector child protection system. For example the "decentralization" of the Child Protection Units of the South African Police Services occurred without consultation with others in the child protection system. This has resulted in poor service delivery to children in need of police protection services, and confusion among many child protection workers in other sectors regarding policing services. Although in theory this process should have brought child protection services closer to children and families at a community level, this has not occurred. Staff are allocated by station commanders to other duties, and inadequate resources, such as vehicles and secure and child friendly interviewing spaces to enable investigations have not been allocated at police stations.

- The need for intra- and inter-sector child protection training remains urgent. Many of those working in this field have had little training in child protection and have little understanding of how to work with other child protection workers. Children and families often experience the child protection system as unpredictable with regard to service delivery. Training initiatives do exist on a small scale, such as the training funded by the Oak Foundation. However, there is an urgent need to ensure that all child protection workers have at least a minimum standard of training that enables them to understand their own role, competently provide the appropriate service, and understand how their role fits with and supports the roles of child protection workers in other sectors. Many in the system do not know of the child protection protocols that do exist, let alone their responsibilities with regard to implementation.

- The need for more material and human resources is urgent. Services require adequate funding for effective implementation. Civil society organizations provide the bulk of child protection services in South Africa. However, funding is partial and unpredictable, dependent on a variety of funding models which vary from one province to another. Inconsistencies in funding result in inconsistent and unpredictable service delivery to children and families in need of child protection services.

Overall, South African law and policy relating to child protection has undergone several positive reforms. Effective implementation remains the biggest challenge.

THE MAJOR CONTROVERSIES IN THE SOUTH AFRICAN APPROACH

What kind of structures best protect the rights of all children equally: In view of South Africa's apartheid history, equal access to resources and services is a high priority. There are continuing debates on how this is best achieved. Equality of access was one of the arguments presented to justify the "decentralization" of the child protection services of the South African Police. However, this has resulted in dilution of an already inadequate pool of specialized skills, and reducing access to a specialized police response.

Fair and equal distribution of scarce resources and where these should be best employed to ensure effectiveness and efficiency. Nevertheless, with the advent of the new Children's Act, collaboration among civil society organizations and government has improved.

PREVENTION STRATEGIES

New law and policy is based on broad prevention ideals, the focus being on the support and strengthening of family life. This includes those community resources that both support the family in raising and protecting their children and those for when the family fails, such as schools and community-based resources.

The new Children's Act focuses on prevention and early intervention in order to prevent the disintegration of family life.. It also promotes the protection of children through early childhood education, partial child care when caretakers are working, and the provision of alternative care when the family has disintegrated or failed. Parenting programmes that support positive parenting and positive discipline are specifically mentioned in the Act as preventive tools. Remedial care is provided for in the legislation when efforts have failed to ensure that maltreated children receive appropriate care and services. As with the child protection services, the implementation of preventive strategies will require intensive planning, training of personnel and a commitment of extensive resources.

CONCLUSIONS

South Africa is a new democracy, bedeviled by deep historical inequalities in service delivery that have compromised the safety and development of the majority of its citizens, including children. Dealing with the impact of this history has been further compromised by poverty, the HIV/AIDS pandemic, high levels of crime, and more recently the outbreaks of xenophobic violence. However, the reform of policy and legislation relating to the protection and the realization of children's rights brings hope, as does the more recent spirit of consultation and partnership between government and civil society.

REFERENCES

[1]   S v Mokoena (CC7/07) and S v Phasmwane (CC 192/07), South African Law Reports 2007

[2]   Andersson N, Sonnekus H, Ho-Foster A. Beyond victims and villains: Evidence-based life skills education. Johannesburg, SA: Educ Workbook, Ciet Trust, 2004.

[3]   Burton P, Leoschut L. How rich the rewards? Results of the 2006 National Youth Victimisation Study. Cape Town, SA: Centre Justice Crime Prev, 2006.

[4]   The Films and Publications Amendment Act no 18 of 2004, Section 11 (b)

[5]   The Criminal Law (Sexual Offences and Related Matters) Amendment Act no 32 of 2007, Section 54

[6]   The Children's Amendment Act, no 30 of 2007, Section 110

[7]   Proudlock P, Dutschke M, Jamieson L, Monson J, Smith C, eds. South African child gauge 2007/8. Cape Town, SA: Children's Inst, Univ Cape Town, 2008.

In: International Aspects of Child Abuse and Neglect
Editors: H. Dubowitz, J. Merrick pp. 231-239

ISBN: 978-1-60876-703-8
© 2010 Nova Science Publishers, Inc.

Chapter 22

SAFEGUARDING CHILDREN:
CHILD PROTECTION SYSTEMS IN ETHIOPIA,
KENYA, TANZANIA AND UGANDA

Azeb Adefrsew and David Mugawe

Programme Department, African Child Policy Forum (ACPF), Addis Ababa, Ethiopia

All societies treasure their children, but the irony is that many of them are subjected to various forms of child abuse and neglect which constitutes violence against children. It is sad and heartbreaking that behind each of the statistics on vulnerable children is a grieving child. Violence against children is unacceptable and it is a violation of their rights. Unfortunately much of the violence remains hidden which further aggravates the suffering of the abused children. It is at the centre of this sad scenario that child protection systems have emerged to operate with a mandate to protect children from risk and/or harm and promote their optimal physical and psychological development. The African Child Policy Forum's (ACPF) assessment of Child Protection Systems in Ethiopia, Kenya, Tanzania and Uganda clearly indicate that issues of child protection remain of serious concern. A large proportion of children in the four countries are suffering from different types of violence, abuse and exploitation in all settings. Serious gaps and limitations in the legal and policy framework were also observed. The suffering of children cannot wait until tomorrow; they need our intervention and response today and now.

INTRODUCTION

All societies treasure their children, but the irony is that many of them are subjected to various forms of child abuse and neglect which constitutes violence against children. According to UNICEF, 40 million children below the age of 15 suffer from abuse and neglect and require health and social care; around 51 million births go unregistered every year in developing countries; an estimated 1.2 million children are trafficked every year; more than 2 million children are estimated to have died as a direct result of armed conflict; more than 1 million children worldwide are detained by law enforcement officials (1) and the list goes on.

It is sad and heartbreaking that behind each of these statistics is a grieving child. Violence against children is therefore unacceptable and it is a violation of their rights. Unfortunately much of the violence remains hidden which further aggravates the suffering of the abused children. It is at the centre of this sad scenario that child protection systems have emerged to operate with a mandate to protect children from risk and/or harm and promote their optimal physical and psychological development.

With that central place of child protection systems in mind, this paper aims to discuss how the child protection systems in four Eastern Africa countries, namely Ethiopia, Kenya, Tanzania and Uganda are safeguarding and responding to the needs of children. It highlights the different types of child abuse and neglect, and further summarises the extent of the problem and the systems that exist in the four countries to address child abuse and neglect. The last section of the paper focuses on the strengths and challenges of the existing child protection systems and the prevention efforts that are in place.

WHAT IS KNOWN ABOUT VIOLENCE AGAINST CHILDREN IN ETHIOPIA, KENYA, TANZANIA AND UGANDA?

African children, especially girls, are highly vulnerable to various forms of violence – physical, psychological and sexual. War, conflict, lack of parental care, poverty and low level of awareness worsen their vulnerability to violence. Children are violated in different settings such as in the home, at school and in the community. The most striking truth is that nine out of ten girls in Eastern Africa are abused by the people who they are supposed to trust most; including close family members, friends and teachers (2).

Harmful traditional practices, especially female genital mutilation (FGM) and early marriage affect children in many African countries. African Child Policy Forum's (ACPF) study on Violence Against Girls in Africa pointed out that around 6,000 African girls are subjected to FGM everyday and 42% of African girls aged 15-24 years were victims of early marriage. They had married before the age of 18 years (3). The table below provides a summary from a UNICEF study on the prevalence of FGM and early marriage in Ethiopia, Kenya, Tanzania and Uganda.

Table 1. Prevalence of FGM(female genital mutilation) and early marriage in Ethiopia, Kenya, Tanzania and Uganda (in percent) (4)

	Ethiopia	Kenya	Tanzania	Uganda
FGM	74	32	15	-
Early Marriage	49	25	41	54

Internal as well as external trafficking in children is prevalent in all four countries. The highest reports were from Uganda (10.2%), followed by Ethiopia (9.3%) and Kenya (5.2%) (3).

Corporal punishment is still widely used to discipline children at home, in schools and institutions, and in the communities in Eastern Africa. Surveys conducted in Ethiopia, Kenya and Uganda reported that more than 90 % of children have suffered from physical and psychological abuse (5).

Although different surveys report varying figures on the prevalence of child labour, all the figures indicate the seriousness of the problem in these countries. According to UNICEF the prevalence of child labour (5-14) in Ethiopia, Kenya, Tanzania and Uganda is 53%, 26%, 36% and 36% respectively (4).

The above statistics are only 'a tip of the iceberg' of the prevalence of violence against children Eastern Africa, but they do serve to highlight the extent of the problem and that it is a growing problem that urgently needs to be addressed. A child experiencing any form of violence cannot wait because violence in the extreme cases can lead to death or permanent injury or have life-time health and psychological effects on the children.

EXISTING SYSTEMS AND INSTRUMENTS TO ADDRESS VIOLENCE AGAINST CHILDREN

All four countries – Ethiopia, Kenya, Tanzania and Uganda - have ratified the United Nations Convention on the Rights of the Child (UNCRC) and the African Charter on the Rights and Welfare of the Child (ACRWC). Tanzania and Uganda have also ratified the two optional protocols to the UNCRC on the Involvement of Children in Armed Conflicts and on the Sale of Children, Child Prostitution and Child Pornography. Kenya ratified the latter one and signed the former. Ethiopia has not yet ratified the two optional protocols to the UNCRC. Kenya has also acceded to the Hague Convention on Inter Country Adoptions, while Ethiopia which is reportedly placing the highest number of children through inter-country adoption in Africa has not yet adopted this essential convention (6).

Ethiopia, Kenya and Uganda have exerted efforts to harmonise domestic legislation with international child rights standards especially after adopting the UNCRC and ACRWC. For Kenya and Uganda this process involved a comprehensive law on child rights issues in the form of the Children Act of 2001 and the Children Act of 2000, respectively. In the case of Ethiopia, on the other hand, harmonisation involved a comprehensive review of major legislations in which child rights standards have been among the major considerations. Though there have been some law reform efforts in relation to the Penal law, the major legislations for children in Tanzania predate the UNCRC (7).

The establishment of effective centralised reporting mechanisms is vital to detection and reporting of violence against children. Especially the requirement for mandatory reporting of child abuse and neglect by professionals such as teachers, doctors, nurses and social workers is essential in protecting children from further abuse and responding to the needs of child victims.

In Uganda reporting of child abuse and neglect involves relevant actors at various levels. These include community child protection committees; child protection working groups, Community Based Organisations (CBOs) and International NGOs (INGOs); Child and Family Protection Units; and the National Monitoring and Reporting Task Force (8). Kenya also has similar reporting desks at the different levels of which the Crisis Desks established at district level by the Department of Children Services are the most significant (9).

In Tanzania, reporting is most often done to the Social Welfare Department, the police or other government officials as well as to community organizations working on children's rights (10). Similarly, in Ethiopia, reporting of abuse cases mostly goes to the Child Protection Units (CPUs) or any Police Station in places where there is no CPU (11).

Most of the reporting in the four countries is voluntarily done; this is because of the absence of an effective system to implement and monitor mandatory reporting systems. This will be further discussed under the challenges being faced.

RESPONSES TO VIOLENCE AGAINST CHILDREN

The fact that major international instruments are ratified and some measures are taken towards harmonisation of laws, are positive steps towards the protection of children. Reporting mechanisms need to be supported by protection structures. According to the CRC, States are obliged to provide comprehensive and multi-sectoral response to all forms of violence against children. All four countries have specific laws criminalising violence against children.

Based on their Children's Acts, Kenya-2001 and Uganda-2000 have provisions to remove children from their abusive parents or guardians (12, 13). Ethiopia and Tanzania are in the process of developing such Acts. Presently, responses are based on provisions in their existing legislation.

In all the four countries over 50% of the child-centred organisations under an ACPF study reported having procedures on what actions to take if there is suspicion of child abuse. Some of them have also conducted staff training on identifying signs of abuse and responding to a child that reports abuse (7).

Unfortunately, laws on violence against children are not effectively implemented in most African countries. Effective enforcement of laws on violence against children requires standard operating procedures for responding to reported incidents or concerns. These should include a consolidated response mechanism, at all levels, that encompasses medical, psychosocial support and legal representation for children in need. Child protection networks at various levels should also be formed to partner with States in responding to violence against children.

Positive prevention and response models such as the establishment of child protection units in police stations, community based correction centres and referral systems are being promoted by INGOs and national NGOs through their local partners. Efforts have been made to introduce child help lines, free legal aid and psychosocial support services. Model protection programmes that provide victim children with rehabilitation programmes, family reunification and reintegration are also being undertaken by child-centred NGOs. Some of the newly established initiatives include the establishment of the steering committees or referral networks for actors working in the area of child protection.

In Uganda, communities, civil society and children are involved in monitoring, reporting and referral of cases of violence against children. The existence of community child protection committees at the grassroots levels is also encouraging (8).

We would like to draw two examples of successful interventions in ensuring the legal protection of children:

In Kenya, The Children's Foundation – Cradle has played a key role in initiating, drafting and presenting legislation. The CRADLE has been instrumental in the development and audit of several laws relating to children. It was one of the key actors in the development of the Children Act and has more recently been involved in the review of this act by the Kenya Law Reform Commission. It took the lead in the development of a draft Sexual Offences Bill together with the Juvenile Justice Network; amongst many other things the final act enhanced the protection of children by outlawing the trafficking of children and child sex tourism, raising the age of sexual consent to 18 years and increasing penalties for abuse of children. This passed into law in 2006 following immense debate and controversy much of it polarised along gender lines and the CRADLE now sits in the Task Force set up by the policy framework and guidelines for the implementation and administration of the act to secure accessible and uniform treatment of offenders. It will also propose measures to secure acceptable programmes for the protection, treatment, and care of victims of sexual violence as well as the treatment, supervision and rehabilitation of sexual offenders. It is also charged with auditing and reviewing all existing policies, laws, regulations, practices and customs relating to sexual offences (14).

In Ethiopia, the Children's Legal Protection Centre of The African Child Policy Forum has been at the centre of legal protection of children. The fact that the UNCRC has not been published in the relevant Ethiopia legal Gazette created ambiguity in the direct application of the instrument in domestic courts. Yet, in 2007 a landmark decision pertaining to a case handled by the Children's Legal Protection Centre (CLPC) resolved this ambiguity by setting precedent for domestic laws.

The Children's Legal Protection Centre (CLPC) has provided legal and psychosocial support to over 3658 children who have come into conflict with the law. It was part of a team of organisations that advocated for the establishment of child-friendly benches in court in Ethiopia. The Centre supports a team of about 30 pro-bono lawyers who offer free legal assistance to children. It has provided training to a number of law enforcement bodies including the judges and police officers. The Centre identifies the media as an important ally in its work. A selected number of media practitioners have been trained in child rights issues and in child-friendly reporting. The Centre has also provided legal assistance to children in prisons and also carried out a study on the state of children in prisons in Ethiopia. The CLPC has also carried out a pioneering study to document the good practice of children's legal protection centres in Africa, Asia and Latin America. A major success for the Centre was when the court in its decision cited article 3/1 of the UNCRC and set a precedent for domestic laws to be interpreted in line with the general principles of the Convention. This was during a case that was successfully handled by the Centre (15).

EFFORTS TO PREVENT VIOLENCE AGAINST CHILDREN

Primary prevention

Prevention efforts at the primary level include awareness raising and advocacy efforts carried out by civil society organisations. Promotion of child protection through workshops, seminars and training as well as dissemination of leaflets, posters and booklets are the usual preventive actions taken in all four countries. Vulnerable children are also targeted for life skill training, self-defence and assertiveness training (8).

Children and youth groups in schools and in local communities are organised in clubs and networks to educate fellow students as well as children and parents in their neighbourhoods. Clusters of such clubs have also been established to form federation level clubs and even children's parliaments with the aim of promoting child protection (8).

Secondary prevention

Identification of children at risk and providing services to children within their family and community setting are instrumental in reducing the vulnerability of children.

Support to economically deprived families and especially to weak and terminally ill parents and guardians are essential in preventing family separation. However, such family support services are limited throughout Africa including the four East African countries. This leaves large proportions of vulnerable children in precarious situations.

Tertiary prevention

The obligation of providing out-of-home care for children, abused by their families, rests with the state. Public social services being inadequate and almost non-existent in most African countries, children in need of care are usually deprived of their rights to care and protection. As a result, children live on the street or in child-headed households with their wellbeing seriously compromised and their rights violated. This is also the reality within the four countries in focus.

However, some support is provided for physically and sexually abused and exploited children through drop-in-centres and safe homes by few child-focused NGOs. These programmes are aimed at rehabilitating victims through the provision of counselling, health, recreational and legal aid services as well as training of peer educators, skills training and apprenticeship. Temporary shelter and economic assistance are also provided by few NGOs (8).

In addition, established child protection units within Police stations handle cases of children in conflict with the law and abused children who are reported by parents, organisations and neighbours and provide the necessary services. In some of the big cities and towns, hospitals provide age determination and medical certificate for victims of sexual and physical abuses and children in conflict with the law upon courts order (8).

CONTROVERSIES IN THE EXISTING CHILD PROTECTION SYSTEMS

One of the major controversies encountered within child protection systems in Ethiopia, Kenya, Tanzania and Uganda include inconsistencies in the implementation of international instruments and national laws. There are ambiguities due to simultaneous application of incompatible standards including national, local, customary and religious laws such as the case in Kenya which is presented above (7).

Another major controversy is related to model projects that are initiated with the intention of getting replicated and incorporated into government structures. The Child Protection Units in Ethiopia initiated over a decade ago are still being supported by NGOs instead of being incorporated into the government structure. Yet, most of these initiatives just continue as projects here and there with very limited impact. Realising the rights of all children to protection in these countries could not be achieved unless actions towards the promotion of good practices are upgraded to the level of comprehensive services with effective coordination at all levels.

GAPS AND CHALLENGES IN THE LEGISLATIVE AND POLICY FRAMEWORK

Analysis of the forms and content of the legislative and policy framework of the four countries reveals the existence of gaps and challenges. Some of the major legislative and policy gaps and challenges include the following (16):

- There are gaps in terms of ratification of some relevant international instruments. Of particular importance in this respect are the two optional protocols to the UNCRC, which have not been ratified by Ethiopia and Kenya.
- There are legislative gaps in relation to the prohibition of corporal punishment. In Tanzania the laws expressly allows corporal punishment in schools and in penal institutions while the Kenyan Penal Code is silent on the issue. In Ethiopia and Uganda, on the other hand, corporal punishment is prohibited in schools but not at home.
- In Ethiopia, the issue of bail right in relation to child sexual offenders is one of the major challenges faced by the Children's Legal Protection Centre. When perpetrators are released on bail, victim children, their families and other children in the community face a wide range of problems. These include the re-traumatization of the victim child; exposure of the victim child and other children to further abuse; and exposure of the victim child and her/his family to threat and even actual revengeful attack. In fact, quite a number of cases are being closed due to the non appearance of suspects who are released with insignificant bail bond.
- Kenyan laws seem to have critical legislative gaps in relation to sexual abuse. The laws give inconsistent definitions of the child. Though the Children Act (2001) defines a child as any human being under the age of 18 years, the Criminal Law Amendment Act (2003) sets the minimum age for sexual consent to 16 years for girls. In addition, the minimum age of marriage, impliedly set at 18 in the Children

Act, has been set at 16 years for girls and 18 years for boys in the Marriage Act and the Hindu Marriage and Divorce Act. The application of Islamic law and various other customary laws creates further inconsistencies as to the minimum age of marriage in Kenya.

- There is a gap in the laws of Tanzania dealing with child trafficking. While the Sexual Offences Act, 2006 outlaws child trafficking [for sexual purposes], the Penal Code does not explicitly criminalise child trafficking.

- Gaps have been identified in the legislative framework for child labour in Kenya in relation to the legality of children working at 16, absence of legal provisions identifying the types of work considered harmful for children, lack of clarity on measures against parents who put their child to work and the lack of a proper legal framework for prosecution of infringements against existing standards.

- The lack of specific laws/standards on child protection applicable to child-centred organisations is a legislative gap in the legal framework in Ethiopia and Tanzania. In Kenya and Uganda the major gap in this respect relates to the limited scope of application of the existing mandatory child protection standards. Their scopes of application do not cover all organisations that directly or indirectly work with children.

CONCLUSIONS

ACPF's assessment of Child Protection Systems in Ethiopia, Kenya, Tanzania and Uganda as well as other reliable sources clearly indicate that child protection is a cause for serious concern for children living in these countries. A large proportion of children in the four countries are suffering from different types of violence, abuse and exploitation in all settings. Serious gaps and limitations in the legal and policy framework are also observed. The following are some of the major actions that could to be considered in order to improve the safety and protection of children:

- Address gaps in substantive laws on violence against children: There are critical gaps as well as existence of laws that fall short of international standards adopted by the respective governments. Critical areas of concern among these include the application of customary laws not consistent with child protection in Kenya, gaps in the prohibition and criminalisation of corporal punishment in all settings in all four countries, and partial criminalisation of child trafficking in Tanzania. Legislative action in these specific areas will strengthen the child protection framework in the concerned countries.

- Address gaps in laws providing for child protection standards for child-centred organisations: There is a need for developing comprehensive, specific and effective child protection laws and administrative measures for child-centred organisations in all four countries. These should focus on mandatory child protection standards, legal duty to put in place adequate organisational child protection policies, codes of conduct, complaint and monitoring procedures as well as the establishment of independent national monitoring mechanisms for child protection within child-centred organisations.

- Strengthen child protection institutional structures and regulatory mechanisms: Advocating for increased capacity and building the capacity of government structures and regulatory mechanisms to effectively oversee and support child protection will lead to more effective interventions to end all forms of child abuse and violence against children. In addition child-centred organisations should put in place and also ensure the implementation of child protection policies within their organisations.
- Establish national forums or networks on child protection: The existence of a national network on child protection could play significant role in promoting child protection issues and also in providing a platform for sharing information and good practices. Such forums and networks will hold child actors accountable.
- Enhance child participation in child protection issues: Child participation is an effective tool for addressing child protection concerns since interventions will be child-informed. The participation of children will lead to the establishment of child-friendly child protection systems.

REFERENCES

[1]   UNICEF. Child Protection from violence, exploitation and abuse. The big picture (available at: http://www.unicef.org/protection/index_bigpicture.html - updated 17 November 2008

[2]   African Child Policy Forum. Violence against girls in Africa. A retrospective survey in Ethiopia, Kenya and Uganda. Presented Second Int Policy Conf on the African Child, 2006

[3]   African Child Policy Forum. Born to high risk: Violence against girls in Africa. A report prepared for the Second International Policy Conference on the African Child, 2006.

[4]   UNICEF. Information by country, 2008 (available at: www.unicef.org/infobycountry/)

[5]   Save the Children Sweden and African Child Policy Forum. Physical and humiliating punishment in Ethiopia, 2005.

[6]   Selman P. Trends in inter-country adoption: Analysis of data from 20 receiving countries. J Populat Res 2006;23(2).

[7]   African Child Policy Forum. Child protection mechanisms in Ethiopia, Kenya, Uganda and Tanzania. Addis Ababa: ACPF, 2008..

[8]   Save the Children Sweden. Regional child protection workshop proceed. Nairobi, Kenya: Save Child, 2009.

[9]   Second CRC Periodic report (2006). Republic of Kenya, CRC/C/KEN/2, 4 July, 2006.

[10]   Second CRC Periodic report (2004). United Republic of Tanzania, CRC/C/70/Add.26, 24 August, 2005.

[11]   Third CRC Periodic report: The Federal Democratic Republic of Ethiopia (2005). CRC/C/129/Add.8, 28 October, 2005).

[12]   Children Act of 2001. Republic of Kenya.

[13]   Children Act of 2000. Republic of Uganda.

[14]   African Child Policy Forum. Exposing realities, children's legal protection centres. Addis Ababa: ACPF, 2008.

[15]   African Child Policy Forum. Programme highlights Addis Ababa: ACPF, 2008.

[16]   African Child Policy Forum. In the best interest of the child. Harmonising laws in Eastern and Southern Africa. Addis Ababa: ACPF, 2007.

In: International Aspects of Child Abuse and Neglect ISBN: 978-1-60876-703-8
Editors: H. Dubowitz, J. Merrick pp. 241-255 © 2010 Nova Science Publishers, Inc.

Chapter 23

A SNAP-SHOT OF CHILD PROTECTION SYSTEMS IN AUSTRALIA

Richard Roylance

Department of Paediatrics, Logan Hospital and School of Medicine,
Griffith University, Queensland, Australia

Australia is a country the size of mainland USA, with an affluent, predominately urban population of 21 million people. Its political, economic and social structures are similar to other developed countries, such as Canada and the United Kingdom. Child Protection statistics for the Australian population as a whole are commensurate with this profile. However, Australian children of Aboriginal and Torres Strait Islander (ATSI) descent are significantly over-represented in the Australian child protection system: more than five times as likely to be the subject of substantiated abuse and neglect; more than seven times as likely to be on care and protection orders; and over eight times as likely to be in out-of-home care than other Australian children. Although interventions to enhance the safety and wellbeing of Australian children (especially Indigenous children) are increasingly recognized by Australian governments (at both state and federal level) as important and fruitful areas for investment, many children and young people continue to live in circumstances of significant relative social disadvantage (including as victims of child abuse and neglect); child protection notifications and substantiations continue to increase; early intervention services are inadequately funded; and child protection agencies in Australia continue to under-perform. The recent very significant investments to prevent and/or reduce the incidence and/or impact of child abuse or neglect in countries such as the United Kingdom have not (to date) been mirrored within the Australian context.

INTRODUCTION

Australia is a physically large nation, similar in size to mainland USA (7,686,850 sq km), but with a relatively small population of approximately 21 million (0-14 years: 19.3%; 15-64 years: 67.4%; 65 years and over: 13.2%) (1). Although this population is primarily concentrated along the costal fringe, there are sufficient numbers living in rural and remote communities to pose significant geographical challenges for the equitable provision of services to vulnerable children and their families, especially indigenous peoples.

Australia is an affluent nation: with a per capita, annual Gross Domestic Product (GDP) on par with the major West European economies (US$ 37,500 per person per annum); a low unemployment rate (4.4%); a high literacy rate (99%); a low infant mortality rate (4.57 deaths/1,000 live births) and a high life expectancy (80.62 years) (2). However, these socio-economic indices of wellbeing are significantly lower for indigenous Australians: with a lower per capita income; twice the rate of unemployment (3); a much higher infant mortality rate (12.2 deaths/1,000 live births) (4), and a much lower life expectancy (nearly 20 years less) (5).

Australia is constituted as a federal parliamentary democracy, with political stability spanning more than a century. There exists a robust system of law (with an independent judiciary) based on English common law: with 6 states (Queensland, New South Wales, Victoria, Tasmania, South Australia, Western Australia) and 2 territories (Northern Territory, Australian Capital Territory).

HOW THE DIFFERENT TYPES OF CHILD ABUSE AND NEGLECT ARE DEFINED?

Within this federal framework, child protection in Australia is predominately managed as a state/territory-based issue, with each State and Territory responsible for its own legislations and policy. Whilst there is therefore no formal, uniform definition of child abuse and neglect (CAN) across the Australian jurisdictions, in practice the following are reasonable 'working definitions' of CAN within the Australian context:

- Physical abuse: Any non-accidental physical act inflicted upon a child by a person having the care of a child;
- Sexual abuse: Any act by a person having the care of the child which exposes a child to, or involves a child in, sexual processes beyond his or her understanding or contrary to accepted community standards;
- Emotional abuse: Any act by a person having the care of a child that results in the child suffering any kind of significant emotional deprivation or trauma;
- Neglect: Any serious omissions or commissions by a person having the care of a child which, within the bounds of cultural tradition, constitute a failure to provide conditions which are essential for the healthy, physical and emotional development of a child (6).

WHAT IS KNOWN ABOUT THE EXTENT OF THE PROBLEM?

Data on child protection have been collected in Australia for many decades. However, jurisdiction-based differences in CAN definitions, legislations and practice guidelines make inter-state and/or national comparisons difficult. Moreover, changes to CAN definitions, legislations and practice guidelines within each individual Australian jurisdiction over past decades make trend analysis even within an Australian jurisdiction problematic.

In this context, the Australian Institute of Health and Welfare (AIHW) has been funded to collate, analyse and publish Australian child protection data annually. The reader is referred to the excellent AIHW "Child Protection Australia/Child Welfare" series of publications for a detailed collation, review and analysis of Australian child protection data from the past decade (7).

At the national level, the AIHW reports on four child protection data collections: 'CAN notifications, investigations and substantiations'; 'care and protection orders'; 'children in out-of-home care'; and 'intensive family support services'.

The most recent AIHW Child Protection Australia Report (2006-07) identified that during 2002-07, child protection notifications in Australia increased by more than 50% (from 198,355 to 309,517); with a commensurate 45% increase in the number of substantiations (from 40,416 to 58,563). In the period 1997-2007, the number of Australian children under care and protection orders (i.e., children for whom state/territory child protection and support services have a responsibility as a result of some formal legal order or an administrative/voluntary arrangement) rose by 87% (from 15,718 to 29,406) – an increase in rate from 3.3 per 1,000 to 6.0 per 1,000 (with significant variations between the States and Territories). During 1997-2007, the number of Australian children in out-of-home care rose by 102% (from 14,078 to 28,441) - with 50% in foster care, 44% in relative or kinship care, and 4% in residential care (8).

It is not easy to quantify the characteristics of child sexual abuse (CSA) within Australia. Jurisdictional differences in how state/territory-based child protection and support services manage allegations of CSA means that significant numbers of allegations of CSA involving persons other than the immediate caregiver are excluded from data state/territory reports to the AIHW. Although there is potential for capture of this some of this data within state/territory based collections of sexual assault data by police services – the separate data inputs are rarely, in practice, combined for analysis.

Aboriginal and Torres Strait Islander children remain significantly over-represented in the Australian child protection system. Across Australia, Indigenous children are more than 5 times as likely to be the subject of CAN substantiations than other children; more than 7 times as likely to be on care and protection orders; and over 8 times as likely to be in out-of-home care (9).

WHAT SYSTEM(S) OR INFRASTRUCTURE EXISTS TO ADDRESS CAN?

Each Australian State and Territory has its individual definitions, laws and practice guidelines in relation to child protection; with each state-based government department having a statutory role to manage allegations of child abuse and neglect (10). An assortment of inter-jurisdictional agreements (mixed legislation and policy protocols) also exist to accommodate the movement of children and their caregivers between states and territories.

Australian Federal laws are primarily concerned with the management of children within the context of family disharmony (i.e. Family Court); or in relation to children within the international context (e.g. Australian citizens involved with sex tourism, international adoptions, child labour agreements, etc.).

The interaction between state/territory-based child protection systems and the federally-based Family Court system has recently been modified. To provide some perspective: of 7757 cases brought before the Family Court of Australia in the 2006-07 period in which Final Orders were sought (i.e., the matter could not be decided by negotiation between the parties, and a Court direction was required), 4965 (64%) of the Court's cases involve parenting disputes (11). Within this context, in 1998 'Project Magellan' was initiated by the Family Court of Australia. Magellan involves a special case management system activated when serious allegations of sexual or physical abuse of a child arise within the Family Court system. Once a Magellan case is identified, it is managed by a designated team consisting of a judge, court registrar and family consultant. An independent children's lawyer is appointed in every Magellan case. A specific goal of Magellan is to foster strong inter-agency coordination, in particular with State and Territory child protection agencies - to ensure that issues in regard to child protection are dealt with efficiently, and that information sharing is of high quality. There have been a total of 734 Magellan cases since the introduction of this case management process, throughout all Australian States and Territories (12).

Within Australia, each State and Territory has a single state/territory-wide police service responsible for the enforcement of its jurisdiction-based Crimes Act (the Australian Capital Territory falls under the auspice of the Australian Federal police). Police services in Australia are involved in child protection when suspected harm to a child is potentially of a criminal nature (i.e. where the allegations are significant sexual or physical abuse or neglect, especially in relation to the injury or death of a child). In most Australian States and Territories, there are laws, protocols or informal arrangements whereby the police are involved in the joint investigation of some allegations of child abuse and neglect with child protection and/or support services.

The Australian Federal Police (AFP) service has a specific role in protecting children living overseas from Australian citizens who travel to other countries and sexually exploit children. The AFP have a federally legislated authority (Crimes Act 1914 Part IIIA) to prosecute Australian citizens and residents of Australia in Australia for child sex offences committed in foreign countries. This legislation aims to supplement foreign law enforcement capacity - by allowing the prosecution of Australian offenders who have escaped the jurisdiction of foreign law enforcement, including those foreign jurisdictions whose laws do not identify these acts as criminal (13). Australian sexual offenders against children living overseas are almost exclusively male, travelling to overseas locations to exploit children sexually by taking advantage of adverse socio-economic factors and lower law enforcement capacity within those jurisdictions – with Thailand, Cambodia and the Philippines being prominent targets (14).

The AFP 'Online Child Sex Exploitation Team' (OCSET) performs an investigative and coordination role within Australia regarding multi-jurisdictional and international 'online' child sex exploitation matters. Referrals come from Australian State and Territory police, government and non-government organisations (including Internet Service Providers and Internet Content Hosts), the Australian High Tech Crime Centre, the Virtual Global Task Force, international law enforcement agencies, Interpol and members of the public. The types of alleged offences investigated include the accessing, sending or uploading of child pornography and/or child abuse material. Grooming and procuring of children over the Internet is also investigated by the AFP (15).

The 'Australian National Child Offenders Register' (ANCOR) monitors the activities of persons convicted in Australia of significant offences against children, including child sex offenders. The objective of the Register is to ensure that persons convicted of sex offences and other serious offences against children can be monitored by police once they have served their sentence. Jurisdictional legislation determines what constitutes a registrable offence (16). In February 2008, there were 6719 offenders registered with ANCOR across Australia (17).

HOW DOES THE SYSTEM WORK REGARDING REPORTING OF POSSIBLE CAN?

Australian children come to the attention of the State and Territory departments responsible for child protection through a number of mechanisms. Reports may be made by an affected child; by a family or community member; by a professional mandated to report suspected abuse and neglect; or by an organisation that has contact with a family or child. There are no national data available regarding the total number of 'reports' of suspicions of CAN made to Australian state/territory child protection services.

Currently, all Australian State and Territory jurisdictions have legislation requiring some level of compulsory (i.e. 'mandated') reporting of suspicions of significant harm (or risk of significant harm) to a child due to child abuse or neglect, but the laws vary widely. In some jurisdictions, specific categories of persons in specific circumstances are mandated to report. In other jurisdictions, anyone who has reason to believe that a child may be abused or neglected must report this to the appropriate authority. In addition, Family Court staff are required to report suspected cases of child abuse or neglect to relevant state/territory-based child protection and support services department (18).

All Australian jurisdictions provide immunity to persons who report suspicions of child abuse or neglect in good faith; regardless of whether the reports are substantiated.

THE "TYPICAL" RESPONSE BY THE RESPONSIBLE AGENCIES

Although there is no uniform or 'typical' response to reports of suspected child abuse or neglect in Australia, there is a broad similarity across jurisdictions.

A 'report' to a state/territory-based department is assessed to determine whether the matter should be dealt with by the child protection and support services department; or referred to another agency.

A report that is deemed appropriate for consideration by the State and Territory child protection and support services is further assessed to determine whether any further action is required by that service.

A report requiring further action is then classified as either a 'family support issue' or a 'child protection notification'.

A 'child protection notification' is assessed by the service to determine whether it requires an 'investigation'; whether it can appropriately be dealt with by other means (such as referral to another organisation); or, whether no further protective action is necessary or possible.

At the end of the 'investigation process', a notification is classified as 'substantiated' or 'not substantiated'. A notification is 'substantiated' where it is concluded after investigation that the child has been, is being, or is likely to be, abused, neglected or otherwise harmed. All Australian jurisdictions 'substantiate' cases where a child has suffered significant harm from abuse and neglect through the actions of parents/guardians. However, in some jurisdictions, the 'substantiation' may be predominately determined by the specifics of the parent's action (or lack of action) itself - i.e., drug use, striking, poor supervision; while in other jurisdictions, the question of 'substantiation' may be determined by whether the child actually suffered harm (or was at predictable risk of suffering harm), rather than what the parent did (or did not) do (19). In cases where a child has suffered significant harm from abuse and neglect through the actions of someone not an immediate parent/guardian(i.e. teacher, neighbour, grandparent, ex-partner etc), the matter may not be recorded within the child protection system as 'substantiated', instead being referred to the state police service as a case of alleged criminal assault. The 'test' in many jurisdictions is whether the parent/ guardian was 'protective' after the allegations came to light and/or whether the parent/guardian was demonstrably 'negligent' to have allowed the situation to have arisen in the first instance.

The State or Territory agency responsible for child protection may apply to a Court to place the child on a 'care and protection' order. This formal Court order/direction might take the form of the relevant authority assuming total responsibility for the welfare of the child (for example, guardianship); responsibility for overseeing the actions of the person or authority caring for the child; responsibility for providing or arranging accommodation; or reporting on the child's welfare (20). Across all Australian jurisdictions, legislation and policy generally dictate that statutory interventions of this type are 'last resorts' – i.e. to be used in situations where supervision and/or counselling is resisted by the family, where other avenues to resolve the situation have been exhausted, or when removal of a child from the home requires that parental rights be overtaken by an external legal authorisation (21).

The State or Territory agency for child protection may seek to divert children and their families into 'family support services.' A family support service may be used instead of a statutory child protection response (that is, as a substitute service) or as a complementary service to a statutory response – with the specifics varying between jurisdictions.

These processes are detailed in the AIHW "Child Protection Australia / Child Welfare" series previously cited.

STRENGTHS IN AUSTRALIA'S APPROACH/SYSTEM

By international standards, Australia should be well placed to provide for the safety and welfare of its children and young people. It is an affluent nation with long-standing social and political stability, a robust legal system (with child protection legislation enshrined in all jurisdictions), and a strong, well-funded public service.

Each of the state and territory jurisdictions have laws regarding the relevant principles of the Convention on the Rights of the Child (CRC): i.e. whole-of-government and community responsibility for child protection (Article 3.1); early intervention (Articles 19.1/19.2);

principles of cultural appropriateness (Article 29.1(c)); principles specific to after care (Articles 26.1 / 27.1); and the best interests principle (Article 3.1) (22).

Australia has for long committed to the provision of an appropriate social safety-net for its vulnerable citizens - including children and their families (e.g. unemployment & sickness benefits, universal healthcare, and housing support, etc.). There has been recent acknowledgement by governments (at both state/territory and Federal levels) of the critical role of early intervention and support services in the prevention and minimisation of the harms arising from child abuse or neglect, with modest new investments in this area (23,24).

There is a growing commitment within government departments and academia in Australia to improve national consistency in legislation and policy related to the protection of children.

There are national initiatives to improve intra-jurisdictional and inter-jurisdictional consistency in child protection data collection in Australia - with the National Child Protection and Support Services (NCPASS) data group established in 1997 to oversee the national child protection data collection.

In the context of a high literacy rate, Australia has an independent media - which has displayed an on-going commitment to pursue issues related to the protection of children. There has been considerable recent public debate within Australia critically reviewing what should appropriately constitute a community response to the abuse or neglect of Australian children and young people – especially in regard to indigenous children, child sexual abuse, the management of offenders, and the documented inadequacy of child protection and support services in all jurisdictions.

New South Wales, Queensland, Tasmania and Western Australia have Commissioners for Children and Young People. South Australia has the Children's Interest Bureau, and Victoria has a Child Safety Commissioner. A Commissioner is soon to be established in the Northern Territory, and the Australian Capital Territory's Disability Commission is expected to be expanded in the near future to encompass a Children's Commissioner. There have been renewed calls for a National Commissioner.

Formal Child Death Review Committees have been established in five of the six Australian state jurisdictions, with plans articulated to establish committees in Tasmania and the Territories in the near future.

There have been recent (sometimes controversial) changes to legislation, policy and funding to try and improve the over-representation of Australia's indigenous children and young people in all the myriad forms of social disadvantage, and specifically within the child protection spectrum (see below).

WEAKNESSES/CHALLENGES IN AUSTRALIA'S APPROACH/SYSTEM

Despite these positive factors in the Australian socio-economic parameters, many children and young people continue to live in circumstances of significant relative social disadvantage (including as victims of child abuse and neglect); child protection notifications and substantiations continue to increase; early intervention services are inadequately funded; and child protection agencies in Australia continue to under-perform.

There have been twenty major inquiries into child protection services in Australia since 2000. The most recent report into child protection services within an Australian jurisdiction (South Australia) was released in 2008 by former Supreme Court Justice Mullighan (25). Mr Mullighan's inquiry follows close on the heels of other inquiries into child protection in Western Australia (2002) (26), Queensland (2004) (27) and the Northern Territory (2007) (28). More recently, a special commission of inquiry into child protection has been commissioned in New South Wales subsequent to concerns raised in that jurisdiction, with its report due later in 2008 (29).

Although Mr Mulligan's report identified significant deficiencies in child protection services within the South Australian jurisdiction, his finding are consistent with the findings of these other Australian inquiries, that "...the State's child protection system, like its counterparts elsewhere in Australia, is in crisis, largely because of poor past practices. The number of children being placed in care has increased; there is a shortage of foster carers and social workers; children tend to be placed according to the availability of placements rather than the suitability.... Such a system cannot properly care for an already vulnerable group of children, let alone protect them from perpetrators of sexual abuse. More resources must be made available to deal with the crisis, as well as to implement necessary reforms for the present and future" (30). He further noted that "...the evidence to the Inquiry indicates that there is a problem with recruiting and retaining social workers, which has resulted in a lack of experience; inexperienced social workers having insufficient professional support and supervision; workloads being too high; and a staff shortage. This is not a recent phenomenon" (31).

Whatever short-falls exist in the broader child protection response in Australia, the outcomes for indigenous children and young people are significantly worse. The inter-generational trauma of Australian Indigenous peoples associated with the cycle of child removal; issues of social and community dislocation; their physical and cultural marginalisation from social services for health, housing, education and policing as well as from family and child welfare services are well documented. Common manifestations of these problems include: alcohol and substance abuse; mental health problems; high levels of family and community violence; inter-generational unemployment and economic deprivation – with significant and pervasive impacts on the health and wellbeing of Indigenous children (32). The over-representation of indigenous children and young people within the Australian child protection system remains inexcusable, especially in the context of the positive gains achieved for indigenous peoples in other jurisdictions with similar socio-economic profiles to Australia (e.g. the First Nation and Native American peoples of Canada and the USA) (33). Although well-intentioned efforts have been made within all Australian jurisdictions to improve outcomes for indigenous children and young people, the concerns raised (by these and earlier reports (34)) remain demonstrably unresolved.

MAJOR CONTROVERSIES

The areas of controversy in regard to the child protection response within the Australian jurisdictions are similar to those of the UK, Canada and the US:

- What is the appropriate balance between family independence and state intervention?

- What is the appropriate balance between under-identification (i.e. false negatives) and over-identification of child abuse and neglect (i.e. false positives)?
- When does a system to monitor and evaluate the child protection bureaucracy become overly intrusive/burdensome?
- How to better identify effective interventions to prevent, minimise and treat child abuse and neglect; and then appropriately resource them?
- How to recruit, train and retain appropriately trained and motivated staff of all disciplines within the child protection sector?
- How to better minimise secondary harm to affected children and their families caught up in criminal and child protection interventions?
- How to better recruit, train and retain alternative care systems for children who can not safely remain at home?
- What is the appropriate balance between approaches to minimise re-abuse and a criminal justice / punitive community response (i.e. offender management)?

A recent controversy within the Australian jurisdiction has brought a number of these issues into sharp focus - 'The Northern Territory Intervention'. In a direct response to the Northern Territory's "Little Children are Sacred" Report (2007) cited above, the Australian government initiated what it called "a number of major measures to deal with what we can only describe as a national emergency in relation to the abuse of children in indigenous communities in the Northern Territory." A number of key measures were announced:

- introducing widespread alcohol restrictions on Northern Territory Aboriginal land for six months. Banning the sale, the possession, the transportation, the consumption and the introduction of broader monitoring of 'take-away' alcohol sales across the Northern Territory;
- undertaking medical examinations of all indigenous children in the Northern Territory under the age of 16 years, with assurances that the government would provide the resources to deal with any follow up medical treatment that will be needed;
- commencing welfare reforms designed to stem the flow of cash going towards alcohol abuse, and to ensure that funds meant to be used for children's welfare are used for that purpose;
- enforcing school attendance by linking income support and family assistance payments to school attendance for all people living on Aboriginal land;
- providing meals for indigenous children at school, with parents paying for the meals;
- taking control of indigenous townships through five year leases to ensure that property and public housing can be improved, and if that involves the payment of compensation on just terms as required by the Commonwealth Constitution then that compensation will be readily paid;
- initiating an intensive on-the-ground clean-up of indigenous communities to make them safer and healthier - by marshalling local workforces through 'Work for the Dole' arrangements;

- banning the possession of x-rated pornography in the proscribed indigenous areas and checking all publicly funded computers for evidence of the storage of pornography;
- immediately increasing policing levels on indigenous communities;
- setting up an Australian Government sexual abuse reporting desk; and
- appointing managers of all government businesses in all indigenous communities.

This intervention by the Federal government in late 2007 was (and continues to be) highly controversial by the indigenous, government, non-government and the broader community – with considerable divergence of opinions as to whether these significant changes should be supported. The results of evaluations of these new policy directions will not be available for some time.

PREVENTION EFFORTS (PRIMARY, SECONDARY, TERTIARY)

Australia's strong social safety-net and historical investment in intervention services in the primary, secondary and tertiary sectors has been noted above. Broadly, the prevention investments in the Australia are similar to those in place within the UK, Canada and the US. However, the recent very significant investments to prevent and/or reduce the incidence and/or impact of child abuse or neglect in the UK have not (to date) been mirrored within the Australian context (35).

It is appropriate that this over-view of the child protection system within the Australian jurisdictions conclude by high-lighting the crucial role that the collection and analysis of high quality data will have in determining how best to invest for the future of Australia's vulnerable children. Systems to improve legislation, policy, professional development, and service infrastructure - so as to better investigate, treat, and above all prevent child abuse and neglect - can only be effective if guided by the evidence of what works, rather than by whims, fancies and 'good ideas' - no matter how well-intentioned they may be!

In this context, the reader is referred to a document recently released by the Australian Institute of Health and Welfare (AIHW). This document outlines a proposal for the collection of key national indicators of the health, development and wellbeing of Australian children (36). These indicators sit under seven broad headings (see table 1):

- How healthy are Australia's children?
- How well are we promoting healthy child development?
- How well are Australia's children learning and developing?
- What factors can affect children adversely?
- What kind of families and communities do Australia's children live in?
- How safe and secure are Australia's children?
- How well is the system performing in delivering quality health, development and well-being actions to Australia's children?

Table 1. Key national indicators of children's health, development and well-being. [a]
Headline indicator

HOW HEALTHY ARE AUSTRALIA'S CHILDREN?
• **Mortality**
o   Infant mortality rate[a]
o   Sudden infant death syndrome (SIDS) rate
o   Death rate for children aged 1–14 years
• **Morbidity**
o   Proportion of children aged 0–14 years with asthma as a long-term condition
o   New cases of cancer per 100,000 children aged 0–14 years
o   New cases of insulin-dependent diabetes per 100,000 children aged 0–14 years
• **Disability**
o   Proportion of children aged 0–14 years with severe or profound core activity limitations
• **Mental health**
o   Proportion of children aged 4–14 years with mental health problems
o   Proportion of children aged 6–14 years with mental health disorders (ADHD, depressive disorder, conduct disorder)
HOW WELL ARE WE PROMOTING HEALTHY CHILD DEVELOPMENT?
• **Breastfeeding**
o   Proportion of infants exclusively breastfed at 4 months of age[a]
• **Dental health**
o   Proportion of children decay-free at age 6 years and at age 12 years
o   Mean number of decayed, missing or filled teeth among primary school children[a]
• **Physical activity**
o   Under development
• **Early learning**
o   Proportion of children aged <1 year old who are read to by an adult on a regular basis
HOW WELL ARE AUSTRALIA'S CHILDREN LEARNING AND DEVELOPING?
• **Transition to primary school**
o   Proportion of children entering school with basic skills for life and learning(a)
• **Attending early childhood education programs**
o   Proportion of children attending an early education program in the 2 years prior to beginning primary school[a]
• **Attendance at primary school**
o   Attendance rate of children at primary school[a]
• **Literacy and Numeracy**
o   Proportion of primary school children who achieve the literacy benchmarks[a]
o   Proportion of primary school children who achieve the numeracy benchmarks[a]
• **Social and emotional development**
o   Under development

Table 1. (continued)

WHAT FACTORS CAN AFFECT CHILDREN ADVERSELY?
• **Teenage births**
o   Age-specific fertility rate for 15–19 year old women[a]
• **Smoking in pregnancy**
o   Proportion of women who smoked during the first 20 weeks of pregnancy[a]
• **Alcohol use during pregnancy**
o   Proportion of women who consume alcohol during pregnancy
• **Birthweight**
o   Proportion of live born infants of low birthweight[a]
• **Overweight and obesity**
o   Proportion of children whose body mass index (BMI) score is above the international cut off points for 'overweight' and 'obese' for their age and sex[a]
• **Environmental tobacco smoke in the home**
o   Proportion of households with children aged 0–14 years where adults smoke inside
• **Tobacco use**
o   Proportion of children aged 12–14 years who are current smokers
• **Alcohol misuse**
o   Proportion of children aged 12–14 years who have engaged in high-risk drinking (5 or more drinks in a row) at least once in the last 2 weeks
WHAT KIND OF FAMILIES AND COMMUNITIES DO AUSTRALIA'S CHILDREN LIVE IN?
• **Family functioning**
o   Under development
• **Family economic situation**
o   Average real equivalised disposable household income for households with children in the 2nd and 3rd income deciles[a]
• **Children in non-parental care**
o   Rate of children aged 0–14 years in out-of-home care
o   Under development - Children in grandparent families
• **Parental health status**
o   Proportion of parents rating their health as 'fair' or 'poor'
o   Proportion of parents with disability
o   Proportion of parents with mental health problems
• **Neighbourhood safety**
o   Proportion of households with children aged 0–14 years where neighbourhood is perceived as unsafe
• **Social capital**
o   Proportion of households with children under 15 years of age where respondent was able to get support in time of crisis from persons living outside the household
HOW SAFE AND SECURE ARE AUSTRALIA'S CHILDREN?
• **Injuries**
o   Age-specific death rates from all injuries for children aged 0–4, 5–9 and 10–14 years[a]
o   Road transport accident death rate for children aged 0–14 years
o   Accidental drowning death rate for children aged 0–14 years
o   Intentional self-harm hospitalisation rate for children aged 0–14 years
o   Assault death rate for children aged 0–14 years
o   Assault hospitalisation rate for children aged 0–14 years

o	Injury hospitalisation rate for children aged 0–14 years
•	**School relationships and bullying**
o	Under development
•	**Child abuse and neglect**
o	Rate of children aged 0–12 years who were the subject of child protection substantiation in a given year[a]
o	Rate of children aged 0–12 years who are the subject of care and protection orders
•	**Children as victims of violence**
o	Rate of children aged 0–14 years who have been the victim of physical and sexual assault
•	**Homelessness**
o	Rate of children aged 0–15 years seeking assistance from the Supported Accommodation Assistance Program (accompanied and unaccompanied)
•	**Children and crime**
o	Rate of children aged 10–14 years who are under juvenile justice supervision
HOW WELL IS THE SYSTEM PERFORMING IN DELIVERING QUALITY HEALTH, DEVELOPMENT AND WELLBEING ACTIONS TO AUSTRALIA'S CHILDREN?	
•	**Congenital anomalies**
o	Under development—Rate of selected congenital anomalies among infants at births
•	**Newborn screening (hearing)**
o	Under development
•	**Immunisation**
o	Proportion of children on the Australian Childhood Immunisation Register who are fully immunised at 2 years of age[a]
•	**Survival for leukaemia**
o	Five-year relative survival rate for leukaemia in children aged 0–14 years
•	**Quality child care**
o	Under development
•	**Child protection re-substantiations**
o	Rate of children aged 0–12 years who were the subject of child protection re-substantiation in a given year

It is hoped that the Australian State, Territory and Commonwealth governments jointly agree to develop and support the systems necessary for the collection and analysis of this data – as a necessary first-step in the enhancement of our capacity to better protect and nurture our children and young people!

REFERENCES

[1]   US Government. The 2008 world factbook. Washington, DC: US Government Printing Office, 2008. Accessed 2008 Feb 10. URL: https://www.cia.gov/library/publications/the-world-factbook/geos/as.html.

[2]   US Government. The 2008 world factbook. Washington, DC: US Government Printing Office, 2008. Accessed 2008 Feb 10. URL: https://www.cia.gov/library/publications/the-world-factbook/geos/as.html.

[3]   Australian Institute of Health and Welfare. Aboriginal and Torres Strait Islander health performance framework, 2006 report: detailed analyses. AIHW cat. no. IHW 20. Canberra: AIHW, 2007.

[4]   Australian Institute of Health and Welfare. Aboriginal and Torres Strait Islander health performance framework, 2006 report: detailed analyses. AIHW cat. no. IHW 20. Canberra: AIHW, 2007.

[5]   Australian Bureau of Statistics (ABS). Deaths Australia, 2004. ABS Cat. No. 3302.0. Canberra: ABS,
        2005.
[6]   Australian Institute of Health and Welfare. Child protection Australia 2006-07. Child Welfare series
        no. 43. Cat. No. Canberra: AIWA; 96, 2008.
[7]   Australian Institute of Health and Welfare (AIHW). Accessed 2008 Feb 10. URL:
        http://www.aihw.gov.au/publications.
[8]   Australian Institute of Health and Welfare. Child protection Australia 2006-07. Child Welfare series
        2008, no. 43. Cat. No. Canberra: AIWA, 2008:x-xi.
[9]   Australian Institute of Health and Welfare. Child protection Australia 2006-07. Child Welfare series
        2008, no. 43. Cat. No. Canberra: AIWA, 2008:x-xi.
[10]   Queensland (Department of Child Safety); New South Wales (Department of Community Services);
        Victoria (Department of Human Services); Tasmania (Department of Health and Human Services);
        South Australia (Families SA / Department for Families and Communities); Western Australia
        (Department for Child Protection); Australian Capital Territory (Office for Children, Youth and
        Family Support); Northern Territory (Department of Health and Community Services).
[11]   Family Court of Australia. Annual Report 2006-07. Pirion Printing, ACT, 2007:39. Accessed 2008
        Feb 10. URL: http://www.familycourt.gov.au.
[12]   Family Court of Australia. Annual Report 2006-07. Pirion Printing, ACT, 2007:19. Accessed 2008
        Feb 10. URL: http://www.familycourt.gov.au.
[13]   Australian Federal Police. Annual Report 2006–07. 2007. Accessed 2008 Feb 10. URL:
        http://www.afp.gov.au.
[14]   Australian Federal Police. Annual Report 2006–07. 2007:26. Accessed 2008 Feb 10. URL:
        http://www.afp.gov.au.
[15]   Australian Federal Police. Annual Report 2006–07. 2007:40. Accessed 2008 Feb 10. URL:
        http://www.afp.gov.au.
[16]   QLD [Child Protection (Offender Reporting) Act 2004]; NSW [Child Protection (Offenders
        Registration) Act 2001]; VIC [Sex Offenders Registration Act 2004]; TAS [Community Protection
        (Offender Reporting) Act 2005]; SA [Child Sex Offenders Registration Act 2006]; WA [Community
        Protection (Offender Reporting) Act 2004]; NT [Child Protection (Offender Reporting and
        Registration) Act 2004]; ACT [Crimes (Child Sex Offenders) Act 2005].
[17]   Commonwealth of Australia, Crimtrac, 2008. Accessed 2008 Feb 10: URL:
        http://www.crimtrac.gov.au.
[18]   Higgins D, Bromfield L, Richardson N. Mandatory reporting of child abuse. National Child Protection
        Clearinghouse (Australian Institute of Family Studies) Resource Sheet Number 3; August 2007.
        Accessed 2008 Feb 10. URL: http://www.aifs.gov.au.
[19]   Australian Institute of Health and Welfare. Child protection Australia 2006-07. Child Welfare series
        no. 43. Cat. No. Canberra: AIWA. 2008; 14.
[20]   Australian Institute of Health and Welfare. Child protection Australia 2006-07. Child Welfare series
        no. 43. Cat. No. Canberra: AIWA. 2008; 97.
[21]   Australian Institute of Health and Welfare. Child protection Australia 2006-07. Child Welfare series
        no. 43. Cat. No. Canberra: AIWA. 2008; 4.
[22]   Australian Institute of Family Studies, National Child Protection Clearinghouse and the Australian
        Institute of Health and Welfare, Children, Youth and Families Unit. International approaches to child
        protection: how is Australia positioned? Sept 2007. Accessed 2008 Feb 10. URL:
        http://www.aihw.gov.au.
[23]   NSW Government. A new direction for New South Wales: state plan 2006. Sydney, 2006.
[24]   NSW Commission for Children and Young People, Commission for Children and Young People
        (QLD), and the National Investment for the Early Years. A headstart for Australia – an early years
        framework. Sydney, 2004.
[25]   Mullighan EP . Children in state care commission of inquiry: allegations of sexual abuse and death
        from criminal conduct 2008. Presented to the South Australian Parliament by the Hon. EP Mullighan
        QC (Commissioner). Adelaide, SA, 2008.

[26] Gordon S, Hallahan K, Henry D. Putting the picture together, inquiry into response by government agencies to complaints of family violence and child abuse in aboriginal communities. Department of Premier and Cabinet, Perth, WA, 2002.

[27] Crime and Misconduct Commission (Queensland). Protecting children: an inquiry into abuse of children in foster care. Government Printer, Brisbane, QLD, 2004.

[28] Wild R, Anderson P. Ampe akelyernemane meke mekarle 'little children are sacred' report of the Northern Territory board of inquiry into the protection of aboriginal children from sexual abuse. Northern Territory Government, Darwin, 2007.

[29] Wood J. Special commission of inquiry into child protection services in New South Wales. NSW Government, Sydney, 2008.

[30] Mullighan EP. Children in state care commission of inquiry: allegations of sexual abuse and death from criminal conduct. Presented to the South Australian Parliament by the Hon. EP Mullighan QC (Commissioner). Adelaide, SA, 2008:15.

[31] Mullighan EP. Children in state care commission of inquiry: allegations of sexual abuse and death from criminal conduct. Presented to the South Australian Parliament by the Hon. EP Mullighan QC (Commissioner). Adelaide, SA, 2008:394.

[32] Stanley J, Tomison AM & Pocock J. Child abuse and neglect in Indigenous Australian communities. National Child Protection Clearinghouse Issues Paper no. 19, Australian Institute of Family Studies, Melbourne, 2003.

[33] Libesman T. Child welfare approaches for indigenous communities: international perspectives. National Child Protection Clearinghouse (NCPC) Child Abuse Prevention Issues no. 20; Autumn 2004.

[34] Commonwealth of Australia. Bringing them home: report of the national inquiry into the separation of Aboriginal and Torres Strait islander children from their families. ACT, 1997.

[35] UK Government. Every child matters: change for children. London: Crown Press, 2004.

[36] Australian Institute of Health and Welfare. Key national indicators of children's health, development and wellbeing: indicator framework for a picture of Australia's children 2009. Cat. no. AUS 100. Canberra: AIHW, 2008.

Chapter 24

ABOUT THE EDITORS

Howard Dubowitz, MD, MS is a professor of pediatrics and director of the Center for Families at the University of Maryland School of Medicine, Baltimore. He is a member of the Council of the International Society for the Prevention of Child Abuse and Neglect (ISPCAN) and a board member of Prevent Child Abuse America (PCAA). He is a founding member and current vice-president of the Helfer Society, an honory society of physicians working in the field of child maltreatment. Dr. Dubowitz is a clinician, researcher, educator and he is active in the policy arena. His main interests are in child neglect and the prevention of child maltreatment. He edited *Neglected Children: Research, Practice and Policy,* co-edited the *Handbook for Child Protection Practice*, and he has over 140 publications. His awards include the "Outstanding Professional" award in 2001 by the American Professional Society on the Abuse of Children. E-mail: hdubowitz@peds.umaryland.edu

Joav Merrick, MD, MMedSci, DMSc, is professor of pediatrics, child health and human development affiliated with Kentucky Children's Hospital, University of Kentucky, Lexington, United States and the Zusman Child Development Center, Division of Pediatrics, Soroka University Medical Center, Ben Gurion University, Beer-Sheva, Israel, the medical director of the Health Services, Division for Mental Retardation, Ministry of Social Affairs, Jerusalem, the founder and director of the National Institute of Child Health and Human Development. Numerous publications in the field of pediatrics, child health and human development, rehabilitation, intellectual disability, disability, health, welfare, abuse, advocacy, quality of life and prevention. Received the Peter Sabroe Child Award for outstanding work on behalf of Danish Children in 1985 and the International LEGO-Prize ("The Children's Nobel Prize") for an extraordinary contribution towards improvement in child welfare and well-being in 1987. E-mail: jmerrick@zahav.net.il; Home-page: http://jmerrick50.googlepages.com/home

About the Division of Child Protection and Center for Families, Department of Pediatrics, University of Maryland School of Medicine, United States

The Division of Child Protection and Center for Families, within the Department of Pediatrics at the University of Maryland School of Medicine, United States of America, is focused on the problem of child abuse and neglect. Our mission is to help ensure the optimal professional response to maltreated children and their families with a special interest in preventing this problem. We have activities in four areas: clinical, research, teaching and advocacy.

Clinical

Our clinical work spans the range from prevention to forensic diagnosis to treatment.

1. The **Safe Environment for Every Kid (*SEEK*)** project involves testing a model of enhanced pediatric primary care focused on identifying and addressing major psychosocial problems (depression, substance abuse, intimate partner violence) families may be facing. *SEEK* aims to strengthen families, support parents and thereby improve children's health, development and safety – and prevent child abuse and neglect. Results thus far have been most encouraging.
2. Our **Child Protection Team (CPT)** provides 24/7 interdisciplinary clinical consultation to hospital staff when concerns of possible abuse or neglect arise. In addition, the CPT offers training and helps develop hospital policies concerning child abuse and neglect.
3. Our **Care Clinic**, funded largely by the Maryland Department of Human Resources provides treatment to abused and neglected children and their families – free of charge. The Clinic also serves as a training site for mental health and medical clinicians.
4. The **Maryland Child Abuse Medical Providers (CHAMP)** program, funded by the Maryland Department of Health and Mental Hygiene, is developing a statewide

network of physicians and nurses, expert in the area of child maltreatment. CHAMP aims to ensure that all children in Maryland suspected of having been abused or neglected receive an optimal medical assessment and care. We also plan to develop preventive activities.

RESEARCH

The Division is committed to developing the knowledge base in the field of child maltreatment and has a rich research program focused on several major issues.

1. **The prevention of child maltreatment.** This is the SEEK project funded by the US Department of Health and Human Services, Administration for Children and Families, the US Centers for Disease Control and Prevention and the Doris Duke Foundation. It is a clinical research project, as described above.
2. **Understanding the antecedents and outcomes of child maltreatment.** This project, LONGitudinal Studies on Child Abuse and Neglect (LONGSCAN), has been funded by the US DHHS, Administration for Children and Families, for almost 20 years. We collaborate with researchers in four other states (see http://www.iprc.unc.edu/longscan/).
3. **Epidemiology of abusive abdominal trauma in young children.** This research project uses a national hospital discharge database to identify the frequency, risk factors, and outcomes for children hospitalized with abusive abdominal trauma. This research is supported by the National Institute on Child Health and Human Development of the NIH.
4. **Epidemiology of occult (masked) abdominal trauma in physically abused children.** Children who are physically abused may have injuries that are clearly identified via history and physical exam. They may also have other injuries that don't show clear signs or symptoms, including injury to the abdominal organs. This research project will examine the frequency of and risk factors for occult abdominal trauma in children who come to the hospital with other child abuse-related injuries. This research is supported by the National Institute on Child Health and Human Development of the NIH.

TEACHING

Our interdisciplinary faculty and staff are actively engaged in teaching on a wide variety of topics related to child maltreatment - within the University of Maryland, locally, within Maryland, nationally and internationally. Residents and students in several disciplines regularly do electives with us.

ADVOCACY

The field of child maltreatment naturally involves advocacy. Our faculty and staff are active in advocating for improved laws, policies and programs concerning child maltreatment – at the local, state, and national levels.

FOR MORE INFORMATION, PLEASE CONTACT

Howard Dubowitz, MD, MS
Professor of Pediatrics,
Head, Division of Child Protection
520 W. Lombard St.,
Baltimore, MD 21201, United States
Tel: (410) 706-6144
E-mail: hdubowitz@peds.umaryland.edu

Chapter 26

ABOUT THE NATIONAL INSTITUTE OF CHILD HEALTH AND HUMAN DEVELOPMENT IN ISRAEL

The National Institute of Child Health and Human Development (NICHD) in Israel was established in 1998 as a virtual institute under the auspices of the Medical Director, Ministry of Social Affairs and Social Services in order to function as the research arm for the Office of the Medical Director. In 1998 the National Council for Child Health and Pediatrics, Ministry of Health and in 1999 the Director General and Deputy Director General of the Ministry of Health endorsed the establishment of the NICHD.

MISSION

The mission of a National Institute for Child Health and Human Development in Israel is to provide an academic focal point for the scholarly interdisciplinary study of child life, health, public health, welfare, disability, rehabilitation, intellectual disability and related aspects of human development. This mission includes research, teaching, clinical work, information and public service activities in the field of child health and human development.

SERVICE AND ACADEMIC ACTIVITIES

Over the years many activities became focused in the south of Israel due to collaboration with various professionals at the Faculty of Health Sciences (FOHS) at the Ben Gurion University of the Negev (BGU). Since 2000 an affiliation with the Zusman Child Development Center at the Pediatric Division of Soroka University Medical Center has resulted in collaboration around the establishment of the Down Syndrome Clinic at that center. In 2002 a full course on "Disability" was established at the Recanati School for Allied Professions in the Community, FOHS, BGU and in 2005 collaboration was started with the Primary Care Unit of the faculty and disability became part of the master of public health course on "Children and society". In the academic year 2005-2006 a one semester course on "Aging with disability" was started as part of the master of science program in gerontology in our collaboration with the Center for Multidisciplinary Research in Aging.

RESEARCH ACTIVITIES

The affiliated staff have over the years published work from projects and research activities in this national and international collaboration. In the year 2000 the International Journal of Adolescent Medicine and Health and in 2005 the International Journal on Disability and Human development of Freund Publishing House (London and Tel Aviv), in the year 2003 the TSW-Child Health and Human Development and in 2006 the TSW-Holistic Health and Medicine of the Scientific World Journal (New York and Kirkkonummi, Finland), all peer-reviewed international journals were affiliated with the National Institute of Child Health and Human Development. From 2008 also the International Journal of Child Health and Human Development (Nova Science, New York), the International Journal of Child and Adolescent Health (Nova Science) and the Journal of Pain Management (Nova Science) affiliated and from 2009 the International Public Health Journal (Nova Science) and Journal of Alternative Medicine Research (Nova Science).

NATIONAL COLLABORATIONS

Nationally the NICHD works in collaboration with the Faculty of Health Sciences, Ben Gurion University of the Negev; Department of Physical Therapy, Sackler School of Medicine, Tel Aviv University; Autism Center, Assaf HaRofeh Medical Center; National Rett and PKU Centers at Chaim Sheba Medical Center, Tel HaShomer; Department of Physiotherapy, Haifa University; Department of Education, Bar Ilan University, Ramat Gan, Faculty of Social Sciences and Health Sciences; College of Judea and Samaria in Ariel and recently also collaborations has been established with the Division of Pediatrics at Hadassah, Center for Pediatric Chronic Illness, Har HaZofim in Jerusalem.

INTERNATIONAL COLLABORATIONS

Internationally with the Department of Disability and Human Development, College of Applied Health Sciences, University of Illinois at Chicago; Strong Center for Developmental Disabilities, Golisano Children's Hospital at Strong, University of Rochester School of Medicine and Dentistry, New York; Centre on Intellectual Disabilities, University of Albany, New York; Centre for Chronic Disease Prevention and Control, Health Canada, Ottawa; Chandler Medical Center and Children's Hospital, Kentucky Children's Hospital, Section of Adolescent Medicine, University of Kentucky, Lexington; Chronic Disease Prevention and Control Research Center, Baylor College of Medicine, Houston, Texas; Division of Neuroscience, Department of Psychiatry, Columbia University, New York; Institute for the Study of Disadvantage and Disability, Atlanta; Center for Autism and Related Disorders, Department Psychiatry, Children's Hospital Boston, Boston; Department of Paediatrics, Child Health and Adolescent Medicine, Children's Hospital at Westmead, Westmead, Australia; International Centre for the Study of Occupational and Mental Health, Düsseldorf, Germany; Centre for Advanced Studies in Nursing, Department of General Practice and Primary Care, University of Aberdeen, Aberdeen, United Kingdom; Quality of Life Research Center,

Copenhagen, Denmark; Nordic School of Public Health, Gottenburg, Sweden, Scandinavian Institute of Quality of Working Life, Oslo, Norway; Centre for Quality of Life of the Hong Kong Institute of Asia-Pacific Studies and School of Social Work, Chinese University, Hong Kong.

TARGETS

Our focus is on research, international collaborations, clinical work, teaching and policy in health, disability and human development and to establish the NICHD as a permanent institute at one of the residential care centers for persons with intellectual disability in Israel in order to conduct model research and together with the four university schools of public health/medicine in Israel establish a national master and doctoral program in disability and human development at the institute to secure the next generation of professionals working in this often non-prestigious/low-status field of work.

CONTACT

Joav Merrick, MD, DMSc
Professor of Pediatrics, Child Health and Human Development
Medical Director, Health Services, Division for Mental Retardation, Ministry of Social Affairs and Social Services, POB 1260, IL-91012 Jerusalem, Israel.
E-mail: jmerrick@inter.net.il

Chapter 27

ABOUT THE BOOK SERIES
"HEALTH AND HUMAN DEVELOPMENT"

Health and human development is a book series with publications from a multidisciplinary group of researchers, practitioners and clinicians for an international professional forum interested in the broad spectrum of health and human development.

- Merrick J, Omar HA, eds. Adolescent behavior research. International perspectives. New York: Nova Science, 2007.
- Kratky KW. Complementary medicine systems: Comparison and integration. New York: Nova Science, 2008.
- Schofield P, Merrick J, eds. Pain in children and youth. New York: Nova Science, 2009.
- Greydanus DE, Patel DR, Pratt HD, Calles Jr JL, eds. Behavioral pediatrics, 3 ed. New York: Nova Science, 2009.
- Ventegodt S, Merrick J, eds. Meaningful work: Research in quality of working life. New York: Nova Science, 2009.
- Omar HA, Greydanus DE, Patel DR, Merrick J, eds. Obesity and adolescence. A public health concern. New York: Nova Science, 2009.
- Lieberman A, Merrick J, eds. Poverty and children. A public health concern. New York: Nova Science, 2009.
- Goodbread J. Living on the edge. The mythical, spiritual and philosophical roots of social marginality. New York: Nova Science, 2009.
- Bennett DL, Towns S, Elliot E, Merrick J, eds. Challenges in adolescent health: An Australian perspective. New York: Nova Science, 2009.
- Schofield P, Merrick J, eds. Children and pain. New York: Nova Science, 2009.
- Sher L, Kandel I, Merrick J. Alcohol-related cognitive disorders: Research and clinical perspectives. New York: Nova Science, 2009.
- Anyanwu EC. Advances in environmental health effects of toxigenic mold and mycotoxins. New York: Nova Science, 2009.
- Bell E, Merrick J, eds. Rural child health. International aspects. New York: Nova Science, 2009.
- Dubowitz H, Merrick J, eds. International aspects of child abuse and neglect. New York: Nova Science, 2010.

- Shahtahmasebi S, Berridge D. Conceptualizing behavior: A practical guide to data analysis. New York: Nova Science, 2010.
- Wernik U. Chance action and therapy. The playful way of changing. New York: Nova Science, 2010.
- Omar HA, Greydanus DE, Patel DR, Merrick J, eds. Adolescence and chronic illness. A public health concern. New York: Nova Science, 2010.
- Patel DR, Greydanus DE, Omar HA, Merrick J, eds. Adolescence and sports. New York: Nova Science, 2010.
- Shek DTL, Ma HK, Merrick J, eds. Positive youth development: Evaluation and future directions in a Chinese context. New York: Nova Science, 2010.
- Shek DTL, Ma HK, Merrick J, eds. Positive youth development: Implementation of a youth program in a Chinese context. New York: Nova Science, 2010.
- Omar HA, Greydanus DE, Tsitsika AK, Patel DR, Merrick J, eds.   Pediatric and adolescent sexuality and gynecology: Principles for the primary care clinician. New York: Nova Science, 2010.
- Chow E, Merrick J, eds. Advanced cancer. Pain and quality of life. New York: Nova Science, 2010.

CONTACT

Professor Joav Merrick, MD, MMedSci, DMSc
Medical Director, Division for Mental Retardation
Ministry of Social Affairs, POBox 1260
IL-91012 Jerusalem, Israel
E-mail: jmerrick@internet-zahav.net

INDEX

D

F

G

H

J

K

L

N